Implant Surgery

Editor

HARRY DYM

DENTAL CLINICS OF NORTH AMERICA

www.dental.theclinics.com

January 2021 • Volume 65 • Number 1

ELSEVIER

1600 John F. Kennedy Boulevard • Suite 1800 • Philadelphia, Pennsylvania, 19103-2899

http://www.dental.theclinics.com

DENTAL CLINICS OF NORTH AMERICA Volume 65, Number 1
January 2021 ISSN 0011-8532, ISBN: 978-0-323-79194-6

Editor: John Vassallo; j.vassallo@elsevier.com
Developmental Editor: Laura Fisher

Dental Clinics of North America (ISSN 0011-8532) is published quarterly by Elsevier Inc., 360 Park Avenue South, New York, NY 10010-1710. Months of issue are January, April, July, and October. Business and Editorial Offices: 1600 John F. Kennedy Boulevard, Suite 1800, Philadelphia, PA 19103-2899. Periodicals postage paid at New York, NY and additional mailing offices. Subscription prices are $313.00 per year (domestic individuals), $846.00 per year (domestic institutions), $100.00 per year (domestic students/residents), $366.00 per year (Canadian individuals), $888.00 per year (Canadian institutions), $100.00 per year (Canadian students/residents) $428.00 per year (international individuals), $888.00 per year (international institutions), and $200.00 per year (international students/residents). International air speed delivery is included in all *Clinics* subscription prices. All prices are subject to change without notice. **POSTMASTER:** Send address changes to *Dental Clinics of North America*, Elsevier Health Sciences Division, Subscription Customer Service, 3251 Riverport Lane, Maryland Heights, MO 63043. **Customer Service (orders, claims, online, change of address): Elsevier Health Sciences Division, Subscription Customer Service, 3251 Riverport Lane, Maryland Heights, MO 63043. Tel: 1-800-654-2452 (U.S. and Canada). Fax: 314-447-8029. E-mail: journalscustomerservice-usa@elsevier.com (for print support); journalsonlinesupport-usa@elsevier. com (for online support).**

Reprints. For copies of 100 or more, of articles in this publication, please contact the Commercial Reprints Department, Elsevier Inc., 360 Park Avenue South, New York, NY 10010-1710. Tel.: 212-633-3874; Fax: 212-633-3820; E-mail: reprints@elsevier.com.

The Dental Clinics of North America is covered in *MEDLINE/PubMed (Index Medicus), Current Contents/Clinical Medicine, ISI/BIOMED* and *Clinahl*.

Contributors

EDITOR

HARRY DYM, DDS, FACS
Chairman of the Department of Dentistry and Oral Surgery, Program Director of the Oral and Maxillofacial Surgery Residency Training Program, The Brooklyn Hospital Center, Clinical Professor, Oral and Maxillofacial Surgery, Columbia University College of Dental Medicine, Consulting Oral and Maxillofacial Surgeon, The Brooklyn VA NY Harbor Healthcare System, Senior Attending, Division of Oral and Maxillofacial Surgery, Woodhull Hospital, Brooklyn, New York, USA

AUTHORS

DAVID R. ADAMS, DDS
Associate Professor, Clinic Chief, Oral and Maxillofacial Surgery, University of Utah School of Dentistry, Salt Lake City, Utah, USA

AMANDA ANDRE, DDS
Oral and Maxillofacial Surgery Intern, The Brooklyn Hospital Center, Brooklyn, New York, USA

NATASHA BHALLA, DDS
Resident, Department of Dentistry/Oral and Maxillofacial Surgery, The Brooklyn Hospital Center, Brooklyn, New York, New York, USA

RICARDO A. BOYCE, DDS, FICD
Director of the General Practice Residency, Chief of General Dentistry/Oral Medicine, The Brooklyn Hospital Center, Brooklyn, New York, USA; Adjunct Clinical Associate Professor, New York University, College of Dentistry, New York, New York, USA

MICHAEL H. CHAN, DDS
Director, Oral and Maxillofacial Surgery, Department of Veterans Affairs, New York Harbor Healthcare System (Brooklyn Campus), Senior Attending, Department of Oral and Maxillofacial Surgery, The Brooklyn Hospital Center, Brooklyn, New York, USA

PETER CHEN, DDS, MS
Departments of Dentistry and Oral and Maxillofacial Surgery, Woodhull Hospital, Brooklyn, New York, USA

EARL CLARKSON, DDS
Chairman of Dentistry, Program Director of Oral and Maxillofacial Surgery, Department of Dentistry, NYC Health + Hospitals/Woodhull, Brooklyn, New York, USA

JENNIFER B. COHEN, DDS
Staff Dentist, Jesse Brown VA Medical Center, Chicago, Illinois, USA

HARRY DYM, DDS, FACS
Chairman of the Department of Dentistry and Oral Surgery, Program Director of the Oral and Maxillofacial Surgery Residency Training Program, The Brooklyn Hospital Center,

Clinical Professor, Oral and Maxillofacial Surgery, Columbia University College of Dental Medicine, Consulting Oral and Maxillofacial Surgeon, The Brooklyn VA NY Harbor Healthcare System, Senior Attending, Division of Oral and Maxillofacial Surgery, Woodhull Hospital, Brooklyn, New York, USA

RAYMOND FAN, DDS
Resident, Department of Oral and Maxillofacial Surgery, Nova Southeastern University, College of Dental Medicine, Fort Lauderdale, Florida, USA; Surgical Arts of Boca Raton, Boca Raton, Florida, USA

YIJIAO FAN, DDS
Department of Dentistry, Division of Oral and Maxillofacial Surgery, Brooklyn Hospital Center, Brooklyn, New York, USA

ALLEN GLIED, DDS
Attending, Oral and Maxillofacial Surgery, St. Barnabas Hospital, Department of Dentistry, Bronx, New York, USA

MARVIN B. GOLBERG, DDS, BS
Assistant Professor, Director of CAD CAM, Department of Prosthodontics, Nova Southeastern University, College of Dental Medicine, Fort Lauderdale, Florida, USA

LESLIE R. HALPERN, DDS, MD, PhD, MPH, FACS, FICD
Professor, Section Head, Oral and Maxillofacial Surgery, University of Utah School of Dentistry, Salt Lake City, Utah, USA

MONICA HANNA, DMD
Resident, Oral and Maxillofacial Surgery, NYC Health + Hospitals/Woodhull, Brooklyn, New York, USA

RAZA A. HUSSAIN, BDS, DMD, FACS
Section Chief, Oral and Maxillofacial Surgery, Jesse Brown VA Medical Center, Clinical Associate Professor, Department of Oral and Maxillofacial Surgery, University of Illinois at Chicago, Chicago, Illinois, USA

EUNSU JUNG, DDS
Department of Dentistry, Chief Resident, Department of Oral and Maxillofacial Surgery, NYC Health + Hospitals/Woodhull, Brooklyn, New York, USA

SPENCER LIN, DMD
Department of Dentistry, Resident, Department of Oral and Maxillofacial Surgery, NYC Health + Hospitals/Woodhull, Brooklyn, New York, USA

MICHAEL MILORO, DMD, MD, FACS
Professor and Department Head, Department of Oral and Maxillofacial Surgery, University of Illinois at Chicago, Chicago, Illinois, USA

NABIL MOUSSA, DDS
Department of Dentistry, Division of Oral and Maxillofacial Surgery, Brooklyn Hospital Center, Brooklyn, New York, USA

JUNAID MUNDIYA, DMD
Resident, Department of Oral and Maxillofacial Surgery, The Brooklyn Hospital Center, Brooklyn, New York, USA

LEVON NIKOYAN, DDS
Attending, Department of Oral and Maxillofacial Surgery, Woodhull Medical Center, Departments of Dentistry and Oral and Maxillofacial Surgery, Woodhull Hospital, Brooklyn, New York, USA; Private Practice, Forward Oral Surgery, Floral Park, New York, USA

YOAV A. NUDELL, DDS, MS
Resident, Department of Oral and Maxillofacial Surgery, The Brooklyn Hospital Center, Brooklyn, New York, USA

ORRETT E. OGLE, DDS
Visiting Lecturer, Mona Dental Program, Faculty of Medicine, University of the West Indies, Kingston, Jamaica; Former Chief, Oral and Maxillofacial Surgery, Woodhull Hospital, Brooklyn, New York, USA

RINIL PATEL, DDS
Chief Resident, NYC Health + Hospitals/Woodhull, Brooklyn, New York, USA

JASON E. PORTNOF, DMD, MD, FACS, FICD, FACD
Adjunct Associate Professor, Department of Oral and Maxillofacial Surgery, Nova Southeastern University, College of Dental Medicine, Fort Lauderdale, Florida, USA; Private Practice, Surgical Arts of Boca Raton, Boca Raton, Florida, USA

GUILLERMO PUIG, DMD
Resident, Oral and Maxillofacial Surgery, NYC Health + Hospitals/Woodhull, Brooklyn, New York, USA

HARVEY A. QUINTON, DDS
Assistant Professor, Department of Cariology and Restorative Dentistry, Nova Southeastern University, College of Dental Medicine, Fort Lauderdale, Florida, USA

JONATHAN ROSENSTEIN, DDS
Former Chief Resident, Department of Oral and Maxillofacial Surgery, The Brooklyn Hospital Center, Brooklyn, New York, USA

DAVID SHEEN, DDS
Department of Oral and Maxillofacial Surgery, Woodhull Medical Center, Brooklyn, New York, USA

Contents

> Advances in dental implant therapy have created choices to enhance the
> expectations of dental practitioners and their patients with respect to oral
> rehabilitation at any age after childhood and regardless of, in most cases,
> medical disabilities. The medical status of the patient however can signif-
> icantly influence the success rate of dental implant therapy. This article ap-
> plies the hierarchy of scientific evidence ranging from case reports,
> retrospective, prospective cohort investigations, systematic reviews, and
> meta-analyses criteria in order to determine whether dental implant place-
> ment in medically compromised patients yields any detrimental sequelae.

> The placement of short implants, which measure less than 10 mm in
> length, requires the practitioner to have a thorough comprehension of
> implant dentistry to achieve acceptable results. Innovation of the rough-
> surface implant and the progression of the implant-abutment interface
> from an external hex to an internal connection have considerably influ-
> enced the longevity of short implants. Dentists are better equipped to
> serve their patients because the utilization of short implants may preclude
> the need for advanced surgical bone-grafting procedures.

> Life-threatening complications of dental implant surgery are rare, but
> include hematoma/hemorrhage of the floor of the mouth, aspiration, and
> ingestion. Prevention of lethal hemorrhagic complications stem from
> knowledge of anatomic structures and precise surgical planning. Preven-
> tion of aspiration and ingestion can be improved by simple techniques
> while understanding clinical settings and factors that put patients at higher
> risk. In the event of these potential lethal situations, early recognition of
> signs and symptoms along with immediate action followed by transfer to
> an emergency department is often necessary.

> As implant placement increases within all dental specialties, it is expected
> that the number of suboptimal results will increase, as well. The goal of this

article is to provide clinicians with an outline of the management of periimplantitis cases, ranging from simple to complex. It will review signs and symptoms, diagnosis, case selection, and armamentarium. In addition, this chapter will discuss basic techniques which can be utilized at various stages to salvage the compromised implant.

Diagnosis and treatment planning are critical in preparation for implant placement. Adequate evaluation, preoperative imaging, and surgical planning minimize early and late-stage soft tissue injuries. Correct placement of dental implants can be challenging with several contributing factors such as lack of proper preoperative soft tissue evaluation and surgical experience in dealing with soft tissue incisions and flap reflection, resulting in injury and complications involving the soft tissues.

Guides used in dental implant surgery add accuracy and an overall predictability. Successful guided implant workflow depends on 3-dimensional image acquisition and precise medical model fabrication. The contemporary process blends acquired images to existing dentition to create implant-specific precise guides. We discuss the overall process, types of guides, and complications to expect during surgery.

In the past, the only way to replace missing teeth was to have a removable appliance. However, these days, dental implants are commonly being used to replace missing teeth. The dental implants are improving as a result of new technological and scientific advances. Different materials have been used in the past for dental implants such as lead, stainless steel, and gold. Currently, the focus is on using Roxolid, surface-modified titanium implants, and zirconia. These materials have superior esthetic and functional characteristics for dental implants.

Immediate implants have become a popular option for replacing teeth. This article describes the surgical and restorative considerations involved in the planning and placement of an immediate implant. Immediate implants require appropriate hard and soft tissue assessment. Virtual planning can help assist in planning of immediate implants. Radiographic and computed tomographic guidance can help in establishing the relationship between the planned implant to the hard tissue and anatomic structures. This article discusses a technique in fabrication of the immediate provisional and final restoration.

Ridge augmentation for implant procedures has been shown to be highly successful. There are several techniques available to the dentist, but they require some degree of surgical expertise and experience. No particular technique has been shown to be superior. This article presents the indications, techniques, and complications of the various procedures for alveolar ridge augmentation. This information will educate the general dental practitioner of the techniques available and provide information on the surgical procedures that could be used to discuss with patients when they are being referred to a specialist.

It is essential for practitioners who place dental implants to be able to diagnose and treat common complications or know when to refer to a specialist. Common complications can include nerve injuries, infections, sinus membrane perforations, and edema. This article discusses these complications, incidence rates, tips to avoid common complications, and management options when a patient returns with a complication.

More patients are requesting fixed prosthesis to replace missing teeth. More than 5 million dental implants are placed annually in the United States. This number will decrease in 2020 owing to the coronavirus disease-19 pandemic. The edentulous patient has a decreased quality of life. Prosthodontic rehabilitation/reconstruction of edentulism improves overall quality of life. Patient-reported outcome measures are subjective reports of patients' perceptions of their oral health status and the impact that it has on their quality of life. This chapter contains a variety of prosthodontic principles for the reader to help satisfy the needs and expectations of the patient.

For successful outcomes in bone grafting, it is important to have a clear and detailed understanding of the fundamentals and basics in regenerative science. This article summarize the grafting materials and growth factors that are now in use to provide an improved understanding of the properties of each material and indications for subsequent use. The article gives an overview of the fundamentals of bone healing, including the physiology of regeneration. It is hoped that clinicians can make improved decisions that are based in literature when considering treatment options for restoring patients' functional dentition.

Implant stability is critical to implant success, and the amount of available bone is vital to achieving that end. Because of low-lying maxillary sinuses, adequate alveolar height on the posterior maxilla is often lacking in many patients in need of implant replacement. This chapter reviews both the traditional lateral sinus lift maxillary approach to achieve vertical augmentation as well as the transcrestal osteotome intraoral approach. A discussion of osseodensification will also be mentioned as an alternative approach.

Over the past 17 years, the All-on-4 treatment concept has been a reliable and predictable modality to rehabilitate edentulous jaws with immediate function as full-arch prostheses. This article highlights clinically relevant data compiled by numerous All-on-4 investigators including complications and their remedies, occlusion and cantilever trends, implant size utilization, and controversial topics. We provide insights for navigating the complexities of medically diverse populations, faced by our daily practice, with a focus on patient avoidance, risk factors for implant and prosthetic failures, in hopes to minimize complications so clinicians would choose this treatment with confidence.

Restoring the dentition of an edentulous patient is often challenging. Endosseous dental implants have allowed for far more versatility in this area but still require adequate maxillary and mandibular alveolar bone. Often, unless significant bone grafting techniques are used, true restoration of the dentition can be impossible with traditional endosseous implants. The advent of zygomatic implants, however, may provide a viable, predictable, and stable alternative for the restoration of the dentition in patients with severe maxillary alveolar bone loss.

DENTAL CLINICS OF NORTH AMERICA

SERIES OF RELATED INTEREST

Atlas of the Oral and Maxillofacial Surgery Clinics
http://www.oralmaxsurgeryatlas.theclinics.com

Oral and Maxillofacial Surgery Clinics
http://www.oralmaxsurgery.theclinics.com

THE CLINICS ARE AVAILABLE ONLINE!
Access your subscription at:
www.theclinics.com

Preface

Implant Surgery

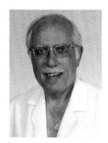

Harry Dym, DDS, FACS
Editor

I have once again been honored with editing another issue of the *Dental Clinics of North America*. However, this preface will not follow the template of my previous ones, as I find myself writing it in extraordinary times. I sit squarely in the epicenter of the COVID-19 novel coronavirus pandemic of the world, New York City. My hospital, The Brooklyn Hospital Center, where I have spent the totality of my career of 35 years and am currently the Chairman of Dentistry/Oral and Maxillofacial Surgery, literally stands at the frontlines and has already been featured multiple times (front page) in the *New York Times*, as well as on CBS's *60 Minutes* news show, discussing our heroic efforts to treat COVID-19 patients.

Hopefully by the time this issue is printed and disseminated, a return to near normalcy will have already occurred, but I share my musings with you, written in the very midst of the pandemic as there are certainly relevant points to be gleaned.

How will the epic pandemic change the way we live and practice? Each and every one of us will certainly have been affected differently. Some may have gotten very sick, even having required hospitalizations and possibly mechanical ventilation. Others may have had milder states of the disease. Almost all of us have had friends or family possibly lost to COVID-19, but certainly sickened by the virus. Most of us had to close our practices for a period of months, and others who did work certainly saw a significant decrease in patient volume and revenue.

As I write this preface, the pandemic still rages around me and there is no light at the end of the tunnel, certainly no bright light that one can see clearly. How long this will last is not certain; the everlasting effects on society and our practices are unknown, but certainly we as a profession will be forever changed and so will the world around us. Our patients may be reluctant to return until there is a real cure or mass immunity via vaccinations, and even then, it seems that return to full normalcy will be in stages and may require an extended period of time.

Dent Clin N Am 65 (2021) xiii–xv
https://doi.org/10.1016/j.cden.2020.09.008
0011-8532/21/© 2020 Published by Elsevier Inc.

In order to restart and rekindle a practice, innovative dentists and oral surgeons will need to change practice patterns and will include all aspects of private practice.

- Offices will need to pay particular attention to practicing safely vis-a-vis Personal Protective Equipment for the doctor, staff, and patients.
- Marketing: patients will need to know that you are back to full operation and fully compliant with all Centers for Disease Control and Prevention and State Department of Health infection control techniques and practices.
- In-office testing for COVID-19 antibodies and for the virus itself will have to become an ongoing standard of care.
- Better appreciation for your staff and for your patients will be necessary to achieve a full return.
- The need to venture out of your comfort zone to provide greater breadth and scope of services in various areas of dentistry/oral surgery/oral medicine/oral pain, and so forth. This means attending high-quality Continuing Dental Education courses, attending online courses, reading textbooks, and attending weekend immersion classes, for only by widening your scope of care can you hope to maintain a fruitful, profitable, and meaningful clinical practice.

This last thought regarding increased exposure to education, especially self-education, is where Elsevier and its *Clinics* journals play such a meaningful role. The *Dental Clinics of North America* series has traditionally played a substantive role in providing high-quality scientific literature to the dental and oral surgery profession with clear, concise, and elucidative articles written by outstanding authors and clinicians. In my opinion, my capable authors for this text have accomplished the above-stated goals. I am forever grateful to them all for their work, dedication, and reliability, even when faced with such turmoil swirling all about them.

I am pleased to have worked once again with my good friend, Mr John Vassallo, the Associate Publisher of the *Dental Clinics of North America*, who is personally dedicated to bringing our readership timely texts on a variety of clinical subjects. My sincere thanks also go to Ms Laura Fisher, my assigned Developmental Editor, and her staff for her outstanding efforts on behalf of this issue.

The pandemic strangely enough provided us with some positive effects.

- It provided our society with the opportunity for valuable teaching lessons—that may have been long overdue—to better value those in our society who devote themselves on a daily basis to the care of others: clinicians, nurses, respiratory therapists, pharmacists, first responders, and all hospital employees, including transporters, housekeepers, and maintenance personnel, who all worked tirelessly despite almost combatlike scenarios during the zenith of the pandemic.
- It clearly elucidated the real meaning of the word hero, which we as a society all too frequently use to describe athletes and Internet influencers, thereby having diminished the very word itself.
- It allowed many to finally understand the real meaning of societal-shared responsibilities, and for each of us individually to be more generous with our charitable gifting and our need for more social involvement.

I wish to acknowledge all my Brooklyn Hospital oral and maxillofacial surgery residents who worked in the trenches throughout the pandemic, working in the COVID-19 surgical SICU and COVID-19 screening tent, and throughout the pandemic nightmare continued to take oral surgical calls in the emergency department treating infections, facial lacerations, and all types of facial and jaw trauma. In fact, five of my oral surgical residents became positive and ill with the virus with one requiring hospitalization—all thankfully fully recovered. I am grateful to the dedication to my young oral and maxillofacial surgery attendings, Drs Joshua Wolf, Jared Miller, and Edward Woodbine, who supervised all the oral and maxillofacial surgical emergency operating room cases. My special gratitude goes to Dr Ricardo Boyce, Director of the General Practice Residency Training Program, who stayed at the hospital every day directing the general practice residents who were redeployed in the service of The Brooklyn Hospital Center as well. Special thanks to Ms Gloria Stallings, my executive assistant and residency coordinator, for her ongoing help.

As parents, my wife and I worried as our youngest son, Akiva (third-year resident in emergency medicine), went daily to work at the largest hospital in Nassau County, Long Island, that at one time simultaneously had 120 COVID-19 patients on ventilators. He, like thousands of others, never wavered in his responsibilities despite the stresses, anxiety, and sheer exhaustion that certainly overwhelmed him at times.

The pandemic brought out the best in us, and hopefully, we will all remember this when COVID-19 becomes but a bad memory. For some it took a pandemic to help concentrate and focus their thoughts and clarify what truly is most essential and meaningful in their lives. For me, it helped reinforce my preexisting notion in what a "meaningful life" means to me: Faith, Family, and Friends.

To my wife, Freidy, who sheltered in place alongside me, and to all my children and grandchildren who ZOOMed and FaceTimed with us, generating light in an otherwise gloomy time, I thank you from the bottom of my heart.

To my dearest friends, Drs Peter Sherman, Earl Clarkson, Orrett Ogle, and Elliot Siegel, who I have known for over 4 decades—thank you and may we continue to speak daily for another 40 years.

To the readers of this issue, I hope it elucidates, clarifies, and brings useful information to your practice. To my capable contributors, once again you humble me with your outstanding work, enthusiasm, and reliability; you all did an outstanding job and delivered the goods.

To The Brooklyn Hospital Center administration, Ms Lizanne Fontaine, Chairperson of the Board of Trustees, Mr Gary Terrinoni, President and CEO, Mr Bob Aulicino, COO, Dr Vasantha Kondamudi, CMO, and Ms Judy McLaughlin, CNO, and to the thousands of employees who tirelessly worked during the pandemic, you have made me proud and have reconfirmed my decision that I made 35 years ago to work and spend my entire career at The Brooklyn Hospital Center.

Finally, I am grateful to God for having protected my family, friends, and colleagues.

Harry Dym, DDS, FACS
Department of Dentistry/
Oral and Maxillofacial Surgery
The Brooklyn Hospital Center
Brooklyn, NY 11201, USA

Oral and Maxillofacial Surgery
Columbia University College of Dental Medicine
New York, NY 12235, USA

E-mail address:
hdym@tbh.org

Medically Complex Dental Implant Patients

Controversies About Systemic Disease and Dental Implant Success/Survival

Leslie R. Halpern, DDS, MD, PhD, MPH, FICD*, David R. Adams, DDS

KEYWORDS

- Dental implants • Medically compromised patients • Diabetes mellitus
- Human immunodeficiency virus • Autoimmune disease • Drug therapy
- Radiation therapy

KEY POINTS

- Dental implant therapy in medically complex patients is predicated on a well-thought-out surgical and restorative foundation that promotes both long-term function and improved health-related quality of life.
- Dental implant therapy in medically compromised patients involves a multiplicity of presurgical and postsurgical and pharmacologic considerations.
- There is no consensus as to whether medically complex patients' risk for early or late implant failure exceeds those of healthy cohorts.
- There is no consensus as to whether dental implant therapy in immunocompromised patients results in an implant survival rate that is comparable with normal healthy cohorts.

INTRODUCTION

Advances in dental implant therapy have created choices to enhance the expectations of dental practitioners and their patients with respect to oral rehabilitation. The bioactivity of implant surface design, as well as the use of hard and soft tissue augmentation, provides a greater opportunity in the rehabilitation of the edentulous and partially edentulous jaw. Well-published studies of long-term dental implant success and survival provide more realistic options for restoration of function and esthetics regardless of postchildhood age, and, in most cases, medical disabilities. The 10-year implant survival is very high in the non–medically compromised patient population.[1–3]

Oral and Maxillofacial Surgery, University of Utah School of Dentistry, 530 South Wakara Way, Salt Lake City, UT 84108, USA
* Corresponding author.
E-mail address: Leslie.halpern@hsc.utah.edu

Dent Clin N Am 65 (2021) 1–19
https://doi.org/10.1016/j.cden.2020.08.001
0011-8532/21/© 2020 Elsevier Inc. All rights reserved.

However, dental implant placement, even in healthy patients, has the potential for adverse outcomes caused by failure of osseointegration or as a result of periimplantitis. Although the past few decades have provided an increased demand by patients for dental implants, failures in treatment are still prevalent because of poor patient selection.

With respect to medically complex patients, doctors must determine whether or not implants are the best option in the functional restoration of a partially or fully edentulous jaw. Controversy still remains with respect to systemic illness and its influence on short-term and long-term dental implant survival and success.[4–6] Systemic morbidity caused by chronic illnesses can significantly compromise treatment planning outcomes. Studies by Scully and colleagues[5] have examined how dental implant therapy can be altered by systemic illnesses in terms of success and survival over time.[2] Vissink and colleagues[1] crafted 6 questions, listed in **Box 1**, to help practitioners determine whether dental implant therapy is a reasonable option in a medically compromised patient. Diz and colleagues[2] and others have written in-depth reviews on implant survival and the risk of periimplantitis in patients with systemic illnesses.[3–6] Many have recommended placing compromising medical conditions into groups of absolute versus relative contraindications when considering dental implant placement (**Box 2**). Full disclosure of the proposed treatment plan and the potential complications and risks versus benefits is essential. This disclosure is the first step in developing a therapeutic alliance between practitioner and patient so that shared decision making can improve surgical outcomes.

This article applies the hierarchy of scientific evidence ranging from case reports, retrospective and prospective cohort investigations, systematic reviews, and meta-analyses that examine relative and absolute contraindications for the placement of dental implants in medically compromised patients. A review of the current literature is used to apply evidence-based criteria that determine whether dental implant placement in medically compromised patients yields significant increased risks of complications and implant failure. Attention is directed toward medically compromised patients who are immunocompromised, such as those with human immunodeficiency virus (HIV), diabetic patients, patients with autoimmune dysfunction, and patients who have been exposed to radiation therapy for malignancies. These systemic conditions are chosen to examine the most current scientific evidence addressing the controversies in dental implant placement in affected patients.

Box 1
Questions for medically compromised patients and dental implants

1. Does implant placement cause a health risk to the patient?

2. Are specific precautions needed when placing the dental implants?

3. Can immediate implant complications be controlled when they occur?

4. Will an implant system be used and a surgical approach applied that has been proved to have favorable long-term outcomes with regard to implant survival and peri-implant health?

5. Is there well-organized postoperative care and long-term follow-up?

6. Is the patient compliant enough to adhere to strict oral care?

From Vissink A, Spijkervet FKL, Raghoebar GM. The medically compromised patient: Are dental implants a feasible option? Oral Dis. 2018;24:253–60; with permission.

Box 2
Absolute and relative contraindications for dental implant therapy

Absolute contraindications: recent myocardial infarction; stroke; organ transplant; valvular prosthetic heart valve; profound immunosuppression; severe bleeding dyscrasia; active malignancy; alcohol and drug abuse; psychiatric illnesses; osteoporosis; oral mucosal diseases; use of intravenous bisphosphonates or antiresorptive agents.

Relative contraindications: titanium allergy; smoking; immunotherapy.

From Vissink A, Spijkervet FKL, Raghoebar GM. The medically compromised patient: Are dental implants a feasible option? Oral Dis. 2018;24:253–60; with permission.

LITERATURE SEARCH

A literature search was undertaken using Medline within the PubMed portal to choose articles within the last 20 years. Only articles in English were chosen for inclusion. Each article's bibliography was evaluated for relevant publications and reviewed by the authors for inclusion. The keywords chosen include "patient assessment," "medically complex patient selection for implants," "medical contraindications for dental implants," "immunocompromised patients and implants," "diabetes and dental implants," "hepatitis and dental implants," "HIV and implants," "radiation therapy and dental implant survival/success," and "medical controversies and dental implants." The level of evidence chosen was based on Sackett's hierarchy of evidence and were predominantly levels 1A, 2A, 3A, 4, and 5 (**Table 1**).[7]

OVERVIEW: MEDICALLY COMPROMISED PATIENTS AND DENTAL IMPLANT THERAPY

Much debate has centered on whether dental implants are a preferred restorative solution in medically compromised patients who most often are candidates in need of complex restorative rehabilitation.[1–6] The challenges faced include increased risk of periimplantitis, recurrence of mucosal disease, poor wound healing, and/or development of osteonecrosis caused by pharmacotherapy (ie, the use of certain drugs for

---

Table 1
Criteria for inclusion of articles chosen from PubMed literature search according to the Sackett hierarchy

Level of Evidence	Description
1A	Systematic review/randomized trials (RCTs)
1B	RCTs with narrow confidence limit
1C	All or none case series
2A	Systematic cohort
2B	Cohort study/low-quality RCT
3A	Systematic review of case-controlled studies
3B	Case-controlled study
4	Case series/poor cohort case-controlled studies
5	Expert opinion

Abbreviation: RCT, randomized controlled trial.
From Sadowsky SJ, Fitzpatrick B, Curtis DA. Evidence-based criteria for different treatment planning of implant restorations for the maxillary edentulous patient. J Prosth. 2015;24(6):433-446; with permission.

osteoporosis/bone cancers), and patients who have been exposed to radiation ther-apy.[1–6] Scully and colleagues[5] suggested the risk/morbidity of dental implant place-ment should be predicated on careful patient work-up because new evidence supports successful implant survival in these patients.[2] Kotsakis and colleagues,[4] in a systematic review evaluating implant placement in the maxilla of medically compro-mised patients, concluded that implant survival is acceptable based on disease type and seems more predictable in the mandible than the maxilla. Vissink and colleagues,[1] in a recent review, differentiated between absolute and relative contraindications for dental implant therapy (discussed earlier). **Table 2** is an adaptation of these consider-ations with measures to improve the feasibility of dental implant placement in patients who are medically challenged.[1,2] The following medical conditions have provided much controversy with respect to long-term implant success and survival in several medically compromised patient populations seen in oral health care practices.

Immunocompromised Patients

Human immunodeficiency virus

Thirty-three million people have been living with HIV for several decades and millions have died of acquired immunodeficiency syndrome (AIDS).[8,9] Within the past decade, the growth rate of HIV infection seems to be plateauing (discussed later).[8] The virus attacks the immune system and causes a reduction in host resistance because of decreased CD4+ T cells that can compromise the normal oral flora. This condition is a concern, especially because there is an increased risk of complications in the oral cavity as a result of oral surgical procedures in patients with HIV. The develop-ment of antiretroviral therapy has saved millions of lives and improved the health-related quality of life of many patients with oral health care concerns. However, ad-vances of antiretroviral therapy have led to adverse events in terms of bone disorders (ie, osteoporosis and osteopenia) because the virus affects osteoblast and osteoclast function.[9] As such, the flora of the mouth in concert with immunosuppression can impede long-term success and survival of dental implants.[8,9] More recent data since the introduction of highly active antiretroviral therapy (HAART) have recharacterized HIV/AIDS as a chronic disease and improved the ability of patients with HIV to become immunologically resistant and, in many cases (discussed later) have viable choices for oral rehabilitation with dental implants.[8–10]

Although no consensus has been reached on recommendations for dental implant therapy in patients with HIV, numerous studies and systematic reviews have attemp-ted to determine whether implants are suitable in the dental rehabilitation of HIV-positive patients.[1,5,6,8,9] Scully and colleagues[5] suggested that immunologically stable HIV-positive patients may be considered as viable candidates to receive implants.[11] A retrospective chart review by Rubenstein and colleagues[8] considered the placement of dental implants in HIV-positive patients to be successful and safe with several ca-veats. They did suggest that low bone mineral density as a result of HAART therapy can lead to increased risk of bone fracture and osteoporosis. Most of the patients in the study were more than 50 years of age, positive for tobacco use, and had low body mass. However, HIV-positive patients who were highly compliant with their oral health care showed an absence of periimplantitis and an increase in the survival of dental implants that were placed.[8] Implants were considered successful in this cohort because of lack of mobility and no fixtures showed signs of infection.[8] Although there were study limitations, such as the small sampling size analyzed, the investiga-tors recommended patient follow-up on a regular basis to measure both changes in crestal bone height and hygiene maintenance as indicators for long-term success of implants placed.

Table 2
Medical illnesses that require consideration for whether dental implant therapy is or is not an option

Condition	(Relative) Contraindication	Implant Survival Rate	Precautions/ Recommendations
Alcoholism	No	Similar	Assure that patients will keep adequate oral health maintenance.
Bleeding disorder	No	Similar	Check coagulation status before placement of implants.
Bone disease			
Osteoporosis	No	Similar	Be aware of a slightly higher risk on MRONJ in patients on oral antiresorptive drugs. Bone augmentation surgery is allowed.
Bisphosphonate use	Yes	Similar/reduced	Antibiotic prophylaxis. Risk of MRONJ is high in patients treated for bone metastasis. When implants in latter patients are indicated, do it early after start of antiresorptive therapy. Also, no augmentation surgery in patients on i.v. administration unless early after start of usage.
Other antiresorptive drugs, for example, denosumab	Yes	Similar/ reduced	Antibiotic prophylaxis. Risk on MRONJ is high in patients treated for bone metastasis. When implants in latter patients are indicated, do it early after start of antiresoprtive therapy. Also, no augmentation surgery in patients on i.v. administration unless early after start of usage.
Cardiac Disease	No	Similar	Assure that patient will keep adequate oral health maintenance. Also with regard to control of cardiac disease.
Diabetes mellitus			
Uncontrolled	No	Similar/ reduced	Antibiotic prophylaxis. Assure that patient will keep adequate oral health maintenance, also with regard to control of diabetes.

(continued on next page)

Table 2
(continued)

Condition	(Relative) Contraindication	Implant Survival Rate	Precautions/ Recommendations
Controlled	No	Similar	Assure that patient will keep adequate oral health maintenance, also with regard to control of diabetes.
Drugs			
Anticoagulants	No	Similar	See bleeding disorder.
Antiresorptive drugs	No	Similar/Reduced	See bone disease.
Biologicals	No	Similar	See Immunocompromised patients.
Chemotherapy	No	Similar	See head neck cancer.
Immunotherapy	Yes	Unknown	Implant treatment often can be postponed until end of therapy.
Xerostomic drugs	No	Similar	See hyposalivation.
Head and Neck Cancer			
Chemotherapy	No	Similar	Assure that patient will keep adequate oral health maintenance during the course of chemotherapy. After completion, the risk of developing peri-implant health problems is comparable to healthy subjects.
Radiotherapy	Yes	Reduced	Preferably place dental implants during ablative surgery. When placed after completion of radiotherapy, implant should be placed under antibiotic coverage (e.g., amoxicillin 500 mg t.i.d. for 2 weeks, starting 1 day before placement of the implants). If cumulative radiation dose in the implant area is >40 Gy, it is recommended to apply hyperbaric oxygen therapy pre- and post-implant placement.
Hypersalivation	No	Similar	
Hyposalivation	No	Similar	Higher risk of per-implant health problems, assure that patient will keep adequate oral health maintenance.

(continued on next page)

Condition	(Relative) Contraindication	Implant Survival Rate	Precautions/ Recommendations
Table 2 *(continued)*			
Immunocompromised patients			
Biologicals	No	Similar	Discuss with physician whether administration of biologicals has to be adjusted or specific precautions are needed.
Crohn's disease	No	Similar/Reduced	Antibiotic prophylaxis. Older studies mention that implant survival is decreased compared to controls. Recent studies indicate that survival is similar.
Mixed connective Tissue disease	No	Similar	Antibiotic prophylaxis. Higher risk of per-implant health problems, Antibiotic prophylaxis.
Rheumatoid arthritis	No	Similar	Higher risk of peri-implant health problems, assure that patient will keep adequate oral health maintenance.
Scleroderma	No	Similar	Antibiotic prophylaxis. Higher risk of peri-implant health problems, assure that patient will keep adequate oral health maintenance.
Sjögren's syndrome	No	Similar	Antibiotic prophylaxis. Higher risk of per-implant health problems, assure that patient will keep adequate oral health maintenance.
Systemic lupus erythematosus	No	Similar	Antibiotic prophylaxis. Higher risk of per-implant health problems, assure that patient will keep adequate oral health maintenance.
Mucosal disease			
Epidermolysis bullosa	No	Similar	Antibiotic prophylaxis. Careful treatment if oral mucosa. Slightly higher risk of peri-implant health problems. Assure that patient will keep adequate oral health maintenance.

(continued on next page)

Condition	(Relative) Contraindication	Implant Survival Rate	Precautions/ Recommendations
Lichen planus	No	Similar	Antibiotic prophylaxis. Slightly higher risk of peri-implant health problems. Assure that patient will keep adequate oral health maintenance. Place implants when mucosal disease is in control.
Others (Crohn, SLE)	No	Similar	Antibiotic prophylaxis. Slightly higher risk of peri-implant health problems. Assure that patient will keep adequate oral health maintenance. Place implants when mucosal disease is in control.
Pemphigoid	No	Similar	Antibiotic prophylaxis. Slightly higher risk of peri-implant health problems. Assure that patient will keep adequate oral health maintenance. Place implants when mucosal disease is in control.
Pemphigus	No	Similar	Antibiotic prophylaxis. Slightly higher risk of peri-implant health problems. Assure that patient will keep adequate oral health maintenance. Place implants when mucosal disease is in control.
Smoking	Yes	Similar/Reduced	Implant survival is reduced, in particular for the maxilla, in heavy smokers. Increased risk of per-implantitis.
Titanium allergy	Yes	Reduced	Use alternative implant material, for example, zirconium.

Table 2 (continued)

Adapted from Scully C, Hobkirk J, Dios PD. Dental endosseous implants in the medically compromised patient. J Oral Rehabil. 2007;34(8):590–9; with permission.

A systematic review by Lemos and colleagues[9] examined the survival and success of dental implants placed in HIV-positive patients. The risk predictors examined were marginal bone loss and complications (ie, periimplantitis, mucositis, and prosthetic failure over a period of 48 months).[9] Three of the studies in the systematic review found no significant differences between HIV-positive and non-HIV study cohorts in terms of implant survival rate.[9,12,13] Significant factors common to these results include HAART therapy, which increases the number of CD4+ T cells. The mean CD4+ T-cell count was greater than 400 cells/mm^3 with a failure rate at less than 200 cells/mm^3 when 2 cohorts for implant placement were compared.[14,15] The other 3 studies of systematic analyses showed no significant difference with respect to CD4+ T cells and implant survival.[9] Another contributory factor for failure seemed to be the lack of prophylactic and postoperative antibiotic medications given.[9,14,15] Antibiotic prophylaxis is recommended, especially for their effect on inflammatory cascades seen in HIV-positive patients, which have the potential to reduce the CD4+ T-cell counts after implants are placed.[9,16]

As stated earlier, other complications most often of concern in the HIV-immunocompromised population are (1) bone loss caused by disorders as a result of viral medications/bone metabolic disorders, and (2) periimplantitis.[8–16] Marginal bone loss, another valid risk predictor for implant success and survival, was measured in these reviews because HAART has the potential to reduce mineral bone density.[8,9] In the HIV-positive population, the most frequent bone metabolic disorders were related to bone demineralization as a result of osteoporosis/osteopenia with a prevalence rate of 48% and 23%, respectively.[9,17,18] Oliveira and colleagues[12] suggested that HAART did not significantly cause marginal bone loss. Ata-Ali and colleagues[17] in their systematic review suggest that bone disturbances may be caused by a combination of factors such as low body weight, suboptimum calcium and vitamin D intake, smoking, alcohol, HIV itself, and HAART. The stimulation of osteoclast and osteoblast activity may be a result of increased production of proinflammatory cytokines secondary to chronic T-cell activation.[10,17] All of the systematic review studies discussed earlier support long-term follow-up over a period of greater than 1 year in order to verify the clinical stability of bone morphology in HIV-positive patients.[9,10,17,18]

Periimplantitis in HIV-positive patients is the most frequently characterized dental implant complication in all systematic reviews examined.[5,6,9,17] Although implant loss was most frequently the result of infection leading to periimplantitis, the periimplant sequela was not caused by immunosuppression but by preexisting periodontal disease. The latter was most often a result of failure to comply with periodontal maintenance.[9,17,18] Several systematic reviews support this finding.[9,17,19] Other risk predictors include tobacco (>10 cigarettes/d) and alcohol use.[9,19] Gherlone and colleagues[20] evaluated the rate of periimplantitis in prosthetic rehabilitation of HIV-positive patients using a prospective longitudinal study. At the 1-year postoperative follow-up, most fixtures placed had good osseointegration and stability and no infection, whereas, in 15 out of 190 implants placed, failures were the result of periimplantitis and concomitant prosthetic dysfunction. However, there were several limitations to this study, such as lack of consistency in the recording of tobacco use, CD4+ T-cell numbers, and oral hygiene.[20] The investigators concluded that a higher incidence of periimplantitis is likely in the first 6 months after implant therapy and, as such, suggest a need to develop a protocol for strict recall appointments and infection control. This finding is supported by other studies.[12,20,21]

The results presented earlier suggest that HIV infection may or may not have an impact on dental implant osseointegration over time. Prophylactic antibiotic treatment, HAART therapy, monitoring of CD4+ T-cell counts, and judicious recall for hygiene maintenance seem to be reliable mitigating risk predictors for success. Future prospective studies are still needed in larger sample sizes with longer follow-up in order to develop a consensus statement when considering HIV positivity to not be a relative or absolute contraindication to dental implant therapy.

Diabetes mellitus

Hyperglycemia (blood glucose level >140 mg/dL) is a frequent condition with a prevalence of 20% to 40% in the general surgery and dental populations. During the perioperative period, it can serve as an independent marker of poor surgical outcomes.[21–23] Patients with diabetes mellitus, whether type 1 or type 2, are at an increased risk of intraoperative and postoperative morbidity caused by hyperglycemia. It is well known that diabetic patients have an increased frequency of periodontitis and tooth loss, as well as delayed wound healing and increase in infections.[21–28] Infections result in compromised wound healing caused by endothelial dysfunction, platelet activation, and synthesis of proinflammatory cytokines, which inhibit fibrinolysis and result in subsequent coronary vessel occlusion with myocardial impairment.[21–25] Chronic hyperglycemia, a potential consequence of surgical stress, can result in significant microvascular and macrovascular disease, such as diabetic neuropathy, retinopathy, cerebrovascular disease, and peripheral vascular disease.

Although there are no prospective randomized trials in relation to blood glucose control during the perioperative period, several laboratory risk predictors can help in perioperative care, such as glycosylated hemoglobin A1c (HbA1c), which is a well-validated variable to monitor the long-term control of diabetes mellitus.[24] In 2018, the American Diabetes Association (ADA) guidelines were updated to reflect limitations in HbA1c measurements caused by hemoglobin variants, ethnicity, age, and altered red blood cell turnover. They have recommended the use of a new term, estimated average glucose (eAG), which expresses the HbA1c in the same units (mg/dL or mmol/L) as the average glucose levels self-monitored by the patients (**Table 3**).[25–28]

Based on the previous medical risk assessment, discussed earlier, diabetic patients who present to an oral health care provider need careful assessment to determine their options for dental implant therapy. Studies in the literature have characterized diabetes as a relative contraindication for implant therapy in a well-controlled patient cohort compared with patients who have poorly controlled glycemic physiology.[27,28] A study by Dowell and colleagues[29] did not find evidence to support implant success in poorly controlled diabetics using HbA1c monitoring, whereas Tawil and colleagues[30] found statistically significant relationships between plasma HbA1c and periimplantitis. In addition, prolonged wound healing was evident in these patient groups, which is not surprising because diabetic patients have impaired macrophage function, collagen

Table 3
The relationship among hemoglobin A1c, blood glucose, and estimated average glucose level

HbA1c (%)	Blood Glucose (mg/dL)	eAG (mmol/L)
6	126	7.0
6.5	140	7.8
7	154	8.6
7.5	169	9.4
8	183	10.1
8.5	197	10.9
9	212	11.8
9.5	226	12.6
10	240	13.4

American Diabetic Association recommends HbA1c less than 7%.
From American Diabetes Association. eAG/A1C conversion calculator. Available at: https://professional.diabetes.org/diapro/glucose_calc; with permission.

production, and fibroblastic innervation, all of which are required for wound healing.[29,30]

Several systematic reviews and meta-analyses have been published to investigate whether dental implant placement in diabetics versus nondiabetics have significantly more postoperative complications; namely, periimplantitis, loss of osseointegration, and implant failure rates. Naujokat and colleagues[28] identified 22 clinical studies and concluded that poorly controlled diabetics were significantly more likely to have impaired osseointegration, increased levels of periimplantitis, and a higher rate of implant failure. However, there was no consensus on whether the length of time a person had diabetes had any effect on implant failure rates.[28,29] They also concluded that dental implants are safe and predictable in diabetics compared with their nondiabetic cohorts over a period of 6 years, but, over a total of 20 years, the rates did differ. However, periimplantitis risk was not significantly different, and data were inconclusive with respect to strict recall in this patient population.[28,29] The HbA1c should be applied as a risk predictor after 1 year in order to monitor whether late changes in glycemic control predict implant failure compared with preoperative levels. In addition, diabetic patients benefit from prophylactic antibiotics preoperatively and postoperatively along with chlorhexidine rinses, which were shown to increase implant success if given at the time of surgery.[28,31]

Chrcanovic and colleagues,[27] in their systematic review of diabetes and oral implant failure using the Preferred Reporting Items for Systematic Reviews and Meta-analyses (PRISMA) guidelines, cautioned against relying on nonsignificant differences in implant success between diabetics and nondiabetics because of several confounders that limit the potential to draw strong conclusions. Examples of confounders included varied sample sizes, as well comparisons along different hierarchy of evidence levels (ie, case studies, retrospective chart reviews, groups not matched appropriately, and incomplete records).[27,28] All systematic reviews agreed that future controlled studies with larger sample sizes and matched cohorts are needed to determine outcomes in diabetic patients as optimal candidates for dental implant therapy.[27,28,30,31] Diabetic patients must still be carefully assessed, especially because of how issues of wound healing affect long-term outcomes for implant survival and successful dental rehabilitation.[27,28,30,31]

Autoimmune diseases

Autoimmune diseases comprise a group of illnesses that produce autoantibodies resulting in a state of self-inflammation. The prevalence of autoimmune disease ranges from 3% in Europe to up to 12.5% in North America.[6] This population presents several dilemmas because they have significant oral manifestations caused by their autoimmune status: ulcers, xerostomia, lichen planus and sclerosis of mucosal tissue, scar formation, and limited mouth opening. Secondary effects include compromised nutrition and swallowing, increased risk of caries and periodontal disease, as well as side effects of pharmacologic management (ie, corticosteroids and immunosuppressive drugs that treat the listed symptoms).[32] In addition, there is an increased risk of caries and severe periodontal diseases that cause a loss of teeth. Dental rehabilitation with removal of prostheses can exacerbate/potentiate the situation and lead to severe mucosal pain and necrosis of oral tissues. Therefore, dental implants have the potential to provide a valid option to improve oral health and health-related quality of life in this patient population.

Oral health care providers see many patients who have systemic autoimmune disease and request a treatment option of dental rehabilitation with implants. Certain considerations must be addressed by practitioners, such as the predisposition of oral mucosal disease, as stated earlier, as well as the pharmacologic therapies that have the potential to affect bone quality, which is most important factor for osseointe-gration (discussed later). Failure to follow oral hygiene protocols can enhance the fail-ure of marginal bone retention around the dental implants placed.[31–35] The risk of periimplantitis is also a consideration, and many studies have supported the correla-tion between oral autoimmune and periodontal disease. This dilemma has prompted clinicians to further examine these risk predictors for dental implants as an option for improved oral and overall health in this patient population. The following studies have examined whether dental implants are a viable option in patients with several autoim-mune disorders.

Scully and colleagues,[5] in their review on dental implants in medically compro-mised patients, suggested that, in patents with Sjögren syndrome (SS), dental implant–retained prostheses have the potential to decrease the oral manifestations of xerostomia and mucositis. A retrospective study on patients with rheumatoid arthritis and other connective tissue diseases that showed xerostomia showed high implant survival rates over a cumulative 3-year period and showed marginal bone resorption with good soft tissue condition.[35] However, patients with other con-nective tissue diseases (ie, scleroderma and SS cohorts with xerostomia) showed increased bone resorption and periimplantitis.[2,35] These investigators stressed that additional systematic reviews were needed with larger sampling cohorts to strongly support the premise of decreased xerostomia and its effect on implant survival. Common side effects of drugs used in patients with autoimmune diseases (dis-cussed later) are xerostomia and gastrointestinal dysfunction. In addition, the accu-mulation of food debris along the cervical areas of teeth caused by hyposalivation can affect periimplant health.[1,5,6] However, hyposalivation itself is not a contraindica-tion to dental implant therapy, and, when good oral hygiene is followed, there should be minimal risk of complications.

Several other systematic reviews have been undertaken to determine whether dental implant rehabilitation is a viable option in patients with autoimmune dysfunction associated with rheumatoid arthritis and SS.[6,32,35,36] Duttenhoefer and colleagues[6] evaluated a series of observational studies that analyzed a total of 236 implants placed into 56 patients with rheumatoid arthritis. The retrospective studies showed 100% sur-vival almost 4 years after implant placement. A prospective study in their systematic review reported a survival rate of 93%. This systematic review concluded that rheuma-toid arthritis did not influence the overall survival rate of dental implants detected.[6] However, the investigators of this systematic review did recommend a careful risk stratification among types of autoimmune status and encouraged more data from ran-domized controlled trials to firmly support the findings. A systematic review by Almeide and colleagues[36] evaluated the dental implant success rate in patients with SS compared with patients without SS using non-randomized controlled clinical and randomized controlled clinical trials. The risk predictors examined were marginal bone loss and biological complications.[36,37] Six studies were chosen for evaluation; however, none were randomized controlled trials. Three of the studies in the system-atic review characterized good bone stability without differences in bone loss when patients with SS were compared with their non-SS cohorts.[36] Other biological compli-cations in this review were characterized by peri-implant parameters. Greater probing depths and bleeding occurred in patients with SS compared with healthy cohorts (non-SS), and another of the 6 studies tabulated a higher incidence of mucositis and periimplantitis in patients with SS.[36] The investigators concluded that implant therapy in patients with SS may have the potential for a high survival rate and an in-crease in the health-related quality of life. The investigators also recommended more prospective studies over a longer period of time to further validate successful implant survival in patients with SS.

A significant risk predictor for implant success in patients with autoimmune disease is pharmacologic therapy. A variety of drug therapies pose challenges with their potential to affect implant osseointegration and long-term survival.[6] It is well documented in numerous studies that corticosteroids can suppress counter-regulatory immune responses to tissue injury and illness.[6,33] Duttenhoefer and colleagues[6] in their systematic review found that the predominant corticosteroid administered was prednisone or cortisone, and neither had a direct effect on implant survival. A review article by Tounta[33] examined oral autoimmune diseases, pharmacologic therapy, and dental implant rehabilitation. Glucocorticoids affected levels of calcium with an increased risk for a decrease in bone mineralization. Glucocorticoids further promoted osteoblast apoptosis and differentiation of bone marrow cells into adipocytes.[33] As such, Tounta[33] concluded that patients who require systemic administration up to 0.5 mg/kg/d of steroids are at a risk for poor bone quality and osteoporosis. However, Petsinis and colleagues,[38] in their review, suggested that glucocorticoid intake did not significantly affect dental implant osseointegration. A study by Lu and Huang[39] provided evidence for successful dental implant placement in a patient with chronic corticosteroid use as long as antibiotic prophylaxis and strict oral hygiene maintenance were followed. This evidence prevents a consensus statement with respect to corticosteroid use and dental implant osseointegration. All investigators recommend that decisions should be based on the individual patient, the duration of steroid therapy, and the type of autoimmune disease present when deciding whether implants are a viable option.

Autoimmune disease can also predispose patients to gastroesophageal issues and this patient population is often prescribed proton pump inhibitors (PPIs).[1,40,41] Adverse effects of PPI therapy include gastrointestinal symptoms, osteoporotic fractures, infection, and thrombocytopenia. Several observational studies have suggested an association between PPI exposure and fractures of the hip and vertebrae.[40–42] In 2010 the US Food and Drug Administration issued an advisory regarding bone fractures if dosing of PPIs was for long durations (ie, >1 year).[42] A retrospective study by Mehmet and colleagues[41] evaluated the effect of PPI use on implant osseointegration and function in 592 patients who had a total of 1918 implants placed. A total of 24 patients were prescribed PPI therapy and, when statistically compared with nonusers of PPI therapy, there was a significant difference ($P<.02$) for implant failure in the PPI cohort before implant loading. The mechanism of action may be a PPI-induced hypochlorhydria leading to malabsorption of calcium in the small intestine. The malabsorption of calcium leads to decrease in bone formation and increased bone resorption, leading to a lower bone mineral density.[41,42] Aghaloo and colleagues[43] in their systematic review suggest that medications such as PPIs and selective serotonin reuptake inhibitors (SSRIs; discussed later) may have a negative effect on implant osseointegration. However, controversy still remains because of study limitations (ie, comorbidities; concomitant medications; dose; duration; and confounders such as sex, age, and social habits). Future prospective trials and randomized controlled studies are needed to validate the outcomes of these studies on the effect of PPIs and dental implant osseointegration.

Depression is most often seen in patients with not only autoimmune diseases but a wide spectrum of chronic illnesses. Within the past few decades, SSRIs have been the drugs of choice in successfully treating depression. In 2011, the American Psychiatric Association (APA) recommended SSRIs as the first-line antidepressant medication.[44,45] It is well documented that depression is associated with low bone mass, and SSRIs are linked to bone loss and bone fractures.[45,46] The mechanism of action may reside in receptors on osteoblasts and osteoclasts that are activated by SSRIs that alter their functions in boney remodeling.[46,47] Several studies have evaluated whether SSRI therapy can be detrimental to dental implant osseointegration and long-term survival/success. A review and meta-analyses by Wu and colleagues[48] evaluated whether there was a decrease in dental implant osseointegration with the use of SSRIs. In a cohort of 916 implants in 490 patients, the cohort that used SSRIs were at an increased risk of implant failure caused by biomechanical alteration in loading. The investigators suggest that SSRIs contribute to bone loss during remodeling of bone under mechanical stress. Study limitations included sample size and biological confounders of parafunctional habits. Further studies were required to maintain their hypothesis. Another retrospective study, by Chrcanovic and colleagues,[49] used a multivariate mixed effects survival analysis to determine whether the intake of SSRIs was associated with increased risk of dental implant failure. Their results using Kaplan-Meir survival curve analysis showed an implant failure rate of 12.5% for SSRI cohorts and 3% for non-SSRI samples ($P<.001$). However, the multivariate model did not show a statistically significant difference between dose of SSRI and implant failure ($P = .125$). There were several significant limitations, including study designs with gaps in data collection, lack of other documented systemic conditions, as well as parafunctional habits that may have affected bone metabolism and osseointegration. The investigators recommended further prospective study designs with larger cohorts of patients to determine a valid association between SSRI use and options for dental implant rehabilitation.

Radiation therapy and dental implants

The treatment of head and neck cancers most often requires surgical intervention, which, depending on staging of the tumor, may include adjunctive radiation therapy (RT) and chemotherapy.[50,51] Ablative surgery involving the jaws most often leaves the patient with a hard and soft tissue foundation that is anatomically imbalanced. Loss of dentition and deformed edentulous ridges make it difficult to rehabilitate these patients with conventional removable prosthetics.[1,50] In addition, RT results in physiologically impaired bony sequelae (ie, a decreased bone vascularity and regenerative ability).[50,52,53] Other adverse events include xerostomia, painful mucositis, thickened saliva, and root caries, all of which complicate prosthetic rehabilitation. The option of a dental implant-supported prosthesis may offer the best hope for functional restoration in many of these patients. However, the placement of implants into irradiated jaws poses many challenges and is without a consensus among oral health care providers (discussed later). Overall, most studies reviewed show that the survival rate of implants is significantly lower in irradiated bone.[1,50–58] There are multiple factors (discussed later) that affect implant failure or success.

1. Placement location. Implants placed in the anterior mandible have a higher success rate than those placed in the maxilla or posterior mandible.[1,50–53,55,56] Most patients irradiated for head and neck tumors do not receive significant doses of radiation to the anterior mandible.[55]
2. Hyperbaric oxygen therapy (HBO). Even though HBO therapy is often used in the treatment and prevention of osteoradionecrosis (ORN), there is no conclusive evidence that its use improves the survival rate of implants placed in irradiated bone.[1,50,52,55,56]
3. Radiation dosage. Although some studies suggested fewer implant failures with doses of less than 50 Gy, others mentioned the increased risk of ORN at more

than 50 to 65 Gy.[53,54] Meta-analysis of multiple studies showed no significant risk of implant failure at higher doses.[52]

4. Timing of implant placement. Most studies indicated preference for waiting after the primary curative treatment (surgery, RT, chemotherapy), usually at least a year, before implant placement.[51,52,55] Implants can be placed at the time of the ablative surgery, which can shorten the time to prosthetic restoration; however, there is a risk of tumor recurrence in the first year. The survival rates of implants placed before or after radiation are not significantly different.[53]

5. Other factors. In addition to the usual considerations for successful implant placement in nonirradiated bone (adequate attached gingiva, bone quality and quantity, placement, prosthesis forces, hygiene, and so forth), there are many challenges beyond the normal. Most patients with oral cancer have a long history of smoking, significant alcohol use, and poor oral hygiene.[52]

Irradiated soft tissues are compromised and adequate attached gingiva often is not available. Xerostomia presents problems for good plaque control. Implant placement in surgical defect areas may result in unusual prosthetic forces in function. In areas where the surgical site was closed with nonmucosal flaps, the tissue thickness over the bone may be much more than is normally encountered.

6. Other potential treatments. Multiple studies over the past several years have shown positive results in the treatment of osteoradionecrosis, chronic osteomyelitis, and medication-related osteonecrosis of the jaw with the combination of pentoxifylline and tocopherol without the use of HBO.[58–60] In reevaluating the pathophysiology of these bone necrosis processes, this medical approach may have some promise in the increased survival rate of implants in irradiated bone.

Many of the articles reviewed on this subject relied on literature reviews of mostly retrospective studies. Of the prospective studies, there were small cohorts. There were few studies with consistent controls as to implant types, surgeon experience, techniques, or postoperative follow-up criteria. Long-term follow-up was mentioned in only a few reviews. A 5-year survival rate of only 50% of these patients makes long-term follow-up especially difficult. In addition, the bottom line, which was not addressed in most studies, is patient function and satisfaction.[52]

FUTURE DIRECTIONS/SUMMARY

Most oral health care practitioners would agree that the medical status of the patient can significantly influence the success rate of dental implant therapy. However, the appropriateness of dental implant therapy in medically compromised patients remains controversial, mostly because there are no clear guidelines with respect to the correlation of health risk and implant efficacy. Optimal timing of bony healing in the early stages of osseointegration is essential for long-term success during biomechanical loading and can be compromised by medical illness and pharmacotherapy. The hierarchy of evidence and controversy presented suggest that, in patients with systemic disease, there may or may not be a significant potential for implant survival. Although the studies presented earlier show successful outcomes in patients, debate remains, with a need for larger sample size populations and prospective clinical trials to better measure risk predictors for implant survival during the early and late phases of osseointegration. Clinicians must be prudent in weighing the issues of disease control as part of a cost-benefit analysis that determines advantages and disadvantages of dental implant therapy. By recognizing systemic conditions that place the patients at a higher probability of failure, practitioners can assist their patients in making informed decisions so that the treatment chosen provides a successful surgical outcome and better health-related quality of life. Immediate-term and long-term follow-up of all patients are essential regardless of disease-related relative or absolute contraindications when deciding whether dental implants are a viable restorative option in medically compromised patients.

CLINICS CARE POINTS

- The clinician must be aware that the medically complex patient may be a candidate for dental implant therapy as long as a thorough medical work-up and well thought-out treatment plan is followed with scheduled recall visits.
- The optimal timing for bony healing in the early stages of osseointegration is essential for implant survival and can be compromised by systemic disease and the pharmacotherapy used in the treatment of disease.
- Immediate and long term follow up is especially important in patients with concomitant illnesses since there are no consensus statements to date that support or refute implant therapy in the medically compromised patient.
- The patient with diabetes and/or autoimmune disease may be a candidate for dental implant therapy based upon careful medical workup, as well as judicious follow-up since they can be susceptible to long term implant complications.
- Patients exposed to radiation therapy must be carefully evaluated for implant therapy due to lack of consistency with respect to long term implant survival.

DISCLOSURE

The authors have nothing to disclose.

REFERENCES

1. Vissink A, Spijkervet FKL, Raghoebar GM. The medically compromised patient: are dental implants a feasible option? Oral Dis 2018;24:253–60.
2. Diz P, Scully C, Sanz M. Dental implants in the medically compromised patient. J Dent 2013;41(3):195–206.
3. Zitzmann NU, Margolin MD, Filippi A, et al. Patient assessment and diagnosis in implant treatment. Aust Dent J 2008;53(1Suppl):S3–10.
4. Kotsakis GA, Ioannou AL, Hinrichs JE, et al. A systematic review of observational studies evaluating implant placement in the maxillary jaws of medically compromised patients. Clin Implant Dent Relat Res 2015;17(3):598–608.
5. Scully C, Hobkirk J, Dios PD. Dental endosseous implants in the medically compromised patient. J Oral Rehabil 2007;34:590–9.
6. Duttenhoefer F, Fuessinger MA, Beckmann Y, et al. Dental implants in immuno-compromised patients: a systematic review and meta-analysis. Int J Implant Dent 2019;5:43, 1-12.
7. Sadowsky SJ, Fitzpatrick B, Curtis DA. Evidence-based criteria for different treatment planning of implant restorations for the maxillary edentulous patient. J Prosthodont 2015;433–46.
8. Rubenstein NC, Jacobson Z, McCausland GL, et al. Retrospective study of the success of dental implants placed in HIV-positive patients. Int J Implant Dent 2019;5:30, 1-5.
9. Lemos CAA, Verri FR, Cruz BS, et al. Survival of dental implants placed in HIV-positive patients: a systematic review. Int J Oral Maxillofac Surg 2018;47: 1336–42.

10. Brown TT, Qaqish RB. Antiretroviral therapy and the prevalence of osteopenia and osteoporosis: a meta-analysis review. AIDS 2006;20:2165–74.
11. Scully C, Watt-smith P, Dios PD, et al. Complications I HIV-infected and non-HIV-infected haemophiliacs and other patients after oral surgery. Int J Oral Maxillofac Surg 2002;31:634–40.
12. Oliveira MA, Gallottini M, Pallos D, et al. The success of endosseous implants in human immunodeficiency virus-positive patients receiving anti-retroviral therapy: a pilot study. J Am Dent Assoc 2011;142:1010–6.
13. Rania V, Pellegrino P, Donati G, et al. Long term efficacy of dental implants in HIV-positive patients. Clin Infect Dis 2015;61:1208.
14. Patton LL, Shugars DA, Bonito AJ. A systematic review of complication risks for HIV-positive patients undergoing invasive dental procedures. J Am Dent Assoc 2002;133:195–203.
15. May MC, Andrews PN, Daher S, et al. Prospective cohort study of dental implant success rate in patients with AIDS. Int J Implant Dent 2016;2:20.
16. Baron M, Gritsch F, Hansy AM, et al. Implants in an HIV-positive patient: a case report. Int J Oral Maxillofac Implants 2004;19:425–30.
17. Ata-Ali J, Ata-Ali F, Di-Benedetto N, et al. Does HIV infection have an impact upon dental implant osseointegration ? A systematic review. Med Oral Patol Oral Cir Bucal 2015;20(3):e347–56.
18. Gay-Escoda C, Perez-Alvarez D, Camps-font O, et al. long term outcomes of oral rehabilitation with dental implants in HIV-positive patients: a retrospective case series. Med Oral Patol Oral Cir Bucal 2016;21:e385–91.
19. Chrcanovic BR, Albrektsson T, Wennerberg A. Smoking and dental implants: a systematic review and meta-analysis. J Dent 2015;43:487–98.
20. Gherlone EF, Cappare P, Tecco S, et al. Implant prosthetic rehabilitation in controlled HIV-positive patients: A prospective longitudinal study with 1-year follow up. Clin Implant Dent Relat Res 2016;18(4):734.
21. Patton LL, Shugards DA, bonito AL. A systematic review of complication rate for HIV-positive patients undergoing invasive dental procedures. J Am Dent Assoc 2002;133:195–203.
22. Kotagal M, Symons RG, Hirsch IB, et al, SCOAP-CERTAIN Collaborative. Perioperative hyperglycemia and risk of adverse events among patients with and without diabetes. Ann Surg 2015;261(1):97–103.
23. Frisch A, Chandra P, Smiley D, et al. Prevalence and clinical outcome of hyperglycemia in the perioperative period in noncardiac surgery. Diabetes Care 2010;33(8):1783–8.
24. Dogra P, Jialal I. Diabetic perioperative management. Available at: https://www.ncbi.nlm.nih.gov/books/NBK540965/?report=reader. Accessed January 1 2020.
25. Soldevila B, Lucas AM, Zavala R, et al. Perioperative management of the diabetic patient. In: Stuart-Smith K, editor. Perioperative medicine-current controversies. Zurich: Springer International Publishing Switzerland; 2016. p. 165–92.
26. American Diabetes Association. Pharmacologic approaches to glycemic treatment: Standards of medical care in diabetes-2018. Diabetes Care 2018; 41(Suppl 1):S73–85.
27. Chrcanovic BR, Albrekisson T, Wennerberg A. Diabetes and oral implant failure: A systematic Review. J Dent Res 2014;93(9):859–67.
28. Naujokat H, Kunzendorf B, Wiltfang J. Dental implants and diabetes mellitus: A systematic review. Int J Implant Dent 2016;2(5):1–10.

29. Dowell S, Oates TW, Robinson M. Implant success in people with type 2 diabetes mellitus with varying glycemic control: a pilot study. J Am Dent Assoc 2007; 138(3):355–61.

30. Tawil G, Younan R, Azar P, et al. Conventional and advanced implant treatment in the type 2 diabetic patient: surgical protocol and long-term clinical results. Int J Oral Maxillofac Implants 2008;23(4):744–52.

31. Guobis Z, Pacauskiene I, Astramskaite I. General disease influence on peri-implantitis development: a systematic review. J Oral Maxillofac Res 2016;7(3): e5–16.

32. Strietzel FP, Schmidt-Westhausen AM, Neurmann K, et al. Implants in patients with oral manifestations of autoimmune or muco-cutaneous diseases- A systematic review. Med Oral Patol Oral Cir Bucal 2019;24(2):e217–30.

33. Tounta TS. Dental implants in patients with oral autoimmune diseases: article. JRPMS 2019;3(1):9–16.

34. Weinlander M, Krennmair G, Piehslinger E. Implant prosthodontic rehabilitation in patient with rheumatic disorders: A case series report. Int J Prosthodont 2010; 23:22–8.

35. Korfage A, Raghoebar GM, Arends S, et al. Dental implants in patients with Sjogren's Syndrome. Clin Implant Dent Relat Res 2016;18(5):937–45.

36. Almeide D, Vianne K, Arriage P, et al. Dental implants in Sjogren's Syndrome patients: A systematic review. PLoS One 2017. https://doi.org/10.1371/journal. 0189507.

37. Misch CA, Perel ML, Wang HL, et al. Implant success, survival and failure: the international congress of Oral Implantologists (ICOI) Pisa consensus conference. Implant Dent 2008;17:5–15.

38. Petsinis V, Kamperos G, Alexandridi F, et al. The impact of glucocorticosteroids administered for systemic diseases on the osseointegration and survival of dental Implants placed without bone grafting : a retrospective study in 31 patients. J Craniomaxillofac Surg 2017;45(8):1197–2000.

39. Lu SY, Huang CC. Resolution of an active periimplantitis in a chronic steroid user by bone augmentation with Pepgen-P-15 and a barrier membrane. J Oral Implantol 2007;33(5):280–7.

40. Korfage A, Raghoebar GM, Slater JJ, et al. Overdentures on primary mandibular implants in patients with oral cancer: A follow up study over 14 years. Br J Oral Maxillofac Surg 2014;529:798–805.

41. Mehmet AA, Sindel A, Ozalp O, et al. Proton pump inhibitor intake negatively affects the osseointegration of dental implants: a retrospective study. J Korean Assoc Oral Maxillofac Surg 2019;46:135–40.

42. Freedberg DE, Kim LS, Yang YX. The risks and benefits of long-term use of proton pump inhibitors: expert review and best practice advice from the American Gastroenterological Association. Gastroenterology 2017;152:706–15.

43. Aghaloo T, Antuns J, Moshaverinia A, et al. The effects of systematic diseases and medications on implant osseointegration: A systematic review. Int J Oral Maxillofac Implants 2019;34:s35–49.

44. American Psychiatric Association. Practice guidelines for the treatment of patients with major depressive disorder. 3rd Edition. Arlington (VA): American Psychiatric Association; 2011.

45. Ouanounou A, Hassanpour S, Glogauer M. The influence of systemic medications on osseointegration of dental implants: a review. J Can Dent Assoc 2016; 82(g7):1–8.

46. Gebara MA, Shea ML, Lipsey KL, et al. Depression, anti-depressants and bone health in older adults: A systematic review. J Am Geriatr Soc 2014;62(8):434–41.
47. Tsapakis EM, Gamie Z, Tran G, et al. The adverse skeletal effects of selective serotonin reuptake inhibitors. Eur Psychiatry 2012;27(3):156–65.
48. Wu Q, Bencaz AF, Hentz JG, et al. Selective serotonin-reuptake inhibitor treatment and risk of fractures: a meta-analysis of cohort and case-controlled studies. Osteoporos Int 2012;23(1):365–75.
49. Chrcanovic BR, Kisch J, Albrektsson T, et al. Is the intake of selective serotonin reuptake inhibitors associated with an increased risk of dental implant failure? Int J Oral Maxillofac Surg 2017;46:782–8.
50. Nobrega AS, Santiago JF, de Faria Almeida DA, et al. Irradiated patients and survival rate of dental implants: A systematic review and meta-analysis. J Prosthet Dent 2016;116:858–66.
51. Koudougou C, Bertin H, Lecaplain B, et al. Post implantation radiation therapy in head and neck cancer patients: Literature review. Head Neck 2020;42:794–802.
52. Chrcanovic BR, Albrektsson T, Wennerberg A. Dental implants in irradiated versus nonirradiated patients: A meta-analysis. Head Neck 2016. https://doi.org/10.1002/hed.23875.
53. Ihde S, Koop S, Gundlach K, et al. Effects of radiation therapy on craniofacial and dental implants: a review of the literature. Oral Surg Oral Med Oral Pathol Oral Radiol Endod 2009;107:56–63.
54. Shugaa-Addin B, Al-Shamiri HM, Al-Maweri S, et al. The effect of radiotherapy on survival of dental implants in head and neck cancer patients. J Clin Esp Dent 2016;8(2):e194–200.
55. Dholam KP, Gurav SV. Dental implants in irradiated Jaws: A literature review. J Can Res Ther 2012;8:85–93.
56. Chambrone L, Mandia J Jr, Shibli JA, et al. Dental implants installed in Irradiated Jaws: A systematic review. J Dent Res 2013;92(suppl no 2):119S–30S.
57. Woods B, Schenberg M, Chandu A. A comparison of immediate and delayed dental implant placement in head and neck surgery patients. J Oral Maxillofac Surg 2019;77:1156–64.
58. Breik O, Tocaciu S, Briggs K, et al. Is there a role for pentoxifylline and tocopherol in the management of advanced osteoradionecrosis of the jaws with pathological fractures: Case reports and review of the literature. J Oral Maxillofac Surg 2019;48:1022–7.
59. Kolokythas A, Rasmussen JT, Reardon J, et al. Management of osteoradionecrosis of the jaws with pentoxifylline-tocopherol: a systematic review of the literature and meta-analysis. J Oral Maxillofac Surg 2019;48:173–80.
60. Aggarwal K, Goutam M, Singh M, et al. Prophylactic use of pentoxifylline and Tocopherol in patients undergoing dental extractions following radiotherapy for head and neck cancer. Niger J Surg 2017;23(2):130–3.

Placement of Short Implants
A Viable Alternative?

David Sheen, DDS[a],*, Levon Nikoyan, DDS[a,b]

KEYWORDS

- Short implant • Rough-surface implant • Bone grafting • Interface

KEY POINTS

- The placement of short implants, which measure less than 10 mm in length, requires the practitioner to have a thorough comprehension of implant dentistry to achieve acceptable results.
- Innovation of the rough-surface implant and the progression of the implant-abutment interface from an external hex to an internal connection have considerably influenced the longevity of short implants.
- Dentists are better equipped to serve their patients because the utilization of short implants may preclude the need for advanced surgical bone-grafting procedures.

HISTORY OF IMPLANTS

Archeologists have discovered that even early civilizations desired to replace missing teeth. Excavations of ruins roughly dating back to approximately 600 AD demonstrate that the Mayan people used a variety of materials to insert into empty tooth sockets, notably carved seashells.[1]

The contemporary age of root form endosseous implants commenced in 1952 when a Swedish physician, Dr. Per-Ingvar Branemark, discovered osseointegration. Subsequently, in 1965, Dr. Branemark placed the first titanium dental implants in a human patient.[2] His extraordinary clinical research and investigations were unparalleled. In 1982, when Dr. Branemark presented his work on osseointegration at a dental conference in Toronto, the field of dental implantology was revolutionized.

IMPLANT LENGTH

Initially, the length of implants ranged from 7 mm to 20 mm. The most common implant diameter accessible to dentists early on was 3.75 mm. The consensus among practitioners at the time was that the length of the implant was considerably more important

[a] Department of Oral and Maxillofacial Surgery, Woodhull Medical Center, Brooklyn, NY, USA;
[b] Private Practice, Forward Oral Surgery, 248-62 Jericho Tpke, Floral Park, NY 11001, USA
* Corresponding author. Department of Oral and Maxillofacial Surgery, Woodhull Medical Center, 760 Broadway, Brooklyn, NY 11206.
E-mail address: dsheen16@gmail.com

Dent Clin N Am 65 (2021) 21–31
https://doi.org/10.1016/j.cden.2020.09.001
0011-8532/21/© 2020 Elsevier Inc. All rights reserved.

dental.theclinics.com

than implant diameter. However, the research had not yet demonstrated a linear relationship with regard to the aforementioned concept.[3]

Numerous researchers have deemed various implant lengths as short. Some assert that implants up to 7 mm or less are short whereas others have proclaimed up to 10 mm or less.[4–9] In the field of dentistry there is no universal agreement on what comprises short and long implants. Throughout this article, long or standard-length implants are 10 mm or longer, whereas short implants are considered to be less than 10 mm.

PARTIALITY FOR LONG IMPLANTS

There were 2 prevailing reasons why long implants were considered superior. First, initial clinical research showed that short Branemark implants with traditional machined surfaces, which were 6 mm to 10 mm in length, had lower success rates than longer implants. Friberg and colleagues[10] investigated 4641 Branemark machined fixtures from the time of implant insertion until prosthetic restoration. Their findings led them to conclude that long implants, ranging from 10 mm to 20 mm in length, were significantly more successful compared with short implants.[10] Wyatt and Zarb[11] reported on a 12-year investigation (mean of 5.4 years) of 230 Branemark machined fixtures. In their study, 25% of short implants, which were 7 mm in length, failed; whereas only an 8% failure rate was associated with 10-mm implants. Longer implants, measuring 13 mm and 15 mm, only failed 5% and 2% of the time, respectively.[11] Bahat reported a 17% failure rate with short implants, measuring 7.0 mm and 8.5 mm, after following 660 fixtures for 5 to 12 years.[12] Attard and Zarb[13] reported that short implants (7 mm) had a 15% failure rate, whereas long implants measuring 10 mm and 13 mm only failed 6% to 7% of the time.

Weng and colleagues[14] conducted a multicenter prospective clinic study for 6 years investigating 1179 3i implants. In their study, short implants were considered to be 10 mm or less in length and comprised 48.5% of all implants evaluated. In 2003, their report showed that short fixtures, measuring 7 mm to 10 mm, had an overall success rate of only 88.7% and were attributed to 60% of all failed fixtures. The 7.0-mm and 8.5-mm implants had a failure rate of 26% and 19%, respectively, whereas the 10-mm implants had a 10% failure rate. Long implants, measuring longer than 10 mm, had an overall success rate of 93.1%.[14] Herrmann and colleagues[5] conducted a multicenter investigation for 5 years following 487 Nobel Biocare implants. In 2005, their report showed that 7-mm implants had a failure rate of 21.8%, whereas 10-mm implants had a 10.1% failure rate.[5]

The second reason why long implants were considered more desirable was based on dental education regarding fixed prosthodontics, which conceivably may have altered the judgment of practitioners. Ante's law states that the total periodontal membrane area of the abutment teeth must equal or exceed that of the teeth to be replaced.[15] Based on this postulate, the crown-to-root ratio was used to determine if a tooth was an appropriate abutment. The literature reports a variety of ratios. Although infrequently found in clinical practice, a crown-to-root ratio of 1:2 was considered ideal.[16] Shillingburg and colleagues[17] stated that a crown-to-root ratio of at least 1:1 was required for an adequate result, and a crown-to-root ratio of 1:1.5 was most favorable. The thought of longer roots serving as more advantageous abutments still endures although Ante's law has subsequently been refuted.[18]

To understand why clinicians and researchers were persistently exploring the concept of short implants, after numerous investigations demonstrated the lower success rate of short fixtures, one must be cognizant of the fact that there are abundant clinical conditions that preclude the application of long implants. Some of the anatomic difficulties encountered are alveolar ridge deficits, maxillary sinus pneumatization with inadequate alveolar ridge height, and the location of the inferior alveolar nerve.[19] Innovative surgical procedures were established to solve these anatomic problems. Block grafting, guided bone regeneration, and maxillary sinus floor grafting were performed to augment alveolar bone height. These advanced surgical techniques can be time-consuming, challenging, costly, can extend total treatment time, and increase surgical morbidity.[19–22]

SURGICAL BONE-GRAFTING PROCEDURES

Milinkovic and Cordaro[21] conducted a systematic review of various surgical techniques that vertically augmented partially edentulous and completely edentulous alveolar ridges. Their report contrasted the mean implant survival rate and the mean complication rate between block grafting, guided bone regeneration, and distraction osteogenesis. Guided bone regeneration in partially edentulous patients had a mean implant survival rate of 98.9% to 100% and a mean complication rate of 6.95% to 13.1%. Block grafts in partially edentulous patients had a mean implant survival rate of 96.3% and a mean complication rate of 8.1%. Distraction osteogenesis yielded the greatest gain in vertical height, but concurrently had the highest mean complication rate of 22.4% while having a mean implant survival rate of 98.2%. Block grafts in completely edentulous patients had a mean implant survival rate of only 87.75%. Its mean complication rate varied widely depending on which donor sites and recipient sites were examined.[21]

Vasquez and colleagues[23] reported both the intraoperative and postoperative complication rate of 200 maxillary sinus floor graft surgeries. Their work showed that sinus membrane perforation was the most common intraoperative complication encountered 25.7% of the time. Prior studies found a sinus perforation rate in the range of 7% to 56%. Postoperative complications occurred 19.7% of the time. They included surgical wound infection at 7.1%, sinusitis at 3.9%, and loss of bone graft at 1.6%.[23]

The posterior segment of atrophic mandibles poses a great challenge to practitioners. When the residual vertical height of posterior mandibular alveolar ridges is not amenable for the placement of implants 10 mm or greater in length, then the only recourse is bone grafting as already stated above or surgical transposition of the inferior alveolar nerve. Hassani and colleagues[22] reported a sensory deficit approaching 100% in the initial postoperative period following transposition of the inferior alveolar nerve. They observed that 84% of patients regained their baseline nerve function, whereas 16% of cases had permanent nerve impairment.[22]

To circumvent the risks associated with advanced surgical procedures, short implants were introduced.[6,7] In 2014, Nisand and Renouard[24] conducted a review of various reports comparing the survival rates of long implants with concurrent bone-grafting procedures with the survival rates of short implants. Similar survival rates were found for both groups being studied; however, the placement of short implants yielded a shorter treatment period, was more cost-effective, and resulted in considerably less morbidity (**Table 1**).[24]

IMPLANT SURFACE

In the late 1980s, it was accepted that there would be 1.5 mm of crestal bone loss in the first year of implant placement and subsequent bone loss not exceeding 0.2 mm during each successive year.[30] Based on this axiom, short implants are inherently at a

Table 1
Short implants versus standard-length implants with various vertical augmentation procedures

Author/Year	Patients/ Implants	Follow-up, mo	Test Implant	Control Implant/Sx	Cumulative Success Rate
Penarrocha-Oltra et al,[8] 2014	37/80	12	5.5 mm (intrabony length)	>10 mm + block vertical graft (>8.5 mm intrabony length)	T: 1 short failed C: 2 long failed (preload); 7 grafts deficient needed to use short implants; 21 needed additional grafting
Gulje et al,[25] 2013	95/208	12	6 mm	11 mm	T: 3 short failed; 2 preloading; 1 postloading C: 1 long failed
Pieri et al,[26] 2012	68/144	36	6 mm	>11 mm + sinus graft	T: 98.6% success C: 96% success
Esposito et al,[27] 2011	60/121	36	6.3 mm	>9.3 mm + vertical bone graft	T: 2 short failed C: 3 long failed; 2 grafts failed
Felice et al,[28] 2011	28/178	5	5.0–8.5 mm	>11.5 mm + vertical bone graft	T: 2 short failed C: 1 long failed; 2 grafts failed
Felice et al,[29] 2010	60/121	12	7 mm	>10 mm + vertical bone graft	T: 1 short failed C: 3 long failed; 2 grafts failed

Abbreviations: C, control; Sx, surgery; T, test.
Adapted from Nisand D, Renouard F. Short implant in limited bone volume. Periodontology 2000;2014;66(1):77; with permission.

disadvantage when considering long-term clinical outcomes. However, when the criteria for success were first published most implant fixtures had a machined/turned surface. As time passed, research on the technology of implant surface advanced and the corollary was rough-surface or textured implants. Through the innovation of rough/textured surfaces, the former criteria were no longer justified.

Renouard and Nisand[24] examined the effect of implant length and diameter on survival rates. During their review of 53 studies, they found that 12 cases demonstrated a higher failure rate with short implants which were associated with machined surface fixtures, preparation of the osteotomy site regardless of bone quality, clinician experience, and placement in regions with inadequate bone density. Twenty-two reports that followed displayed similar survival rates between short and long implants when rough-surface fixtures were placed and a modified osteotomy technique corresponding to bone quality was used.[7]

When published in 2011, a meta-analysis conducted by Pommer and colleagues[4] showed that the failure rates of rough-surface fixtures were significantly lower compared with machined surface fixtures. Balshe and colleagues[31] conducted a retrospective analysis of 2425 rough-surface fixtures and 2182 machined surface fixtures and found that there was no statistical difference in the 5-year survival rates. The rough-surface implants had a survival rate of 94.5%, whereas the machined surface implants had a survival rate of 94%. In addition, the survival rates for rough-surface and machined surface implants were 93.7% and 88.5%, respectively, when implants measuring 10 mm or less were studied separately.[31] Nedir and colleagues[32] reported on a 7-year life table analysis of success rates between short and long rough-surface implants. In their prospective study, they found that the cumulative success rate of short rough-surface fixtures measuring 8 to 9 mm was equivalent to long rough-surface fixtures measuring 10 to 13 mm when loaded for at least 1 year.[32]

IMPLANT-ABUTMENT INTERFACE

The progression of the implant to abutment interface from an external hex to an internal connection, such as a Morse taper or conical design, has considerably influenced the longevity of short implants. De Castro and colleagues[33] reported that abutments with the Morse taper connection sustain less marginal bone resorption than ones with an external hex connection. Furthermore, their study found that the internal conical connection might allow for bone growth over the shoulder of the fixture in close proximity to the abutment.[33]

Weng and colleagues[34] reported on crestal bone loss among fixtures with an internal connection and those with an external hex. In their study, they placed implants with an internal conical connection at the level of the bony crest and also 1.5 mm subcrestal, and then compared the amount of crestal bone loss incurred by those implants with that of the external hex implants that were correspondingly placed at the bony crest level and 1.5 mm subcrestal. They found that the implant-abutment interface with an internal connection had significantly less crestal bone loss than the external hex implants. In addition, external hex fixtures that were placed subcrestal sustained the largest amount of crestal bone loss.[34] These findings demonstrate that crestal bone loss is not a substantial component in the survival of short implants.

IMPLANT-BONE INTERFACE

The implant-to-bone interface can be analyzed via a computer program, called Finite Element Analysis, that is capable of anticipating how the amount of stress that is applied to an implant will affect it and also how the applied stress will affect the association between the implant and adjacent bone. The program generates a lattice of points in the form of the fixture that encompasses data about the fixture which can be analyzed at all points. Finite Element Analysis enables clinicians to try to predict what will occur to the implant-bone interface during various situations as they modify aspects such as bone density, implant diameter, and length.

Using 3-dimensional computer models created by Finite Element Analysis, Himmlova and colleagues[35] investigated the stress that occurs at the implant-bone interface. The diameters of their simulated fixtures ranged from 2.9 mm to 6.5 mm and the lengths ranged from 8 mm to 18 mm. When comparing an 8-mm implant with a 17-mm implant, there was not much variance in area affected by maximum stress, and the maximum amount of stress was concentrated at the superior 5-mm to 6-mm portion of the implant. Only a 7.3% difference in stress was noted. In addition, there was a negative correlation between implant diameter and stress. The narrow 2.9-mm implant had maximum stress values that were 60% higher than those of the wider 6.5-mm implant.[35] Therefore, implant diameter was a more significant factor than length regarding stress distribution.

Using the computer program with 5 commercially accessible fixture designs, Baggi and colleagues[36] evaluated the impact of fixture diameter and length on stress distribution. The simulated implants had lengths of 7.5 mm to 12 mm and diameters of 3.3 mm to 4.5 mm. The results of their study led them to conclude that implant diameter had greater efficacy than implant length in withstanding biomechanical stress.[36]

IMPLANT-CROWN RATIO

There have been numerous case series and studies that have investigated crown-to-implant length ratios specifically concerning short implants. Blanes[37] conducted a systematic review of the effect of crown-implant ratios on implant survival rates and peri-implant crestal bone resorption. The analysis, which included rough-surface and machined implants, showed that implants with crown-implant ratios greater than or equal to 2 had a 94.1% survival rate after a mean follow-up of 6 years. Furthermore, the study found that crestal bone resorption was not affected by crown-implant ratios.[37]

Tawil and Younan[38] conducted a prospective clinical study following 269 machined surface fixtures for a period of 12 to 92 months. In the study, standard-length fixtures measured 10 mm, whereas short fixtures had lengths of 6 mm to 8.5 mm. The diameters of the fixtures ranged from 3.3 mm to 5 mm. The survival rates for the short and standard-length fixtures were 93.1% and 97.4%, respectively. These findings were not statistically significant. In addition, they found that the 3.75-mm-diameter fixtures had a survival rate of 96.3%, the 4-mm-diameter fixtures had a survival rate of 96.0%, and the 5-mm-diameter fixtures had a survival rate of 94.5%. Again, the findings were not statistically significant when analyzing survival rates based on the various diameters. The 3.3-mm-diameter fixtures were not evaluated. Furthermore, the average peri-implant crestal bone resorption was 0.71 mm.[38]

Nedir and colleagues[32] conducted a 7-year life table study of 528 rough-surface fixtures with regard to their crown-implant ratios. In their analysis, the crown-implant ratios ranged from 1.45 to 1.97 for the short implants which had lengths of 6 mm to 9 mm. The crown-implant ratios ranged from 1.05 to 1.3 for the long implants which had lengths of 10 mm to 13 mm. Their findings demonstrated a cumulative success rate of 99.4% and showed that short implants did not have a higher failure rate compared to long implants although the short implants had greater crown-implant ratios.[32]

A systematic review of 33 studies conducted by Atieh and colleagues[39] focused on short implant placement in the posterior regions of the maxilla and mandible. A total of 3573 short implants measuring 8.5 mm or less in length were studied. Fifty-one percent of the implants were in the mandible, 38% were in the maxilla, and it was unknown where the other 11% of implants were placed. The mean follow-up was 3.9 years with a range of 1 to 7 years. In total, there were 67 implants that failed, and 71% of the failures occurred before implant loading.[39] The finding of implant failure before loading is congruous with other analyses,[6,10,38] and indicates that forces concomitant with loading of implants and a decrease in the implant-bone interface are not the predominant factors in the definitive failure or success of short implants.

RISK FACTORS

Contemporary literature supports the placement of short fixtures; however, there are risk factors such as low-quality bone, smoking, and the experience of the clinician. A systematic review of 29 studies conducted by Telleman and colleagues[40] focused on short implant placement in the posterior regions of the maxilla and mandible. A total of 2611 short implants measuring 5.0 mm to 9.5 mm in length were studied. They evaluated several factors including the type of implant surface, implant length, if the patient was a smoker or not, and whether the implants were placed in the maxilla or mandible. Their study found that rough-surface implants had a 29% higher success rate than machined implants. The overall survival rate enhanced as the length of the implants increased. The 5-mm implants had a survival rate of 93.1%, the 6-mm implants had a survival rate of 97.4%, the 7-mm implants had a survival rate of 97.6%, the 8-mm implants had a survival rate of 98.4%, the 8.5-mm implants had a survival rate of 98.8%, the 9-mm implants had a survival rate of 98.0%, and the 9.5-mm implants had a survival rate of 98.6%. The heavy smoker group, composed of patients who smoked at least 15 cigarettes per day, had a 57% higher failure rate compared with nonsmokers. The study also found that implants placed in maxilla, which generally has low-quality or low-density bone, had a twofold increase in their failure rate in contrast to implants placed in the mandible.[40]

In 2014, Nisand and Renouard[24] conducted a review of various reports comparing the survival rates of long implants with short implants. Short implants were considered to have a length of 8 mm or less. In their analysis of long implants, they evaluated 5 reviews that consisted of 58,953 implants, and found an overall survival rate ranging from 93.1% to 99.1%. In their analysis of short implants, they evaluated 29 case series that consisted of 9780 implants, and found an overall success rate of 96.67%. The findings are congruent with other studies that validate the effectiveness of short implants when placed in suitable clinical conditions.[24]

Several studies that have evaluated short implants demonstrate promising success rates (**Table 2**). A total of 493 short implants were analyzed in these 4 studies with an average follow-up ranging from 2 years to 10 years. The studies included rough-surface and machined implants, implants that were placed in high-density and low-density bone in both the maxilla and mandible, implants with lengths that ranged from 5.5 mm to 10 mm, and implants that were placed in patients who were smokers and nonsmokers. The short implants had an overall success rate of 95.5%.

The experience of the practitioner and the surgical protocol also need to be considered when assessing the efficacy of short implants. Various clinicians and researchers have proposed modified surgical guidelines to enhance the primary mechanical stability of short implants, including Nisand and Renouard,[24] Fugazzotto and colleagues,[45] and Tawil and Younan.[38] Although minor distinctions exist in the details, the general

Table 2
Recent studies with favorable success rates

Author/Year	Mean Follow-up (mo)	No. of Patients/ Implants	CSR (%)	No. of Failed Implants	Prosthesis Failures
Anitua et al,[41] 2014	24	34/45 <6.5 mm	100	0	0
Anitua et al,[42] 2014	123.3	75/111 (94 were splinted to longer implants)	98.90	1	NR
Lai et al,[43] 2013	86 (range 60–120)	168/231	98.7 at 5 y 98.3 at 10 y	4	11
Sanchez-Garces et al,[44] 2012	81	136/273 (total) 167 10 mm 106 short	92.67 92.82 92.5	20 (total) 12 8	NR — —

Abbreviations: CSR, cumulative success rate; NR, not recorded.
Adapted from Nisand D, Renouard F. Short implant in limited bone volume. Periodontology 2000;2014;66(1):77; with permission.

concept of increasing primary stability is the same. The experience of the practitioner is perhaps the toughest factor to measure. Clinical experience with placement of short implants has been cited as an explanation for the varied results among studies evaluating short implants.[7]

Short implant placement should not be regarded as a less complex procedure when compared with placement of long implants. Novice practitioners need to bear in mind that they have to be absolutely confident in the fundamentals of surgical implant placement, as there is a learning curve associated with short implants. A sound understanding of implant surgery is required to be able to effectively alter the surgical protocol as needed to account for difficulties that may be encountered with 3-dimensional positioning and bone density.[7,24]

Because research has demonstrated adequate success rates for implants measuring as short as 6 mm, determining the minimum amount of residual bone in the maxilla and mandible required for accommodating these implants is possible.[39,40] Without the utilization of surgical bone-grafting procedures when placing short implants in the maxilla, the minimum height of alveolar bone inferior to the maxillary sinus has to measure 6 to 7 mm. If at least 6 mm of bone in the vertical dimension is not available, then maxillary sinus graft surgery is recommended. In addition, the practitioner has to consider other risk factors, such as periodontal disease, bone density, patient age, and smoking. When placing a 6-mm implant in the mandible, the minimum height of bone above the inferior alveolar nerve canal required is 8 mm. This measurement accounts for not only the length of the short implant, but also for a safety zone of 2 mm superior to the inferior alveolar nerve canal. If at least 8 mm of bone height is not available, then a surgical transposition of the inferior alveolar nerve or a bone-grafting procedure is indicated.

SUMMARY

The placement of short implants, which measure less than 10 mm in length, require the practitioner to have a thorough comprehension of implant dentistry to achieve acceptable results. Dentists are better equipped to serve their patients because the utilization of short implants may preclude the need for advanced surgical bone-grafting procedures.

DISCLOSURE

The authors have nothing to disclose.

REFERENCES

1. Ring ME. Dentistry: an illustrated history. New York: Harry N Abrams; 1985.
2. Branemark PI, Zarb GA, Albrektsson T. Tissue-integrated prostheses: osseointegration in clinical dentistry. Quintessence (IL): 1985.
3. Lee JH, Frias V, Lee KW, et al. Effect of implant size and shape on implant success rates: a literature review. J Prosthet Dent 2005;94:377–81.
4. Pommer B, Frantal S, Willer J, et al. Impact of dental implant length on early failure rates: a meta-analysis of observational studies. J Clin Periodontol 2011;38: 856–63.
5. Herrmann I, Lekholm U, Holm S, et al. Evaluation of patient and implant characteristics as potential prognostic factors for oral implant failures. Int J Oral Maxillofac Implants 2005;20:220–30.
6. Neves FD, Fones D, Bernardes SR, et al. Short implants—an analysis of longitudinal studies. Int J Oral Maxillofac Implants 2006;21:86–93.
7. Renouard F, Nisand D. Impact of implant length and diameter on survival rates. Clin Oral Implants Res 2006;17(Suppl 2):35–51.
8. Penarrocha-Oltra D, Aloy-Prosper A, Cervera-Ballester J, et al. Implant treatment in atrophic posterior mandibles: vertical regeneration with block bone grafts versus implants with 5.5-mm intrabony length. Int J Oral Maxillofac Implants 2014;29:659–66.
9. Hagi D, Deporter DA, Pilliar RM, et al. A targeted review of study outcomes with short (<7 mm) endosseous dental implants placed in partially edentulous patients. J Periodontol 2004;7 5:798–804.
10. Friberg B, Jemt T, Lekholm U. Early failures in 4,641 consecutively placed Branemark dental implants: a study from stage 1 surgery to the connection of completed prostheses. Int J Oral Maxillofac Implants 1991;6:142–6.
11. Wyatt CC, Zarb GA. Treatment outcomes of patients with implant-supported fixed partial prostheses. Int J Oral Maxillofac Implants 1998;13:204–11.
12. Bahat O. Branemark system implants in the posterior maxilla: clinical study of 660 implants followed for 5 to 12 years. Int J Oral Maxillofac Implants 2000;15:646–53.
13. Attard NJ, Zarb GA. Implant prosthodontic management of partially edentulous patients missing posterior teeth: the Toronto experience. J Prosthet Dent 2003; 89:352–9.
14. Weng D, Jacobson Z, Tarnow D, et al. A prospective multicenter clinical trial of 3i machined-surface implants: results after 6 years of follow-up. Int J Oral Maxillofac Implants 2003;18:417–23.
15. Ante IH. The fundamental principles of abutments. Mich State Dent Society Bulletin 1926;8:14–23.
16. Dykema RW, Goodacre CJ, Phillips RW. Johnston's modern practice in fixed prosthodontics. 4th edition. Philadelphia: WB Saunders; 1986. p. 8–21.
17. Shillingburg HT Jr, Hobo S, Whitsett LD. Fundamentals of fixed prosthodontics. 3rd edition. Chicago: Quintessence Publishing; 1997. p. 89–90.
18. Lulic M, Bragger U, Lang NP, et al. Ante's (1926) law revisited: a systematic review on survival rates and complications of fixed dental prostheses (FDPs) on severely reduced periodontal tissue support. Clin Oral Implants Res 2007; 18(Suppl 3):63–72.

19. Kotsovilis S, Fourmousis I, Karoussis I, et al. A systematic review and meta-analysis on the effect of implant length on the survival of rough-surface dental implants. J Periodontol 2009;80:1700–18.
20. Esposito M, Grusovin M, Felice P, et al. The efficacy of horizontal and vertical bone augmentation procedures for dental implants–a Cochrane systematic review. Eur J Oral Implantol 2009;2(3):167–84.
21. Milinkovic I, Cordaro L. Are there specific indications for the different alveolar bone augmentation procedures for implant placement? A systematic review. Int J Oral Maxillofac Surg 2014;43:606–25.
22. Hassani A, Motamedi M, Saadat S. Inferior alveolar nerve transpositioning for implant placement, a textbook of advanced oral and maxillofacial surgery. Rijeka (Croatia): InTech Publishing; 2013. p. 659–93.
23. Vasquez JC, Rivera AS, Gil HS, et al. Complication rate in 200 consecutive sinus lift procedures: guidelines for prevention and treatment. J Oral Maxillofac Surg 2014;72:892–901.
24. Nisand D, Renouard F. Short implant in limited bone volume. Periodontol 2000 2014;66:72–96.
25. Gulje F, Abrahamsson I, Chen S, et al. Implants of 6 mm vs. 11 mm lengths in the posterior maxilla and mandible: a 1-year multicenter randomized controlled trial. Clin Oral Implants Res 2013;24:1325–31.
26. Pieri F, Aldini N, Fini M, et al. Preliminary 2-year report on treatment outcomes for 6-mm-long implants in posterior atrophic mandibles. Int J Prosthodont 2012;25: 279–89.
27. Esposito M, Cannizzaro G, Soardi E, et al. 3-year post-loading report of a randomized controlled trial on the rehabilitation of posterior atrophic mandibles: short implants or longer implants in vertically augmented bone? Eur J Oral Implantol 2011;4(4):301–11.
28. Felice P, Soardi E, Pellegrino G, et al. Treatment of the atrophic edentulous maxilla: short implants versus bone augmentation for placing longer implants. Five-month post-loading results of a pilot randomized controlled trial. Eur J Oral Implantol 2011;4(3):191–202.
29. Felice P, Pellegrino G, Checchi L, et al. Vertical augmentation with interpositional blocks of anorganic bovine bone vs. 7-mm-long implants in posterior mandibles: 1-year results of a randomized clinical trial. Clin Oral Implants Res 2010;21: 1394–403.
30. Smith DE, Zarb GA. Criteria for success of osseointegrated endosseous implants. J Prosthet Dent 1989;62:567–72.
31. Balshe AA, Assad DA, Eckert SE, et al. A retrospective study of the survival of smooth-and rough-surface dental implants. Int J Oral Maxillofac Implants 2009; 24:113–8.
32. Nedir R, Bischof M, Briaux JM, et al. A 7-year life table analysis from a prospective study on m implants with special emphasis on the use of short implants. Results from a private practice. Clin Oral Implants Res 2004;15:150–7.
33. De Castro D, De Araujo M, Benfatti C, et al. Comparative histological and histomorphometrical evaluation of marginal bone resorption around external hexagon and Morse cone implants: an experimental study in dogs. Implant Dent 2014;23: 270–6.
34. Weng D, Nagata M, Bosco A, et al. Influence of microgap location and configuration on radiographic bone loss around submerged implants: an experimental study in dogs. Int J Oral Maxillofac Implants 2011;26:941–6.

35. Himmlova L, Dostalova T, Kacovsky A, et al. Influence of implant length and diameter on stress distribution: a finite element analysis. J Prosthet Dent 2004; 91:20–5.
36. Baggi L, Cappelloni I, Di Girolamo M, et al. The influence of implant diameter and length on stress distribution of osseointegrated implants related to crestal bone geometry: a three-dimensional finite element analysis. J Prosthet Dent 2008; 100:422–31.
37. Blanes RJ. To what extent does the crown-implant ratio affect survival and complications of implant-supported reconstructions? A systematic review. Clin Oral Implants Res 2009;20(Suppl 4):67–72.
38. Tawil G, Younan R. Clinical evaluation of short, machined-surface implants followed for 12 to 92 months. Int J Oral Maxillofac Implants 2003;18:894–901.
39. Atieh M, Zadeh H, Stanford C, et al. Survival of short dental implants for treatment of posterior partial edentulism: a systematic review. Int J Oral Maxillofac Implants 2012;27:1323–31.
40. Telleman G, Raghoebar GM, Vissink A, et al. A systematic review of the prognosis of short (<10 mm) dental implants placed in the partially edentulous patient. J Clin Periodontol 2011;38:667–76.
41. Anitua E, Alkhraist M, Pinas L, et al. Implant survival and crestal bone loss around extra-short implants supporting a fixed denture: the effect of crown height space, crown-to-implant ratio, and offset placement of the prosthesis. Int J Oral Maxillofac Implants 2014;29:682–9.
42. Anitua E, Pinas L, Begona L, et al. Long-term retrospective evaluation of short implants in the posterior areas: clinical results after 10–12 years. J Clin Periodontol 2014;41:404–11.
43. Lai HC, Si MS, Zhuang LF, et al. Long-term outcomes of short dental implants supporting single crowns in posterior region: a clinical retrospective study of 5–10 years. Clin Oral Implants Res 2013;24:230–7.
44. Sanchez-Garces MA, Costa-Berenguer X, Gay-Escoda C. Short implants: a descriptive study of 273 implants. Clin Implant Dent Relat Res 2012;14:508–16.
45. Fugazzotto P, Beagle J, Ganeles J, et al. Success and failure rates of 9 mm or shorter implants in the replacement of missing maxillary molars when restored with individual crowns: preliminary results 0 to 84 months in function. A retrospective study. J Periodontol 2004;75:327–32.

How to Avoid Life-Threatening Complications Associated with Implant Surgery

Earl Clarkson, DDS, Eunsu Jung, DDS*, Spencer Lin, DMD

KEYWORDS

- Life-threatening implant complications • Hematoma • Hemorrhage • Floor of mouth
- Aspiration • Ingestion

KEY POINTS

- Life-threatening complications of dental implants are hematoma, hemorrhage of floor of the mouth, aspiration, and ingestion.
- The key to preventing hemorrhagic complication is knowing anatomic structures relevant to the implant position and proper planning.
- Aspiration and ingestion can be better prevented by understanding clinical settings and patient risk factors.

INTRODUCTION

Ever since the discovery of dental implants, its surgery has become more prevalent and now routinely done in a clinical setting due to its high success rate and safety. Although many methods and technological advances have emerged in the recent decades, complications still occur as described in previous chapters (periimplantitis, mucositis, infection, nerve damage). Although unfortunate, these complications often do not pose lethal consequences. These adverse outcomes are often preventable and are typically able to be managed in a clinical setting. Despite being uncommon, life-threatening complications can occur in some situations. Such emergencies include hemorrhage/hematoma formation of the floor of mouth, aspiration, and ingestion of foreign bodies, that is, implant parts. These complications can happen during routine dental implant surgery and can cause lethal events such as airway obstruction, perforation of organs, and infection. Management of these life-threatening conditions can be more challenging and have life altering consequences to the patient in addition to both legal and financial loss to the practitioner. It is crucial for clinicians to be able to promptly recognize life-threatening emergencies and take appropriate

Department of Dentistry, Department of Oral and Maxillofacial Surgery, NYC Health + Hospitals/Woodhull, 760 Broadway, Brooklyn, New York 11206, USA
* Corresponding author.
E-mail address: vcleaner7@gmail.com

Dent Clin N Am 65 (2021) 33–41
https://doi.org/10.1016/j.cden.2020.09.002
0011-8532/21/

measures. With pertinent preparation, knowledge of anatomic structures, and preventative protocols, these adverse events can be prevented.

HEMORRHAGE/HEMATOMA IN THE FLOOR OF THE MOUTH

One of the common complications in implant surgery is hemorrhage. Minor bleeding is frequently encountered during and after the procedure and is relatively well managed with local measures in a clinical setting. However, significant hemorrhage and hematoma formation in anterior mandible can be life threatening, as it can lead to airway obstruction. In general, the incidence of severe implant related hemorrhage was found to be ~ 24%. Reported causes included soft tissue damage, violation of arteries, and osteotomy perforations.[1] Regarding the site of injury, life-threatening consequences via airway obstruction originated more commonly from bleeding in the anterior mandible compared with other parts of the mouth. This is due to perforation of the lingual cortex causing vascular injury within soft tissue.[2]

The lingual aspect of the anterior mandible has a rich vasculature as it is supplied by the sublingual, submental, and incisive arteries. These arteries also supply the muscles and soft tissues of the floor of the mouth. The sublingual artery originates from the lingual artery, anastomosing with the submental artery that branches from the facial artery. These arteries run along the lingual side of the anterior mandible parallel to the mylohyoid muscle. In most of the cases (80%–90%) sublingual arteries run through the lingual foramen in the midline, penetrating through the lingual cortical plate.[2–4] These vessels anastomose with the incisive arteries that are branches of the inferior alveolar artery These vessels together form a highly vascularized network in the lingual aspect of mandible (**Fig. 1**). Damaging vessels in this area during implant surgery can cause significant hemorrhage with blood loss rate of 14 mL/min. This bleeding can spread through the loose adipose and connective tissues of the floor of the mouth to involve facial spaces such as sublingual, submental, and

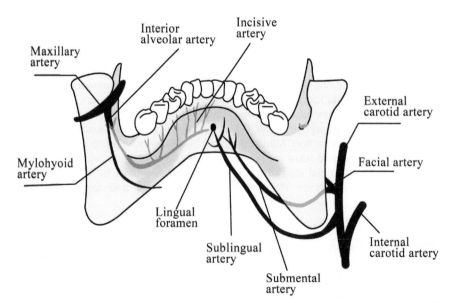

Fig. 1. The lingual aspect of the anterior mandible, showing complex vasculature with anastomoses.

submandibular spaces. As this hemorrhage worsens, it can cause posterior displacement of the tongue. This will apply direct pressure against the soft palate into the pharynx, leading to rapid upper airway obstruction.[1,5] In such circumstances, often aggressive airway management may be necessary. Law and colleagues found that in 25 reported cases, lingual cortex perforation was the most common cause of severe hemorrhage, resulting in 68% of patients requiring intubation or tracheostomy due to airway obstruction.[6] Therefore, knowing key anatomic structures in the anterior mandible combined with precise surgical planning is crucial to preventing life-threatening consequences.

Management

The definitive procedures to control airway obstruction due to severe hemorrhage/hematoma in the floor of the mouth are limited in a dental office setting. Initial recognition of such symptoms should prompt the clinician to consider transfer and immediate airway management. Clinical findings of hemorrhage progressing to airway obstruction may present with evident bleeding in the oral cavity, severe pain, protrusion of the tongue, bruising, and swelling of the floor of the mouth. The patient can show symptoms of dysphagia, dyspnea, and cyanosis with inadequate oxygen saturation, eventually resulting in respiratory arrest.

Local hemostatic measures are crucial; however, initial treatment options are limited in an ambulatory clinic in the event of severe hemorrhage in the floor of the mouth. In such event, one should immediately terminate the surgical procedure and apply direct pressure. Bimanual compression inferiorly at the floor of the mouth and lingual surface of the mandible in conjunction with upward force against the submental region is recommended. The goal is to decrease bleeding and expansion of the hematoma to ultimately prevent airway obstruction. In addition, compression with ice can aid in hemostasis.[7] Hemostatic agents such as resorbable gelatin sponges, oxidized cellulose, or bovine collagen plugs combined with pressure can be applied to osteotomy and/or extraction sites. If available, electrocautery can aid in hemostatic efforts. If hemorrhage/hematoma expansion remains uncontrolled or signs of airway obstruction are present despite attempting local measures, activate 911 response and rapid transport to the nearest hospital emergency department. Meanwhile, vital signs should be monitored and oxygen may be supplied through nasal canula to lessen dyspnea stress. Moreover, efforts should be made to reduce patient anxiety to prevent further bleeding due to hypertension.[2] Endotracheal intubation or tracheostomy may be required if the patient is unable to breath adequately, demonstrating signs of oxygen desaturation.

Emergency evacuation of the hematoma can be considered if the clinician is adequately trained to do so. However, an inexperienced practitioner attempting this procedure can worsen the bleeding and create more soft tissue destruction.[6] Moreover, experienced clinicians can attempt to ligate the damaged vessel. Studies suggest that ligating the facial or sublingual artery can control floor of the mouth hemorrhage. If unsuccessful, ligation of the lingual artery can be attempted.[5] However, without adequate anesthesia or specialized training, attempting to ligate the damaged vessel might worsen the situation due to multiple anastomoses of nearby arteries and a limited visual field in an office setting. Hence, prompt transport to an emergency department is crucial as definitive treatment involves airway management and complex operations that require the expertise of a skilled surgeon. If direct intraoral approach is unsuccessful, angiographic e-embolization or ligation of the carotid artery via extraoral approach can be considered in conjunction with using vascular angiography or computed tomographic (CT) scans.[3]

Prevention

Severe hemorrhage in the floor of the mouth can put the patient's life at risk, requiring invasive treatment. The importance of using preventive measures cannot be overemphasized. One of the simple and easy preventive methods is obtaining a preoperative cone-beam computed tomographic (CBCT) scan. Compared with conventional 2-dimensional radiographs, CBCT is superior, as it can reveal the position and diameter of intrabony vascular canals that may contain significant vessels, especially in anterior mandible. This can be advantageous to the clinician in avoiding or preparing to control any incidental arterial hemorrhage during implant placement. In the studies of 25 reported cases of hemorrhage, most of the bleeding was caused by lingual cortex perforation.[6] Only one case used preop 3-dimensional imaging before implant placement. This demonstrates the importance of obtaining preop CT. In addition, CBCT allows one to visualize mandibular atrophy and its angulation. This encourages ideal implant position by engaging more bone, leading to better primary stability while avoiding perforation of the lingual plate, protecting sublingual soft tissue.

Injecting local anesthesia multiple times in anterior mandible, especially it the lingual aspect, is suboptimal, as it can cause bleeding from nicks in vessels that do not cease spontaneously. These local injections with a vasoconstrictor can delay the symptoms of a hematoma of the floor of the mouth. Therefore, inferior alveolar nerve blocks are preferred to avoid direct damage to vessels in that region.[8]

Favoring a narrower diameter implant in anterior mandible can be another method to prevent hemorrhagic complications. The occlusal load of the anterior mandible is one-third of the posterior and generally has a bone dense enough to resist occlusal forces. The clinician can opt for narrow diameter implants that can be placed a few millimeters away from the midline to possibly avoid a single large sublingual artery.

In patients with severely angulated and/or atrophic mandibles, there is an increased risk of perforating the lingual cortical plate, which is in close vicinity to a vascular plexus that has great potential to cause severe bleeding. Avoiding lingual subperiosteal tears is of utmost importance, as its injury can lead to detrimental bleeding, as the main vascular osseous supply of the anterior mandible is provided by the facial artery via periosteal vasculature in the atrophic mandible. Injury of mandibular lingual vascular canals itself is less concerning due to their small diameter. CBCT and surgical stents can decrease the chance of perforating the lingual cortical plate by encouraging correct implant positioning. In addition, digital palpation on the lingual mandible should be applied for tactile feedback to avoid perforation while gently advancing the bur. Furthermore, lingual subperiosteal flap enhances visualization to prevent lingual perforation.[5] On the contrary, some claim that flapless implant placement in the anterior mandible may have fewer complications compared with open flap procedures.[7] However, if excessive bleeding occurs while using the flapless technique, blood can expand into the floor of the mouth and deep neck region rather than draining into the oral cavity. Therefore, manual palpation of the lingual mandible in conjunction with proper preop planning of implant position with CBCT should be considered.

ASPIRATION AND INGESTION

Aspiration and ingestion of instruments and/or materials can occur during any stage of implant surgery and may lead to life-threatening consequences. The foreign object can be either aspirated or swallowed, depending on the route taken beyond the pharynx. It is evident in the literature that aspiration was observed more often during implantation, prosthodontics, and restorative dentistry, whereas prosthodontics and root canal treatment was more related to ingestion.[9] In general, aspiration or ingestion is an infrequent occurrence, the latter happening more often as a direct result of the strong coughing that occurs when there is a foreign object in the patient's airway. Although aspiration has lower incidence, it poses a higher risk for lethal complications, as an aspirated object can lead to acute airway obstruction and lung infections including abscess formation or pneumonia. Similarly, an ingested foreign object can also be life threatening, as objects can become entrenched through its passage through the gastrointestinal (GI) tract and lead to severe inflammation, obstruction, and infection.[10]

There are various risk factors related to a patient's medical history in addition to modifiable clinical factors that can facilitate aspiration and ingestion of a foreign body during implant surgery. Patients with psychological disorders, mental retardation, excessive gag reflex, alcoholism, small oral cavity, and macroglossia; those who are obese or pregnant; and the elderly should be considered at higher risk for complications. In a clinical setting, the patient's risk of aspiration and ingestion of foreign objects may also be increased by local anesthesia, supine positioning, inadequate lighting, ineffective assistants, and airway protection.[11] Evidently, these complications can be detrimental to the patient but can also create potential for legal action against the clinician and related economic costs. Thus, it is crucial to thoroughly evaluate a patient's medical history for aspiration/ingestion risk factors and be mindful of adjustable clinical settings to prevent complications.

Symptoms

The symptoms of aspiration and ingestion can be varied. In general, patients commonly present with coughing, gagging, and dyspnea following aspiration of a foreign body. If larger objects are aspirated, immediate airway obstruction is possible, which can present as inspiratory stridor, paradoxic breathing, and cyanosis with inadequate oxygen saturation. On physical examination, one may notice tachypnea, tachycardia, stridor, unilateral or bilateral decreased breath sounds, localized wheezing, and/or crackles. It is possible for a patient to not present with any initial discomfort or symptoms. However, even asymptomatic patients who had potentially aspirated a foreign body, necessary protocol should be taken, because chronic retention of foreign bodies in the airway can manifest as serious consequences including infection, pneumothorax, vocal cord paralysis chronic cough, hemoptysis, pneumonia, unexplained fever, and even death.

In contrast, patients with ingested foreign bodies are often asymptomatic. Nevertheless, signs and symptoms can still develop, commonly presenting as coughing, gagging, dysphagia, odynophagia, cramps, nausea, and vomiting. In the event of an asymptomatic patient who has ingested foreign body, adequate treatment protocol is still necessary, as complications can progress to bowel obstruction, infection, and perforation.

Management and Prevention

Consequences of aspiration and ingestion may lead to lethal complications that require invasive treatment, and thus prevention is key. A simple yet important preventative technique is applying a gauze screen. Often times, the practitioner negates this method for various reason; however, there is no superior way to prevent accidents. The gauze screen should be applied posterior to the surgical site to block entry of a foreign body passing the oropharynx. Tying floss or sutures to small instruments such as an implant screwdriver can prevent aspiration and ingestion, as it provides the clinician a fast way to retrieve the fallen object. In addition, controlling variables such as inadequate lighting, the lack of assistance, or proper instrumentation such as high-speed suction should be addressed before any implant-related procedure. This becomes crucial especially when placing implants in posterior regions where visibility and accessibility can be compromised. Controlling chair position can be advantageous especially when patients have an unfavorable gag reflex and are unable to tolerate a gauze screen. In this circumstance, patients seated upright with their head turned sideways is beneficial. Also, adequate suction to evacuate excessive saliva and blood can help reduce the gag reflex, leading to unpredictable movements.[12]

If an object is lost beyond the oropharynx while in a supine position, the patient should be kept supine, turned to their right side, and attempt to "cough up" the foreign body. Slow inhalation followed by a forceful cough can minimize aspirating the object deeper.[13] Because the adult right bronchus diverges at a more acute angle from the trachea compared with the left side and also has a greater diameter than the left bronchus, the right side is the more common path for aspirated objects (**Fig. 2**).[14,15] This right-sided Trendelenburg positioning decreases the effect of gravity pushing the foreign body deeper while helping keep the aspirated object to the right mainstem bronchus. Spontaneous or endoscopic retrieval is easier in the right mainstem bronchus, as its diameter is wider and provides a straight passage. If aspiration occurs while the patient is upright, the patient should be lowered to the favored right-sided Trendelenburg position, unless they are violently coughing.[13] In contrast, there are conflicting views, as some experts believe that the patient should be placed into reverse Trendelenburg position before being encouraged to cough. They believe this maneuver may aid in regurgitating the foreign body.[11] Regardless, if the object is visible, the clinician may use forceps or high-volume suction to retrieve the object while being careful not to dislodge it further. Immediate action must be taken to prevent respiratory failure if the patient shows signs of airway obstruction such as choking, dyspnea, stridor, and using accessory muscles to breathe. In this instance, abdominal thrusts in conjunction with finger sweeps and suction can be performed. If unsuccessful, cricothyroidotomy may be considered by emergency personnel while the patient is being arranged for immediate transfer to the closest emergency department. It is also important to reassure asymptomatic

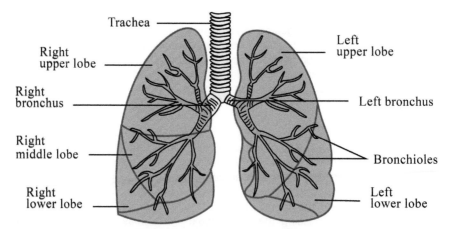

Fig. 2. The lung, showing difference between right and left mainstem bronchus. Right bronchus branches at a more acute angle and has a wider diameter.

and stable patients who have aspirated or ingested foreign body that the situation is manageable. At the same time, patients must seek immediate medical attention and determine whether the object was aspirated or ingested by taking a series of radiographs of the abdomen and chest. The treatment modality depends on the location of the foreign body.

Aspiration
If radiographic examination reveals aspiration, it is a medical emergency that requires immediate intervention. Patient will require evaluation for urgent bronchoscopy. Retrieval of the object can be accomplished via bronchoscopy in conjunction with a suctioning or grasping device. Intubation may be required before bronchoscopy in the event of complex cases such as deeply dislodged foreign bodies. Literature suggests that bronchoscopy has been extremely effective in foreign body removal, reaching a 99% success with a complication rate ranging from 2.4% to 5%.[12] In severe cases where the retrieval has failed with bronchoscopy, thoracotomy with bronchotomy may be indicated.

Ingestion
Most foreign body ingestions are asymptomatic and fortunately, once an objects reaches the stomach, there is a greater than 90% chance of the object being passed from the GI tract without complications, usually over a 7 to 10-day period.[16] If an ingested object is radiographically confirmed to be passing, conservative monitoring is possible as long as the foreign body is blunt and is less than 2.5 cm in diameter and is less than 6 cm in length.[17] In this case, patients must be informed about their situation in addition to instructions for examining their stools. Mandatory daily inspection of stool combined with a high-bulk, high-fiber diet may be helpful, although no literature specifically demonstrates increased success with any specific diet. Laxatives are contraindicated as excessive peristalsis can lead to mucosal perforations. If passage of a blunt foreign object is not confirmed within 7 days or if the patient becomes symptomatic, additional CT scan and endoscopic removal might be necessary.

In cases of an ingested sharp object or if acute symptoms of obstruction occur, immediate intervention is required. Sharp objects pose the risk of organ perforation, whereas larger object greater than 6 cm have greater risk of obstruction and perforation. In these circumstances, immediate transfer to an equipped facility and endoscopy is indicated. The most common location for obstruction is the upper esophagus, which can lead to esophageal perforation with subsequent mediastinitis. Esophageal obstruction can eventually transition into aspiration, further adding to the urgency of the situation. Although some experienced clinicians may attempt to retrieve the foreign body via direct visualization using a laryngoscope and forceps, this can risk dislodging the object deeper. Hence, endoscopy is considered as the treatment of choice due to its relatively low complication rate, its high success rate, and because it often does not require postoperative hospital admission. If the foreign body is unable to be removed via endoscopy, does not progress along the GI tract in 72 hours, or if severe symptoms such as vomiting, continuous abdominal pain, hematemesis, or melena occur, more invasive measures such as cervical esophagectomy might be necessary.[17]

CLINICS CARE POINTS

- Use caution and precise surgical planning when working near the lingual aspect of the anterior mandible as it contains rich vasculature.

- Activate 911 response and rapid transport to the nearest hospital emergency department if uncontrolled hemorrhage in the floor of the mouth.
- Thoroughly evaluate a patient's medical history for aspiration/ingestion risk factors and be mindful of adjustable clinical settings to prevent complications.
- Radiographic examination is crucial to determine location of ingested/aspirated foreign body, even if asymptomatic.

DISCLOSURE

The authors have nothing to disclose.

REFERENCES

1. Misch K, Wang HL. Implant Surgery Complications: Etiology and Treatment. Implant Dent 2008;17(2):159–68.
2. Schiegnitz E, Moergel M, Wagner W. Vital Life-Threatening Hematoma after Implant Insertion in the Anterior Mandible: A Case Report and Review of the Literature. Case Rep Dent 2015;2015:531865.
3. Limongelli L, Tempesta A, Crincoli V, et al. Massive Lingual and Sublingual Haematoma following Postextractive Flapless Implant Placement in the Anterior Mandible. Case Rep Dent 2015;2015:839098.
4. Saquib Mallick M, Rauf Khan A, Al-Bassam A. Late Presentation of Tracheobronchial Foreign Body Aspiration in Children. J Trop Pediatr 2005;51(3):145–8.
5. Tarakji B, Nassani MZ. Factors associated with hematoma of the floor of the mouth after placement of dental implants. Saudi Dent J 2012;24(1):11–5.
6. Law C, Alam P, Borumandi F. Floor-of-Mouth Hematoma Following Dental Implant Placement: Literature Review and Case Presentation. J Oral Maxillofac Surg 2017;75(11):2340–6.
7. Peñarrocha-Diago M, Balaguer-Martí JC, Peñarrocha-Oltra D, et al. Floor of the mouth hemorrhage subsequent to dental implant placement in the anterior mandible. Clin Cosmet Investig Dent 2019;11:235–42.
8. Sakka S, Krenkel C. Hemorrhage Secondary to Interforaminal Implant Surgery: Anatomical Considerations and Report of a Case. J Oral Implantol 2013;39(5):603–7. Allen Press, Available at: meridian.allenpress.com/joi/article/39/5/603/7243/Hemorrhage-Secondary-to-Interforaminal-Implant.
9. Hou R, Zhou H, Hu K, et al. Thorough documentation of the accidental aspiration and ingestion of foreign objects during dental procedure is necessary: review and analysis of 617 cases. Head Face Med 2016;12:23.
10. Santos Tde S, Antunes AA, Vajgel A, et al. Foreign Body Ingestion During Dental Implant Procedures. J Craniofac Surg 2012;23(2):e119–23.
11. Pingarrón Martín L, Morán Soto MJ, Sánchez Burgos R, et al. Bronchial impaction of an implant screwdriver after accidental aspiration: report of a case and revision of the literature. Oral Maxillofac Surg 2010;14(1):43–7.
12. Fields RT Jr, Wolford LM. Aspiration and Ingestion of Foreign Bodies in Oral and Maxillofacial Surgery: A Review of the Literature and Report of Five Cases. J Oral Maxillofac Surg 1998;56(9):1091–8.
13. Bosack R, Lieblich S. Anesthesia complications in the dental office. Hoboken: John Wiley & Sons; 2015.
14. Lee EJ, Yang HR, Cho JM, et al. Two Cases of Colonoscopic Retrieval of a Foreign Body in Children: A Button Battery and an Open Safety Pin. Pediatr Gastroenterol Hepatol Nutr 2017;20(3):204–9.

15. Warshawsky ME. "Foreign Body Aspiration." Background, Pathophysiology, Epidemiology. Medscape 2015. Available at: emedicine.medscape.com/article/298940.
16. Webb WA. Management of Foreign Bodies of the Upper Gastrointestinal Tract. Gastroenterology 1988;94(1):204–16.
17. Abusamaan M, Giannobile WV, Jhawar P, et al. Swallowed and aspirated dental prostheses and instruments in clinical dental practice: a report of five cases and a proposed management algorithm. J Am Dent Assoc 2014;145(5):459–63.

An Update on the Treatment of Periimplantitis

Raza A. Hussain, BDS, DMD[a,b,*], Michael Miloro, DMD, MD[c], Jennifer B. Cohen, DDS[d]

KEYWORDS

- Dental • Implants • Failing • Salvage • Periimplantitis • Inflammation

KEY POINTS

- Increased dental implant placement equates to an increased number of long-term maintenance issues.
- Discussion of methods to avoid short- and long-term issues in relation to dental implants.
- Techniques for management of early, intermediate, and late stage issues that can arise from periimplantitis.
- Algorithm for when to attempt implant repair/salvage versus removal and replacement.

INTRODUCTION

Dental implants have been used to replace natural dentition since the 1960s. Branemark discovered that when titanium was implanted into a patient's bone, it would lead to a process termed "osseointegration." Gosta Larsson was the recipient of the first dental implant, placed by Branemark himself in 1965. When Larsson died in 2006, several implants were still in function. It can be assumed that he was a motivated patient who was diligent in maintaining his newly acquired dentition for decades. Many of the authors' medical colleagues wonder how it is possible to implant a foreign body in the oral cavity without the constant risk of infection and rejection. The capacity of surgical grade titanium to promote bony fusion and acceptance is critical in the success of dental implants. The excellent vascularity of the head and neck area and rapid bony/oral epithelial turnover is also paramount. In addition, the constant flow of saliva, with its protective properties, is necessary in maintaining a healthy microbiological

[a] Oral and Maxillofacial Surgery, Jesse Brown VA Medical Center, 820 South Damen Avenue, 4th Floor Damen Pavilion, Chicago, IL 60612, USA; [b] Department of Oral and Maxillofacial Surgery, University of Illinois at Chicago, Chicago, IL, USA; [c] Department of Oral and Maxillofacial Surgery, University of Illinois at Chicago, 801 South Paulina Street, M/C 835, Chicago, IL 60612, USA; [d] Jesse Brown VA Medical Center, 820 South Damen Avenue 4th Floor Damen Pavilion, Chicago, IL 60612, USA
* Corresponding author. Jesse Brown VA Medical Center, 820 South Damen Avenue, 4th Floor Damen Pavilion, Chicago, IL 60612.
E-mail address: raza.hussain@va.gov

Dent Clin N Am 65 (2021) 43–56
https://doi.org/10.1016/j.cden.2020.09.003
0011-8532/21/Published by Elsevier Inc.
dental.theclinics.com

environment for the titanium and synthetic fixtures associated with the implant. It has been well established, however, that a significantly smaller amount of bacteria is needed to create inflammation, and subsequently infection, around a dental implant compared with a natural tooth.[1]

Bacteria such as streptococci, lactobacilli, staphylococci, and corynebacteria along with large numbers of anaerobes, such as the bacteroides species, which normally make up the healthy oral flora of most humans, can turn into pathologic entities resulting in acute or chronic infection. The groves, threads, and irregularities, essential in osseointegration, could begin to harbor bacteria and then spill their toxic bioproducts into the periimplant space.[2]

DIAGNOSIS OF PERIIMPLANTITIS

Unlike periodontal disease, which is well defined and organized into specific categories, periimplantitis is an ambiguous, and often controversial, term. It is typically used to describe any "less-than-ideal" condition surrounding a dental implant fixture. A survey by J. Thakkar and colleagues from the University of Michigan Department of Oral and Maxillofacial Surgery reported that approximately 62% of respondents considered periimplantitis a serious issue. Furthermore, 50% thought they did not receive sufficient training on this subject matter during residency.[3] Many clinicians believe the most important criteria for a diagnosis of periimplantitis are exposure and gingival recession. Occasionally, a patient may present as asymptomatic with exposed implant threads, yet inflammation is minimal to nonexistent. This is often seen in patients who maintain excellent oral hygiene. Conversely, smokers with poor oral hygiene and a history of periodontal disease are particularly prone to developing periimplant issues.

In a recent article, Tolstunov describes a situation of progressive buccal bone loss, occurring in the anterior maxilla after implant placement.[4] The clinical presentation is blueish in color and with granulation tissues or purulent discharge. In the absence of inflammation, this case does not meet the traditional definition of periimplantitis. Rather, Tolstunov refers to this presentation as "periimplantosis," a noninflammatory diseased state.

The term periimplant mucositis can be used to describe a compromised implant in its earliest stage. It is often associated with exudate, increased pocket depth, and

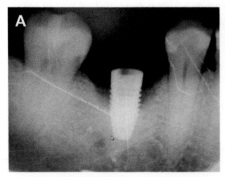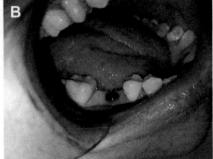

Fig. 1. It is obvious from the radiographic appearance of the implant that a diagnosis of periimplantitis is warranted. Based on the clinical images, however, there is lack of inflammation and the gingival tissue seems healthy and pink, even considering the visible exposed threads. (*Courtesy of* Raza A. Hussain, BDS, DMD, FACS, Chicago, IL.)

progressive bone loss. With early intervention, it may be possible to avoid severe bone loss, infection, and mobility leading to implant failure (**Fig. 1**, **Table 1**).

CONTRIBUTING FACTORS
Keratinized Tissue

The role of keratinized tissue, in relation to both natural dentition and dental implants, is a controversial topic among clinicians and the absolute necessity is still unknown.[4–22] This type of tissue tends to be more resistant to abrasion and more resilient when considering its susceptibility to gingival recession. In many cases, its presence results in decreased probing depths and less plaque accumulation, which limits bacterial penetration into the periimplant space. Additional benefits include easier cleansability and increased patient comfort. Alternatively, there are several studies that confirm implant success in regions with little to no keratinized tissue.[11,12,23] Therefore, it can be concluded that an implant with healthy keratinized tissue is preferable. Those without are not guaranteed to become compromised but it is more likely and even more diligent home care is required.

Table 1
Periodontal disease chart

Type	Subtype
Gingival diseases	Dental plaque-induced gingival diseases Non–plaque-induced gingival lesions
Chronic periodontitis (previously adult periodontitis)	Slight (1–2 mm CAL) Moderate (3–4 mm CAL) Severe (>5 mm CAL) Localized (<30% of sites involved) Generalized (>30% of sites involved)
Aggressive periodontitis[11] (previously early onset periodontitis)	Slight (1–2 mm CAL) Moderate (3–4 mm CAL) Severe (>5 mm CAL) Localized (<30% of sites involved) Generalized (>30% of sites involved)
Periodontitis as a manifestation of systemic diseases	Associated with hematological Disorders Associated with genetic disorders Not otherwise specified
Necrotizing periodontal diseases	Necrotizing ulcerative gingivitis Necrotizing ulcerative periodontitis
Abscesses of the periodontium	Gingival abscess Periodontal abscess Pericoronal abscess
Periodontitis associated with endodontic lesions	Combined periodontic-endodontic lesions
Developmental or acquired deformities and conditions	Localized tooth-related factors that modify or predispose to plaque-induced gingival diseases/periodontitis Mucogingival deformities/conditions around teeth Mucogingival deformities/conditions on edentulous ridges

From Nair SC, Anoop KR. Intraperiodontal pocket: An ideal route for local antimicrobial drug delivery. J Adv Pharm Technol Res. 2012;3(1):9–15; with permission.

Implant Surface

A rough, hydroxyapatite-coated implant surface, combined with an absence of keratinized gingiva, has been associated with periimplantitis and subsequent bone loss. An insufficient amount of attached tissue leaves the rough surface exposed, increasing the chances of implant failure.[24,25] A meta-analysis by Esposito and colleagues[26] revealed 20% fewer cases of periimplant complications among implants with smooth surfaces compared with those with rough surfaces.

Implant Location

It has been well established that posterior implants experience greater bone loss than their anteriorly placed counterparts. The difference amounts to 3.5 times more bone loss in the posterior, with these implants losing approximately 0.14 mm of bone annually. Conversely, anterior implants only lose 0.04 mm of bone on average.[27] In addition, the amount of keratinized tissue more profoundly affects implants in the posterior in terms of soft tissue health.

Restorative Factors

Prosthetic design can play a significant role in both the short- and long-term health of an implant. Home care can prove to be challenging, even for patients with excellent oral hygiene, if the restoration is poorly designed.[28] Bulky crowns and nonhygienic embrasures, for example, are extremely difficult to maintain. The crown-to-implant ratio must also be considered when treatment planning in order to avoid excessive occlusal and lateral forces. Clinicians should reevaluate the occlusal scheme and consider the placement of additional implants to decrease the occlusal loading if the fixture becomes compromised. The progression from periimplant mucositis to periimplantitis and to eventual implant failure is more gradual in cases with these unfavorable restorations. If recognized early, interventions to impede the periimplant disease process can be initiated (**Figs. 2–4**).

Alcohol

The relationship between alcohol and periimplantitis was investigated by Carr and colleagues.[29] He concluded that mild to moderate consumption led to fewer occurrences of periimplantitis (12% and 6%, respectively) than heavy consumption, which resulted in 42% of cases. Based on this study, it was presumed that mild to moderate alcohol consumption decreases inflammatory markers, leading to improved overall periimplant health. The investigators could not determine why heavy consumption of alcohol led to a nearly 3-fold increase in the rate of periimplantitis. Since the data were inconclusive, it remains uncertain whether a topical application of alcohol would be beneficial or if the improved periimplant environment was a systemic effect.

PREVENTION OF PERIIMPLANTITIS
Education and Home Care

Implant candidate selection and patient education are paramount in the long-term success of the final restoration. Establishing realistic expectations with the patient before initiating implant therapy is extremely important. It must be made clear that health and maintenance of an implant is distinctly different from that of a natural tooth. For example, removal of supragingival plaque is even more critical in maintaining an implant. Oral hygiene instructions, including various brushing techniques, should be emphasized and demonstrated by the clinician. Certain anatomic presentations must also be taken into consideration. Posterior implants frequently lack adequate

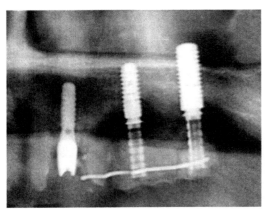

Fig. 2. A crown-to-implant ratio of 1:1 and posterior maxillary position of these implants makes them prone to periimplantitis and eventual failure. (*Courtesy of* Raza A. Hussain, BDS, DMD, FACS, Chicago, IL.)

keratinized, which can make oral hygiene challenging for the patient. If this is the case, a pulsatile oral irrigation device should be provided. The patient must be instructed to use the lowest setting possible to removal all supragingival debris. The goal of this device is to decrease bacterial burden rather than remove intrasulcular calculus, which can be accomplished during hygiene visits.[30]

In-Office Implant Maintenance

The hygiene team must understand the armamentarium and techniques necessary in maintaining dental implants. Instruments used in routine care, such as ultrasonic and metallic scalers, should be avoided as they have been proved to damage the delicate implant surface.[31] Any imperfections created can promote bacterial growth, which

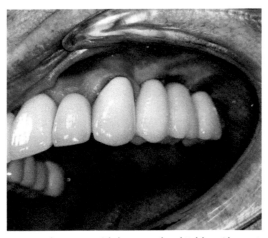

Fig. 3. Large, overcontoured crowns with large occlusal tables. Also note the frenal attachments and lack of keratinized tissue. (*Courtesy of* Raza A. Hussain, BDS, DMD, FACS, Chicago, IL.)

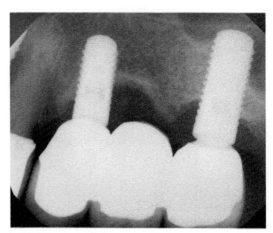

Fig. 4. Close-up image of the same implants after restoration. Note the bulky crowns and progressive bone loss. (*Courtesy of* Raza A. Hussain, BDS, DMD, FACS, Chicago, IL.)

subsequently results in periimplantitis, bone loss, and possible implant failure. Alternatively, ultrasonic scalers with plastic sleeves or nonmetallic tips are preferred for implant maintenance. Hand instruments made of graphite, nylon, or plastic, along with those coated in Teflon are also recommended. In addition, titanium curettes are appropriate for scaling, and the implant can be polished with a rubber cup and pumice.[32–34] A smooth, flawless implant surface is important in the prevention of plaque accumulation and periimplant bacterial colonization.

In the case of the patient with clinically evident perimucositis, without associated bone loss, a deep pseudopocket often exists. Typically, the tissue is flaccid with poor tone, allowing food and plaque to collect along the implant surface. Unlike a healthy implant, which requires gentle maintenance, these pockets require a deeper, more extensive debridement, similar to scaling and root planing, with the instrumentation listed earlier. Once the deposits are removed, the desired outcomes are increased tissue tone, decreased bacterial burden, and elimination of a passage in which bacteria can accumulate. In some instances, however, tissue redundancy recurs and must be treated through surgical methods, such as gingivectomy or gingivoplasty (**Fig. 5**).

Intervention
The International Congress of Oral Implantologists (ICOI) developed a table to delineate and evaluate the health of a functional dental implant. It categorizes an implant as having either (1) optimal health, (2) satisfactory health, (3) compromised health, or (4) failure. If an implant falls into group II or III, clinical intervention may be possible in order to decrease progression of periimplantitis and thereby salvage the ailing implant (**Table 2**).

Patients with implants of satisfactory health experience no discernible pain or tenderness on function, palpation, or percussion. There is no mobility in any direction with loading forces of 500 g or less. Radiographs typically reveal between 2 mm and 4 mm of bone loss from the time of implant placement. The coinciding probing depths are usually in excess of this due to the pseudopocket that often forms in these circumstances. Intervention for these cases include occlusal stress reduction, frequent hygiene visits, and possible reduction surgery.

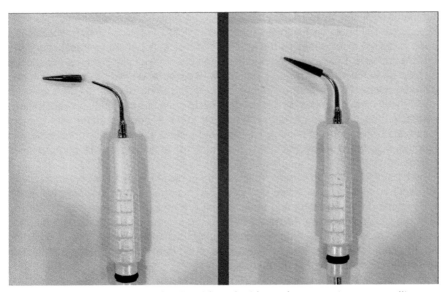

Fig. 5. A standard ultrasonic scaler tip with and without the protective nonmetallic cover. (*Courtesy of* Raza A. Hussain, BDS, DMD, FACS, Chicago, IL.)

Table 2
Health scale for dental implants[a]

Implant Quality Scale Group	Clinical Conditions
I. Success (optimum health)	a. No pain or tenderness on function b. 0 mobility c. <2 mm radiographic bone loss from initial surgery d. No exudates history
II. Satisfactory survival	a. No pain on function b. 0 mobility c. 2–4 mm radiographic bone loss d. No exudates history
III. Compromised survival	a. May have sensitivity on function b. No mobility c. Radiographic bone loss >4 mm (<1/2 of implant body) d. Probing depth >7 mm e. May have exudates history
IV. Failure (clinical or absolute failure)	Any of following: a. Pain on function b. Mobility c. Radiographic bone loss >1/2 length of implant d. Uncontrolled exudate e. No longer in mouth

[a] International Congress of Oral Implantologists, Pisa. Italy. Consensus Conference. 2007.
From Misch CE, Perel ML, Wang H-L, et al. Implant success, survival, and failure: the International Congress of Oral Implantologists (ICOI) Pisa Consensus Conference. Implant Dent. 2008;17(1):8; with permission.

Implants classified by the quality scale as "compromised survival" often exhibit mild to moderate periimplantitis with associated bone loss of up to 50% radiographically. These cases are also defined by the presence of bleeding, periimplant pocketing, and purulent drainage. Despite these conditions, the patient typically does not experience any pain on function and may only present with slight tenderness to percussion and palpation. Bone loss is greater than 4 mm, and probing depths are in excess of 7 mm. These circumstances can be mitigated with open debridement, implantoplasty, chemical/antibiotic applications to the implant surface, and regrafting with primary closure and return for reexposure. The patient must be appropriately consented and informed that these measures are a final attempt at salvaging the compromised implant.

The type of intervention necessary should be considered on a case-by-case basis, with factors, such as age, taken into account. In certain situations, removal of the failing implant with regrafting and replacement is a more predictable option. For patients who cannot tolerate invasive salvage surgery, the use of titanium tubes has proved to be beneficial. J. Woo and colleagues[35] described the technique of sliding this smooth titanium sleeve over the exposed rough threads in an attempt to maintain the severely compromised implant.

Based on guidelines set forth at the 2007 ICOI, the scenario discussed earlier would fall into the category of compromised health. The patient was not in pain and no movement was noted, yet the bone loss and exudate would indicate that some type of intervention to prevent disease progression would be indicated. In the past, the likely course of treatment would have involved implant removal, regrafting, and reimplantation (**Figs. 6–8**).

TECHNIQUE FOR IMPLANT SALVAGE

Before initiating implant salvage, the prosthetic fixture and abutment will need to be removed. Ideally, this has been completed by the restorative dentist and only a surgical cover screw will be in place. The purpose of this cover screw is to promote soft tissue coverage over the compromised implant. The role of soft tissue coverage is critical in obtaining primary closure over the implant after salvage has been attempted.

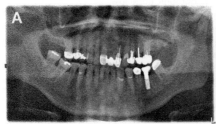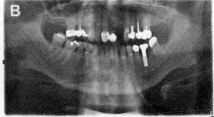

Fig. 6. These images clearly depict how an implant is more prone to structural bone loss as compared with natural dentition. The images were taken approximately 2 years apart. The teeth show stable bone level; however the implant fixture has been preferentially affected by the process of periimplantitis. At presentation the implant was stable and the patient had little to no complaints from the region. The bone loss was discovered incidentally on routine follow-up radiographs. On probing there was bleeding and exudate expressed from the sulcus. (*Courtesy of* Raza A. Hussain, BDS, DMD, FACS, Chicago, IL.)

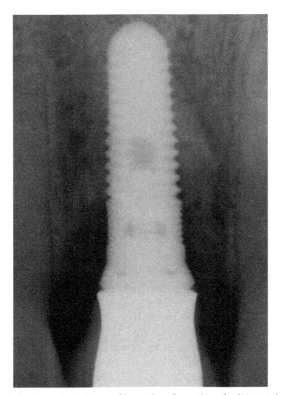

Fig. 7. Radiograph depicting 3 to 4 mm of bone loss from CEJ of adjacent dentition. Implant has no associated mobility, pain, and minimal periimplant inflammation. CEJ, cemento-enamel junction. (*Courtesy of* Raza A. Hussain, BDS, DMD, FACS, Chicago, IL.)

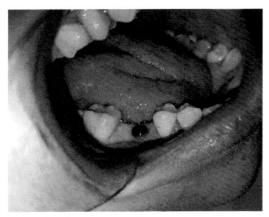

Fig. 8. Appearance 2 weeks after removal of restorative components and placement of cover screw. Note the improved gingival health and lack of inflammation. (*Courtesy of* Raza A. Hussain, BDS, DMD, FACS, Chicago, IL.)

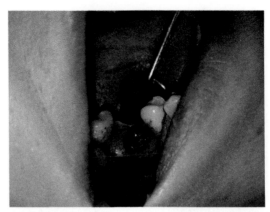

Fig. 9. All granulation tissues should be removed before implant surface preparation. Some noted on distal in this image. (*Courtesy of* Raza A. Hussain, BDS, DMD, FACS, Chicago, IL.)

Once the patient presents with healed soft tissue and minimal inflammation, the clinician can proceed with implant salvage surgery. The initial step involves wide exposure of the entire surgical field. The defect is typically circumferential, and significant reflection of both the buccal and lingual flaps is required. After the soft tissue is reflected and the implant can be visualized completely, all granulation tissue must be debrided. This may be challenging, as this tissue is particularly adherent to the implant surface and grows into every thread and porosity. Aggressive mechanical curettage with hand instruments, and often ultrasonic scalers, should be used in order to ensure complete removal. The high-volume irrigation from the ultrasonic assists in decreasing the bacterial burden around the implant. Once the implant surface has been cleansed of all visible granulation tissue, the next step is surface decontamination and biofilm removal. The biofilm of a compromised typically consists of Bacteroides,

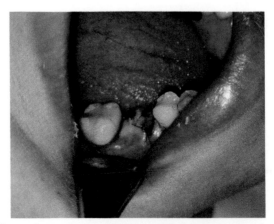

Fig. 10. Tension-free, primary closure achieved. Note the placement of a resorbable membrane to bolster and protect against any perforations. (*Courtesy of* Raza A. Hussain, BDS, DMD, FACS, Chicago, IL.)

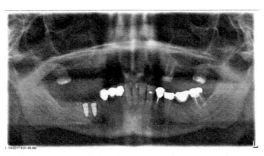

Fig. 11. Radiograph of titanium mesh in place around attempted salvage site. (*Courtesy of* Raza A. Hussain, BDS, DMD, FACS, Chicago, IL.)

Fusobacterium, Aggregatibacter actinomycetemcomitans, Porphyromonas gingivalis, and Prevotella intermedia.[36] Removal can be accomplished with citric acid 40% ph1 application or an antibiotic slurry with proxy brush to prevent release of antigens and reaction with local tissues.

In addition, the surrounding bone should be prepared in anticipation of bone graft placement. Before insertion of the grafting material, the clinician must ensure adequate soft tissue mobilization. Tension-free primary closure is imperative and may require significant undermining of the flap and periosteal releasing incisions. This must be completed in order to prevent displacement of these devices. The membrane, composed of nonresorbable titanium mesh or titanium reinforced polytetrafluoroethylene, allows for rigid protection of the newly grafted site. Significant soft tissue laxity is required to minimize exposure of this membrane and prevent the salvage surgery from becoming compromised.

The type of grafting material used for implant salvage varies widely among clinicians. Autogenous, allogenic, bovine, and synthetic are all suitable options in cases where periimplantitis has induced bone loss. After all granulation tissue, compromised bone, and biofilm have been removed, the graft material is worked along and pressed into all available spaces. The entire implant should be covered by the graft and then the selected nonresorbable membrane is placed over top. The mobilized soft tissue can then be reapproximated and tension-free, primary closure achieved.

Occasionally, the clinician may observe small voids or fenestrations in the soft tissue, which can be remedied by laying a resorbable collagen membrane over the titanium mesh, thereby decreasing the chances of propagation (**Figs. 9–12**).

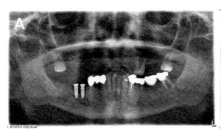
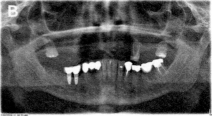

Fig. 12. (*A*) Presalvage. (*B*) Postsalvage in function 3 years. (*Courtesy of* Raza A. Hussain, BDS, DMD, FACS, Chicago, IL.)

SUMMARY

Dental implants have become a routine solution for replacing missing teeth over the years, yet it is important for patients to understand they are not equivalent to their natural dentition. Reasonable expectations should be established before placement and patients should be provided with the tools they need to maintain their new teeth. Clinicians must be prepared for complications, however, that may arise over time. Each compromised implant case, whether simple or complex, requires an individualized and well-organized plan of action to resolve the issue. Although further research is warranted, considering the diagnosis and management of periimplantitis remains controversial, various degrees of intervention have proved to be effective, leading to many successful outcomes for ailing implants.

CLINICS CARE POINTS

- Periimplantitis is a complex and more commonly arising issue.
- Patient education and involvement are paramount.
- Early recognition and interceptive treatment can improve outcomes.
- In cases where implant stability is present salvage of the compromised fixture may be attempted.
- Implant mobility requires removal and possible replacement.

DISCLOSURE

Dr M. Miloro is a consultant for Axogen. The other authors have nothing to disclose.

REFERENCES

1. Quirynen M, deSote M, Steeberghe D. Infectious risks for oral implants: a review of the literature. Clin Oral Implants Res 2002;13:1–19.
2. Nevins M, Langer B. The successful use of osseointegrated implants for the treatment of the recalcitrant periodontal patient. J Periodontol 1995;66:150.
3. Thakkar J, Oh J, Inglehart S, et al. Etiology, Diagnosis and Treatment of Peri-Implantitis- a National Survery of AAOMS Members. J Oral Maxillofac Surg 2017; 75(10):e355–6.
4. Tolstunov L. Peri-implant disease: peri-implantitis versus "peri-implantosis". J Oral Maxillofac Surg 2020;78(5):680–1.
5. Lang NP, Loe H. The relationship between the width of keratinized gingiva and gingival health. J Periodontol 1972;43:623–7.
6. Wennstrom JL. Lack of association between width of attached gingiva and development of soft tissue recession: a 5 year longitudinal study. J Clin Periodontol 1987;14:181–4.
7. Kennedy J, Bird W, Palcanis K, et al. A longitudinal evaluation of varying widths of attached gingiva. J Clin Periodontol 1985;12:667.
8. Miyasato M, Crigger M, Egelberg J. Gingival condition in areas of minimal and appreciable width of keratinized gingiva. J Clin Periodontol 1977;4:200–9.
9. Stetler K, Bissada NF. Significance of the width of keratinized gingiva on the periodontal status of teeth with subgingival restoration. J Periodontol 1987;58: 696–700.
10. Valderhaug J, Birkeland JM. Periodontal conditions in patients 5 years following insertion of fixed prostheses. Pocket depth and loss of attachment. J Oral Rehab 1976;3:237–43.

11. Schroeder A, Pohler O, Sutter F. Tissue reaction to a titanium hollow cylinder implant with titanium plasma sprayed surface. Schweiz Monatsschr Zahnmed 1976;86:713–27.

12. Becker W, Becker BE, Newman MG, et al. Clinical micro-biologic findings that may contribute to dental implant failure. Int J Oral Maxillofac Implants 1990; 5:31–8.

13. Strub JR, Gaberthuel TW, Grunder U. The role of attached gingiva in the health of peri-implant tissue in dogs: clinical findings. Int J Periodontics Restorative Dent 1991;11:317–33.

14. Wennstrom JL, Bengazi F, Lekholm U. The influence of the masticatory mucosa on the peri-implant soft tissue condition. Clin Oral Implants Res 1994;5:1–8.

15. Krekeler G, Schilli W, Diemer J. Should the exit of the artificial abutment tooth be positioned in the region of the attached gingiva? Int J Oral Surg 1985;14:504–8.

16. Adell R, Lekholm U, Rockler G, et al. Marginal tissue reactions at osseointegrated titanium fixtures. I. A 3- year longitudinal prospective study. Int J Oral Maxillofac Implants 1986;15:39–52.

17. Lekholm U, Adell R, Lindhe J, et al. Marginal tissue reactions at osseointegrated titanium fixtures. II. A cross-section restrospective study. Int J Oral Maxillofac Surg 1986;15:53–61.

18. Consensus report: implant therapy II. Proceedings of the 1996 World Workshop in Periodontics. In: Nevins M, Kenney E, van Steenberghe D, et al, editors. Ann Periodontol 1996;1:816–20.

19. Warrer K, Buser D, Lang NP, et al. Plaque-induced peri-implantitis in the presence of absence of keratinized mucosa: an experimental study in monkey. Clin Oral Implants Res 1995;6:131–8.

20. Kirsch A, Ackermann KL. The IMZ osteointegrated implant system. Dent Clin North Am 1989;33:733–91.

21. James RA, Schultz RL. Hemidesmosomes and the adhesion of junctional epithelial cells to metal implants: a preliminary report. J Oral Implantol 1974;4:294.

22. Listgarten M, Lang NP, Schroeder HE, et al. Periodontal tissues and their counterparts around endosseous implant. Clin Oral Implants Res 1991;2:81–90.

23. Rapley JW, Mills MP, Wylam J. Soft tissue management during implant maintenance. Int J Periodontics Restorative Dent 1992;12:373.

24. Adell R, Lekholm U, Rockler B, et al. A 15 year study of osseointegrated implants in the treatment of the edentulous jaw. Int J Oral Surg 1981;10:387–416.

25. Block MS, Kent JN. Factors associated with soft- and hard tissue compromise of endosseous implants. J Oral Maxillofac Surg 1990;48:1153–60.

26. Esposito M, Coulthard P, Thomsen P, et al. The role of implant surface modification, shape and material on the success of osseointegrated dental implants: a Cochrane systemic review. Eur J Prosthodont Restor Dent 2005;13:15–31.

27. Kirsch A, Mentag P. The IMZ endosseous two phase implant system: a complete oral rehabilitation treatment concept. J Oral Implantol 1986;12:576–89.

28. Chung DM, OH TJ, Shotwell JL, et al. Significance of keratinized mucosa in maintenance of dental implants with different surfaces. J Periodontol 2006;77: 1410–20.

29. Carr B, Boggess W, Coburn J, et al. Is alcohol consumption associated with protection against peri-implantitis? a retrospective cohort analysis. J Oral Maxillofac Surg 2020;78:76–81.

30. Yukna R. Optimizing clinical success with implants: maintenance and care. Compend Contin Educ Dent 1993;15:554–61.

31. Rapley JW, Swan RH, Hallmon WW, et al. The surface characteristics produced by various oral hygiene instruments and materials on titanium implant abutments. Int J Oral Maxillofac Implants 1990;5:47–52.
32. English C. Hygiene, maintenance, and prosthodontic concerns for the infirm patient: clinical report and discussion. Implant Dent 1995;4:166–72.
33. Brough Muzzin K, Johnson R, Carr P, et al. The dental hygienist's role in the maintenance of osseointegrated dental implants. J Dent Hyg 1988;62:448–53.
34. Meschenmoser A, d'Hoedt B, Meyle J, et al. Effects of various hygiene procedures on the surface characteristics of titanium abutments. J Periodontol 1996; 67:229–35.
35. Woo J, Kwon J, Kim B. Titanium Tube around Implant Fixture as Salvage Treatment for Peri-Implantitis: Pilot Study. J Oral Maxillofac Surg 2019;77(9):e73–4.
36. Mombelli A, Van Oosten MAC, Schurch E, et al. The microbiota associated with successful or failing osseointegrated titanium implants. Oral Microbiol Immunol 1987;2:145–51.

Soft Tissue Injury in Preparation for Implants

Earl Clarkson, DDS[a], Monica Hanna, DMD[b],*, Guillermo Puig, DMD[b],*

KEYWORDS

- Grafting • Incision • Soft tissue • Split-thickness • Tissue

KEY POINTS

- Proper medical and clinical evaluations of patients is imperative to avoid soft tissue complications in implant planning.
- Several grafting techniques are available, and proper clinical judgment should be used to evaluate which technique patients may benefit most from.
- Patient anatomy should be taken into consideration when planning for soft tissue grafting.
- Soft tissue grafting may be indicated before, at time of, or after implant placement in order to reduce risk of soft tissue complications.

OVERVIEW OF GRAFTING PRINCIPLES
Soft Tissue Evaluation

Evaluation of adequate quality and quantity of soft tissue is imperative before implant placement in order to optimize success. Attached tissue around dental implants allows for increased soft tissue stability, a decreased risk of soft tissue complications, and a favorable esthetic outcome. Evaluation begins with the gingival biotype as described by Olsson and Lindhe[1]: thin scalloped versus thick flat (**Fig. 1**). Gingival biotype is determined by variances in soft tissue, bone, and tooth morphology. Thin scalloped biotype reacts to insult with recession as opposed to thick flat biotype that reacts with pocket formation. The underlying buccal plate in thin biotype is thin with frequent fenestration and dehiscence type of defects, whereas the underlying bone of thick flat biotype is typically much thicker and rarely has dehiscences or fenestrations. The bony architecture in thin biotype tends to extensively remodel after extraction of teeth including increased loss of height and buccal plate and socket dimension, whereas thicker plates tend to undergo lesser remodeling. In thin biotype, teeth tend to be more triangular in shape with narrow contact areas in the incisal one-third, whereas in thick biotype, teeth are squarer in shape with long contact areas

[a] NYC Health + Hospitals/Woodhull, 760 Broadway, Brooklyn, NY 11206, USA; [b] Oral and Maxillofacial Surgery, NYC Health + Hospitals/Woodhull, 760 Broadway, Brooklyn, NY 11206, USA
* Corresponding authors.
E-mail addresses: Mhanna0113@gmail.com (M.H.); guillermo_puig@outlook.com (G.P.)

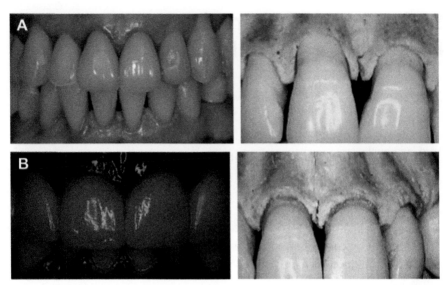

Fig. 1. (*A*) Thin scalloped gingival biotype with triangular teeth, thin buccal plate, fenestrations, and scalloping of the bony architecture. (*B*) Thick flat gingival biotype with square teeth, thick buccal plate, and flat bony architecture. (*From* Batal H, Yavari A, Mehra P. Soft tissue surgery for implants. Dent Clin North Am. 2015;59(2):472–3; with permission.)

extending to the cervical one-third with a more pronounced emergence profile.[2] Soft tissue grafting in patients with thin scalloped biotype results in improved esthetic outcomes and improves long-term soft tissue stability.[3]

General Principles

Following the general principles in soft tissue grafting increases the chances of success and decreases complications. These principles involve the proper creation of recipient site, recipient site vascularity, adequate operative hemostasis, good graft adaptation to recipient site, graft thickness, proper immobilization, and closure.

During the initial healing stages (first 24 hours), a graft receives its nutrients by plasmatic diffusion, a process known as imbibition. This plasmatic diffusion is guided by the hypoxic gradient between graft and recipient site, providing initial nutrition to the graft. Following this, during days 2 to 3, the process of inosculation takes place and vessels from the graft anastomose with vessels from the recipient site. As graft healing proceeds during days 3 to 7, revascularization begins and ingrowth of new vessels into the graft takes place. After vascularity is achieved, remodeling takes place restoring normal histologic architecture.[4]

Early graft mobility disrupts revascularization and increases chances of necrosis. Failure to achieve intimate adaptation of the graft to the recipient bed decreases plasmatic diffusion and increases capillary travel distance; similarly uncontrolled hemostasis can cause hematoma or blood clot formation hindering adequate nutrient support. Graft thickness also plays an important factor in healing. Thin and intermediate-thickness grafts tend to have higher survival rates. Thicker grafts also have less secondary contracture leading to better clinical outcomes.

Timing of soft tissue grafts can be variable, depending on several factors including the type of graft being used. No difference has been seen in outcome between simultaneous and phased soft tissue augmentation in implant placement when keratinized tissue width and soft tissue thickness are considered.[5] They may be performed before, during, or after bone grafting, during or after implant placement, during second-stage abutment placement, or after crown placement. However, successful outcomes decrease when soft tissue grafting procedures are performed after crown placement.[2]

Types of Soft Tissue Grafts

There are various options for soft tissue grafting, including connective tissue autografts, vascularized interpositional periosteal connective tissue flaps, palatal roll technique, and epithelialized palatal grafts.

Connective soft tissue autografts are commonly harvested from the hard palate or alternatively the maxillary tuberosity. The palate provides maximum volume, whereas the maxillary tuberosity provides a greater thickness. Palatal soft tissue is composed of 3 layers: epithelium, subepithelial connective tissue, and submucosa. Connective tissue grafts can be categorized as either subepithelial connective tissue grafts or epithelial connective tissue grafts.[6]

Subepithelial connective tissue grafts are typically harvested between the palatal root of the first molar and the canine tooth for optimal thickness.[7] Careful consideration should be given to the location of the greater palatine artery in this region to avoid injury. Reiser and coworkers reported the greater palatine artery enters the palate in the area of the greater palatine foramen and travels anteriorly in the direction of the incisive foramen[8] (**Fig. 2**A). The greater palatine foramen most commonly is at the junction of the horizontal and vertical shelf of the palatine bone corresponding with the position between the second and third molar.[2] The neurovascular bundle is located between 7 and 17 mm from the cementoenamel junction of the teeth with an average of 12 mm distance, with the distance being shorter in patients with a shallow palatal vault and longer in patients with a higher palatal vault[2] (**Fig. 2**B). Dissection should therefore be limited to 8 mm in height to avoid injuring the greater palatine artery.

Vascularized interpositional periosteal connective tissue flaps were initially described by Sclar.[9] The technique involves a rotation of a pedicled subepithelial finger flap to the anterior maxilla with a random pattern blood supply.[2] This technique has several advantages as compared with free soft tissue grafts: it allows for effective simultaneous hard and soft tissue augmentation, provides superior soft tissue augmentation in both vertical and horizontal directions, and provides greater stability

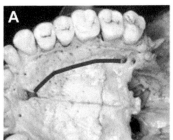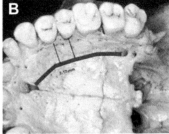

Fig. 2. (*A*) Course of the greater palatine artery exiting the greater palatine foramen, crossing the palate in the direction of the incisive canal. (*B*) The greater palatine artery is located between 7 and 17 mm from the cementoenamel junction of teeth. (*From* Batal H, Yavari A, Mehra P. Soft tissue surgery for implants. Dent Clin North Am. 2015;59(2):475; with permission.)

with decreased secondary shrinkage. It is ideal to correct large defects, and it is an optimal graft for compromised tissue beds.[2] The main disadvantages are that this flap cannot be used with concomitant temporization or if the implant is not submerged.

The palatal roll technique as first described by Abrams is a split-thickness palatal flap that is reflected separating the epithelium from the connective tissue.[10] The connective tissue is reflected from the palate and rolled onto the buccal to correct deficiencies in the buccolingual direction.[2] The palatal roll technique was modified by Scharf and Tarnow in 1992 and is commonly indicated to correct minor buccal soft tissue defects during the time of implant placement or placement of the healing abutment.[11]

The epithelialized palatal graft was first described by Bjorn and coworkers[12] and was later modified by Sullivan and colleagues[13] to describe full-thickness versus split-thickness grafts. Full-thickness grafts consist of epithelium and the entire zone of lamina propria, whereas split-thickness grafts contain epithelium and only partial thickness of lamina propria.[13] Split-thickness grafts are further divided into thick, intermediate, or thin based on the width of lamina propria included. Epithelialized palatal grafts are indicated for mucogingival defects as well as the need to increase the zone of keratinized tissue.

SOFT TISSUE COMPLICATIONS DURING IMPLANT PREPARATION

Soft tissue injuries and complications can result without proper evaluation of soft tissue sites before implant placement. An adequate preoperative medical evaluation also plays an important role in decreasing risk of complications, especially in smokers, alcoholics, immunocompromised patients, or those suffering from cancer, cardiovascular, or hematologic disorders. Although sometimes inevitable, surgical complications can be minimized through ensuring adequate planning and preparation of the soft tissue of the implant recipient site. Injuries and complications may occur before implant placement, after grafting, during implant placement, or after implant placement.

Infection

Surgical site infection can arise during the initial postoperative days and present as excessive edema, pain, erythema, and discharge. Adequate use of surgical asepsis may decrease the risk of this complication. Additional preventive measurements such as the use of preoperative antibiotics, appropriate oral hygiene, and the use of chlorhexidine 0.12% rinses during the first 2 weeks has also shown benefits. A study by Lambert and colleagues reported that there is a significant reduction in infectious complications when chlorhexidine rinses were used perioperatively during implant surgery. With chlorhexidine, there was a reduction of infection complications from 8.7% in the control group to 4.1% infection rate in the study group.[14] Use of antibiotics is advised; however, they are not indicated in every case.

Edema

Swelling is caused by excess plasma fluid (transudate) accumulation in the interstitial space of tissues, defined as at least a 10% increase. It is correlated with the extent of surgical trauma and to the duration of surgery,[15] and can cause severe discomfort to the patient and may negatively affect overall healing. Minimizing traumatic damage, the use of postoperative cold compresses postoperatively (<48 hours) and warm compress (after >48 hours), and corticosteroids may prevent or decrease edema after implant surgery.

Bleeding

Bleeding can occur due to traumatic handling of soft tissue during implant placement. This bleeding can be caused by failure to stabilize the flap, tearing of soft tissue caused by placing too much tension on soft tissue during closure, or a sharp suture material. Other causes of soft tissue bleeding include masticatory trauma from the opposing dentition or failing to appropriately modify a prostheses to be used after implant placement. Eliminating the cause of bleeding and use of local measures to promote hemostasis are included in treatment. Continuous bleeding after local measures are used will require reevaluation of the flap and exploration, followed by reapproximation of the flap to fully immobilize the soft tissue in order to promote clot formation and stabilization.

Ecchymoses and Hematomas

Ecchymoses are blood effusions infiltrating surface tissues, and hematomas are circumscribed blood collections. These can be dramatic and more prominent in elderly patients due to their increased capillary fragility. Several factors can contribute to these injuries such as longer and more complex surgical time, lack of surgical experience, traumatic surgical techniques, lack of postoperative patient compliance, elderly patients, and failure to discontinue antiplatelets medications (if indicated) before surgery. Intraoperative and postoperative ecchymoses and hematomas can be extensive if there is poor hemostasis during the surgical procedure.

Soft tissue ecchymoses typically resolve on their own, but the use of intermittent ice packs in the first 24 hours followed by moist heat after 48 hours can aid in resolution.[15] If a hematoma is present between bone and the mucoperiosteal flap, it should be drained and external compression applied on soft tissue to avoid relapse.

Loss of the Graft

Partial or complete loss of connective tissue grafts is possible despite their high success rates (**Fig. 3**). Adequate healing of graft sites depends on vascularity, thus immobilization of the graft at the time of surgery is imperative. Creating a flap at the recipient site allowing for primary closure may also decrease the risk of graft necrosis. Immediately postoperatively, the grafted site may seem pale and may turn grayish after

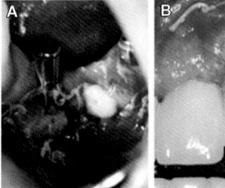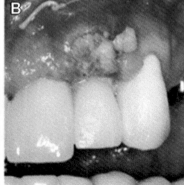

Fig. 3. (*A*) Partial loss of subepithelial connective tissue graft. (*B*) Partial loss of subepithelial connective tissue graft. (*From* Batal H, Yavari A, Mehra P. Soft tissue surgery for implants. Dent Clin North Am. 2015;59(2):490; with permission.)

48 hours due to tissue ischemia. If adequate neovascularization is achieved by day 14, tissue will return to normal pink color and edema will resolve.[16] Observation or conservative debridement is recommended depending on the extent of graft necrosis. The use of local measures such as gentle saline irrigations may also be beneficial.

Subcutaneous Emphysema

Emphysema results from a sudden increase in intraoral pressure that may occur if a patient sneezes, and air is forced through the mucoperiosteal flap into connective tissues or fascial planes. Patients present with facial swelling and crepitus on palpation. Massage and cold compresses will help resorb air that is trapped in the tissues, resulting in spontaneous resolution of the emphysema. The use of antibiotics should be considered, as these may prevent secondary infection from oral bacteria.

Avoiding the use of high-velocity instruments for osteotomy preparation, using copious irrigation, and ensuring adequate and proper closure of flap margins when suturing may contribute to minimizing the risk of developing emphysema. More severe complications can arise with extensive emphysema, as it dissects fascial planes into the mediastinum. Subcutaneous emphysema can be life-threatening in the presence of air embolism. Severe infections may also arise due to microbial dissemination through emphysematous tracts.

Flap Dehiscence

Dehiscence results when surgical wound edges separate, exposing the dental implant or bone (**Fig. 4**). Contributing factors include thin gingival mucosa, excessive tension causing soft tissue necrosis, failure to adequately reapproximate flap margins, cover screw loosening, mechanical irritation, edema or hematomas, premature use of prosthodontic appliances, trauma from the opposing dentition, subperiosteal debris, and smoking due to its vasoactive and cytotoxic effects. As previously mentioned, there are 2 distinct gingival biotypes: thin scalloped and thick flat. Thin scalloped gingival biotype tends to react to insult with recession. The underlying buccal plate is typically thin with frequent fenestration and dehiscence type of defects.

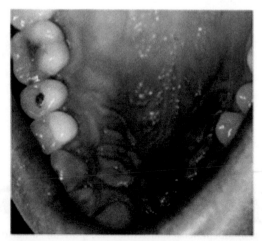

Fig. 4. Dehiscence of soft tissue at palatal donor site. (*From* Batal H, Yavari A, Mehra P. Soft tissue surgery for implants. Dent Clin North Am. 2015;59(2):490; with permission.)

The extent of the exposure and bone health determines treatment[17]:

- Small exposures usually do not require correction; the presence of granulation tissue compensates the opening and promotes healing by secondary intention.
  - A small exposure within the first 24 to 48 hours can be resutured.
  - If the granulation tissue formation process lasts longer than 2 weeks, and there is no necrotic bone, the epithelial wound margins may be refreshed and re-sutured.
- Large exposures or a time lapse greater than 48 to 72 hours and no necrotic bone require removing sutures, refreshing epithelial wound margins, and resuturing.
- Recurring exposures in healthy, young, and nonsmoking patients may require debridement thorough irrigation and mouthwash with chlorhexidine. Denuded bone should also be covered with dressing, gradually reducing dressing size and monitoring region for 3-6 weeks until healed.
- Nonresolving dehiscence with necrotic bone requires bone removal until fresh bleeding bone is reached. Consider implant removal if there is infection present or if the implant is mobile, as these can interfere with tissue closure. Excision of wound margins and mobilization of a large mucoperiosteal flap buccally and lingually are also indicated. An antibiotic regimen should also be prescribed for 7 to 10 days.

Wound dehiscence can be prevented by tension-free closure using a buccal releasing incision and adequate preoperative assessment of the soft tissues. Assessing the amount of keratinized mucosa present and planning of augmentation procedures when appropriate are imperative. Minimally invasive flap elevation and reflection, proper reapproximation and suturing of the flap, copious irrigation of subperiosteal debris, and delaying use of prosthodontic appliances until soft tissue healing is completed may also reduce the risk of wound dehiscence.

Deficient Attached Gingiva

When using open flap implant surgery versus the flapless technique, particular care is given to the esthetics zone in order to enhance soft tissue appearance. Flapped procedures are indicated when the ridge is narrow in a buccal/lingual dimension or there is limited attached gingiva that would be lost using a punch at the crest. In order to conserve the attached gingiva, the crestal incision should be placed palatally in order to provide greater thickness of keratinized tissue on the facial aspect of the flap. This also enhances papilla height by allowing more interproximal tissue to be elevated.

A narrow zone of attached gingiva surrounding implant restoration is associated with a higher risk of gingival inflammation, gingival recession, and decreased resistance to plaque accumulation. Sufficient keratinized gingiva around dental implants offers resistance to forces of mastication and external trauma and provides a barrier to inflammatory infiltrates.

Patients with thin gingival biotypes may benefit from soft tissue grafting. The increased thickness provides more esthetic outcomes, especially at the level of the buccal gingival margin. Epithelialized palatal grafts are indicated for mucogingival defects and to increase the zone of keratinized tissue.[18]

Thicker grafts are more ideal for increasing the zone of attached gingiva and provide better outcomes as they contract less than split-thickness grafts.

Mucoperiosteal Perforation

Screw exposure is a common complication and can be associated with excessive prosthetic pressure compromising vascularity, trauma, thin mucosal soft tissues, or cover screw loosening. Exposure of implant screws can lead to plaque buildup, inflammation, and eventually bone loss around the implant surface. Cehreli and colleagues[19] confirmed that there is a direct relation between spontaneous early cover screw perforations and early crestal bone loss. He also concluded that early placed implants experienced more spontaneous perforations and associated bone loss in comparison with conventionally placed submerged implants. Typically mucoperiosteal perforations do not require treatment because tight closure of the soft tissue flap is not indispensable for implant osseointegration. In some cases, in order to decrease plaque accumulation and inflammation, areas of exposure may be extended and the implant cover screw may be replaced by a healing abutment. In early exposure of crestal bone, flap elevation or soft tissue grafting should be considered to cover the defect.

Adequate preoperative evaluation can decrease the frequency of this complication. If soft tissue thickness is deficient, a connective tissue graft should be planned alongside implant placement. A study by Linkevicius and colleagues[20] reported that initial gingival tissue thickness at the crest of implants may have significant influence on marginal bone stability around implants. If there is soft tissue thickness of 2.0 mm or less, crestal bone loss up to 1.45 mm may occur, despite a supracrestal position of the implant-abutment interface.

Maxillary Sinus Perforation

In cases where there is a severe degree of resorption that may preclude placement of a short implant or the primary stability of the implant would be compromised, the maxillary sinus must be augmented. Bone regenerative procedures for implant preparation are encompassed by 2 main approaches: the lateral sinus window and the transalveolar or crestal approach. Although each procedure is very different, perforation of the maxillary sinus is one of the complications that both procedures share. Maintaining the integrity of the sinus membrane is important to decrease bacterial contamination and infection to the grafting site. This could lead to a further decrease in potential future complications, but in some cases it may be unavoidable despite adequate presurgical evaluation.

Management of maxillary sinus perforations changes according to the extent of damage to the sinus membrane[21]:

- Small perforations of less than 1 mm, the membrane may self-repair by folding over or through clot formation.
- Perforations of less than 5 mm may benefit from the use of fibrin glues, collagen tapes, bioabsorbable membranes, or suturing the membrane defect, which are usually sufficient to allow for simultaneous implant placement.
- Perforations larger than 5 mm may require the use of bioabsorbable membranes, lamellar bone plates, suturing alone or in combination with fibrin glue, or ultimately aborting the procedure.
- Larger perforations are even more challenging to repair and may require more specific management with the use of collagen membranes to cover all internal sinus walls, local flaps, or autogenous bone blocks.

Perforation of the membrane may also occur during the implant placement itself. If this happens, implants that penetrate inside of the sinus cavity less than 2 mm do not require further intervention, as spontaneous covering of the implants with the sinus mucosa may occur. However, if the implant extends into the maxillary sinus more than 2 mm, chances of spontaneous mucosal repair are diminished and accumulation of debris around the implant surface could lead to maxillary sinusitis. In a study by

Corbella and colleagues,[22–26] it was observed that there were no statistically signifi-cant differences in implant survival between implants penetrating less than or equal to 4 mm or greater than 4 mm with long-term survival rates of 99.5% and 98.5%, respectively. Complications associated with maxillary sinus perforations such as epistaxis, sinusitis, and membrane thickening are common.

SUMMARY

Several soft tissue injuries and complications may be prevented with proper presurgi-cal evaluation. A detailed medical and clinical evaluation also play an important role in decreasing the risk of future complications.

Soft tissue grafting may be indicated before, at the time of, or after implant place-ment in order to minimize risks of injury. Thus, a rigorous examination of soft tissues before implant placement is always recommended. Proper evaluation and preparation of soft tissue sites, surgeon experience, and careful postoperative care may contribute to reducing these soft tissue injuries and complications.

CLINICS CARE POINTS

- Most of the implant placement surgeries complications can be avoided as long as the case has been properly diagnosed, planned and adequate surgical princi-ples are followed.
- Failure to follow proper surgical techniques can have detrimental effects in an im-plants sucess.
- Care during retraction and proper soft tissue management can help avoid com-plications such as flap tearing and tissue dehiscence.

DISCLOSURE

The authors have nothing to disclose.

REFERENCES

1. Olsson M, Lindhe J. Periodontal characteristics in individuals with varying form of the upper central incisors. J Clin Periodontol 1991;18(1):78–82.
2. Dym H. Implant Procedures for the General Dentist. Dent Clin North Am 2015; 59(2). https://doi.org/10.1016/j.cden.2014.12.002.
3. Bhat V, Shetty S. Prevalence of different gingival biotypes in individuals with vary-ing forms of maxillary central incisors: a survey. J Dent Implants 2013;3(2): 116–21.
4. Greenwood J, Amjadi M, Dearman B, et al. Real-time demonstration of split skin graft inosculation and integra dermal matrix neovascularization using confocal laser scanning microscopy. Eplasty 2009;9:e33.
5. Cho-Ying L, Zhaozhao C, Whei-Lin P, et al. Impact of timing on soft tissue augmentation during implant treatment: A systematic review and meta-analysis. Clin Oral Implants Res 2018;29(5):508–21.
6. Rees TD, Brasher WJ. A technique for obtaining thin split-thickness grafts in peri-odontal surgery. Oral Surg Oral Med Oral Pathol 1970;29(1):148–54.
7. Dibart S, Karima M. Practical Periodontal plastic surgery. Danvers (MA): Black-well; 2006.
8. Reiser GM, Bruno JF, Mahan PE, et al. The subepithelial connective tissue graft palatal donor site: anatomic considerations for surgeons. Int J Periodontics Restorative Dent 1996;16(2):130–7.

9. Sclar A. Soft tissue and esthetic considerations in implant therapy. Quintessence Publishing; 2003.

10. Abrams L. Augmentation of the deformed residual edentulous ridge for fixed prosthesis. Comp Contin Educ Gen Dent 1980;1(3):205–13.

11. Scharf DR, Tarnow DP. Modified roll technique for localized alveolar ridge augmentation. Int J Periodontics Restorative Dent 1992;12(5):415–25.

12. Bjorn H. Free transplantation of gingival propria. Sven Tandlak Tidskr 1963;22: 684–5.

13. Sullivan HC, Atkins JH. Free autogenous gingival grafts. I. Principles of successful grafting. Periodontics 1968;6(3):121–9.

14. Lambert PM, Morris HF, Ochi S. The influence of 0.12% chlorexidine digluconate rinses on the incidence of infectious complications and implant success. J Oral Maxillofac Surg 1997;55(suppl 5):25–30.

15. Annibali S, Ripari M, LA Monaca G, et al. Local complications in dental implant surgery: prevention and treatment. Oral Implantol (Rome) 2008;1(1):21-33.

16. Pippi R. Post-surgical clinical monitoring of soft tissue wound healing in periodontal and implant surgery. Int J Med Sci 2017;14(8):721–8.

17. Sadig W, Almas K. Risk factors and management of dehiscent wounds in implant dentistry. Implant Dent 2004;13(Issue 2):140–7.

18. Greenstein G, Cavallaro J. The clinical significance of keratinized gingiva around dental implants. Compend Contin Educ Dent 2011;32(8):24–31.

19. Cehreli MC, Kökat AM, Uysal S, et al. Spontaneous early exposure and marginal bone loss around conventionally and early-placed submerged implants: a double-blind study. Clin Oral Implants Res 2010;21(12):1327–33.

20. Linkevicius T, Apse P, Grybauskas S, et al. The influence of soft tissue thickness on crestal bone changes around implants: a 1-year prospective controlled clinical trial. Int J Oral Maxillofac Implants 2009;24(4):712–9.

21. Alper S, Mustafa Özarslan M, Özalp Ö. Management of the complications of maxillary sinus augmentation, challenging issues on paranasal sinuses. London: Tang-Chuan Wang, IntechOpen; 2018. https://doi.org/10.5772/intechopen. 80603.

22. Corbella S, Taschieri S, Del Fabbro M. Long-term outcomes for the treatment of atrophic posterior maxilla: a systematic review of literature. Clin Implant Dent Relat Res 2015;17(1):120–32.

23. Lauc T, Kobler P. Early post-operative complications in oral implantology. Coll Antropol 1998;22:251–7.

24. Ragucci GM, Elnayef B, Suárez-López del Amo F, et al. Influence of exposing dental implants into the sinus cavity on survival and complications rate: a systematic review. Int J Implant Dent 2019;5:6.

25. Schwarz L, Schiebel V, Hof M, et al. Risk factors of membrane perforation and postoperative complications in sinus floor elevation surgery: review of 407 augmentation procedures. J Oral Maxillofac Surg 2015;73(7):1275–82.

26. Hernández-Alfaro F, Torradeflot MM, Marti C. Prevalence and management of Schneiderian membrane perforations during sinus-lift procedures. Clin Oral Implants Res 2008;19(1):91–8.

Guided Implant Surgery
A Technique Whose Time Has Come

Peter Chen, DDS, MS[a,b,]*, Levon Nikoyan, DDS[a,b,c]

KEYWORDS

- Dental implants • Guided implant surgery
- Computed tomography/cone-beam computed tomography
- Computer-aided design and manufacturing • Computer-aided manufacturing
- Virtual implant surgery planning
- In-office/desktop stereolithographic 3D printed surgical guides
- Dynamic navigated guided surgery

KEY POINTS

- Indications of guided implant surgery include avoiding vital anatomic structures, minimized flap, accurate implant placement, placement in limited access, and maintaining esthetic needs.
- Implant surgical techniques: free-handed, static-guided (tooth-, mucosa-, or bone-supported guides), or dynamic guided surgery.
- The workflow of guided implant surgery: Conventional compared with modern simplified.
- Selection and fabrication of implant surgical guide: 3D printed, dental laboratory, or manufacturer.

INTRODUCTION

Guided implant surgery has advanced to become nearly routine for implant placement alongside the availability and widespread use of in-office technology. Technology like cone-beam computed tomography (CBCT) has readily become more common for in-office use.[1] CT-guided surgery has become even more accessible with the increased availability of virtual implant planning software.[2] Adjunctive technology like intraoral scanners and 3-dimensional (3D) printers have both helped streamline the implant planning and surgical guide fabrication while decreasing patient chair time. Dental laboratories and manufacturers have also become fully capable of fabricating guides

[a] Department of Oral and Maxillofacial Surgery, Woodhull Hospital, 760 Broadway, Brooklyn, NY 11206, USA; [b] Department of Dentistry, Woodhull Hospital, 760 Broadway, Brooklyn, NY 11206, USA; [c] Private Practice, Forward Oral Surgery, 248-62 Jericho Tpke, Floral Park, NY 11001, USA
* Corresponding author. Department of Oral and Maxillofacial Surgery, Woodhull Hospital, 760 Broadway, Brooklyn, NY 11206, USA
E-mail address: peterchenoralsurgery@gmail.com

Dent Clin N Am 65 (2021) 67–80
https://doi.org/10.1016/j.cden.2020.09.005
dental.theclinics.com
0011-8532/21/© 2020 Elsevier Inc. All rights reserved.

specific to the wide range of implant systems available, so it is not required to have a full in-office setup of CBCT and 3D printer.

GUIDED IMPLANT SURGERY

Plain film radiographs (periapical and panoramic) have been mainstays in the preoperative planning of free-handed implant surgery. Two-dimensional images have clear limitations in the planning of dental implants. Although free-handed implant surgery requires less planning and lead time to insertion, results are highly variable. Guided surgery, on the other hand, is a dependable, reproducible, and safe method of doing implant surgery.[3,4] The surgeon commonly uses guided surgery when operating in the proximity of vital anatomic structures. Many types of guides will provide vertical stops to avoid excessive osteotomy, whereas others will even allow insertion of the implants through the guides. Those practitioners in favor of minimally invasive surgery will use guides to provide smaller flaps or eliminate them in favor of flapless surgery. Using surgical guides will require less effort to ensure implant parallelism and angulation, which will save significant intraoperative time.

As the technology for guide fabrication is advanced and digital software is improved, the cost of doing guided surgery decreases. This treatment modality is now broadly available, with significantly decreased planning and wait times. Dental implant guides can be classified broadly into static and dynamic, as shown in **Table 1**.[5,6] Static guides are fabricated ahead of time and provide no surgical feedback during the surgery. So, if the guide does not fit during the surgery, for example, the surgeon has very few options in continuing the surgery guided. Dynamic guide, on the other hand, is a "navigation" type setup that uses the patient's skeletal structure superimposed on CT and provides the surgeon with real-time feedback. Dynamic guided surgery is developing technology and requires substantial investment and has an increased learning curve.[7]

Dynamic guided surgery systems use optical technologies to track the patient and the handpiece with real-time image display on the monitors. The optical technology uses active or passive tracking arrays.[6] The passive system uses a light source that reflect light emitted (from an overhead source) back to the cameras. While the active system emits light that is tracked by the cameras. Navigation is achieved with the triangulation of the extraoral overhead array, intraoral markers, and handpiece arrays. The intraoral markers consist of a clip that contains metallic markers that fit onto the patient's teeth. The intraoral clip must be in place during CBCT scan and saved for use again during surgery.

Static guides have a long history of evolution in dentistry. In contemporary dentistry, when one refers to guides, it is usually understood that this is a radiographic type of static guide. It is not uncommon, however, to encounter suck down stents as a communication method between the general dentist and the surgeon. From the surgical point of view, these guides are of minimal use and are quite often used for the first few minutes of the surgery to mark the osteotomy and are rapidly discarded afterward (**Fig. 1**). Furthermore, these guides did not account for local anatomy or bone resorption and provided no vertical control for the fixture. Occasionally, the general dentist places radiopaque material within the proposed path of the osteotomy. When combined with cone-beam, these guides would confirm the position of alveolar bone along the osteotomy path. The most significant limitation of these guides is the lack of flexibility. Mainly the guide has limited value if the alveolar bone is not within the marked path, as modifications to the surgical protocols are not possible.

Table 1
Implant surgical techniques

Implant Surgical Technique	Advantages	Disadvantages	Indications	Accuracy[5,6]
Free-handed surgery:	Surgeon-dependent accuracy, most cost-effective	Least accurate when compared with guided surgery with similar surgeon experience	For less-complex implant cases (adequate access, low esthetic demands, sufficient bony dimensions)	Least accurate 2.7 mm deviation (at entry), 2.9 mm (at apex), 9.9 degrees angulation
Static-guided surgery: tooth-, mucosa-, bone-supported				0.6–1.15 mm (at entry) 0.6–1.22 mm (at apex) 2.5–5 degrees angulation
Tooth-supported	More accurate less invasive flap compared with bone-supported	Requires adjacent dentition	Simple to complex cases	Tooth-supported Slightly more accurate than mucosa- and bone-supported
Mucosa-supported	Least-invasive flap and hence less morbidity to patient	Least stable; can be combined with tooth-borne or bone-bore as initial pilot drill followed by bone-supported	Complex partial or full-edentulous cases	
Bone-supported	Stable with adequate bone, good accuracy	Most invasive flap (can be minimized with initial pilot drill guide with mucosa-supported)	Required for full edentulous, recommended for long-spanning partial-edentulous patients	
Dynamic guided surgery	Perioperative real-time adjustment Higher accuracy than static and free-hand	High equipment cost Training required Difficulty in the edentulous mandible due to mobility of mandible	Complex cases Limited access due to limited opening or positioning of second molar	Most accurate, but less data than static-guided surgery, 0.4-mm deviation at entry, 4 degrees of angulation.

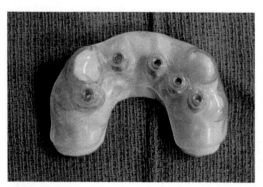

Fig. 1. Simple pilot-only guide.

Currently, the most popular types of guides combine dentition scans (obtained either conventionally or by scanning the dentition with an intraoral scanner) with the 3-D imaging. These guides usually have an opening to accept manufacturer-specific metal cylinders to control precise width (**Fig. 2**). It is also possible to obtain the pilot only guide to accommodate the pilot drill only. Regardless of which of these options was chosen, these guides provide information gathered from a patient-specific 3D radiograph. Currently, many dental implant companies have guided surgical kits that allow different sizes of cylinders to be inserted into the surgical guide with a specific goal of controlling the width and direction from the very first drill until the placement of the implant. Furthermore, the guided surgical kits also provide control of the vertical position as well as the depth of implant placement. The control of vertical depth and angulation of the implant are critical. Both factors are critical for successful implant-retained prosthesis, and also if any temporization is intended.

Cases requiring multiple dental implants with extractions and immediate temporization are the most complex implant procedures. The success of the immediate temporary is directly dependent on precise dental implant placement in the vertical and

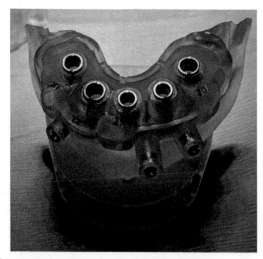

Fig. 2. Radiographic surgical guide to be used with guided kit.

horizontal planes and the quality of the initial impression. Although it is possible to free-hand these surgeries and then use trial and error to find appropriate multiunit abutments, the predictability of such an approach is quite limited.

WORKFLOW OF GUIDED IMPLANT SURGERY

The contemporary workflow for guided implant surgery (**Fig. 3**) incorporates new technology such as optical intraoral scanners, in-office CBCT, virtual implant planning software, and in-office 3D printers. Which of these advanced modalities the practitioner chooses to use will depend on the availability of equipment and experience level. At the time of the first consultation, the dentist should review pertinent medical history, indication, and risks of implant surgery. For complex cases, the practitioner should obtain impressions and CBCT of the patient in the desired occlusion. For straightforward cases with stable posterior occlusion, this can be achieved with patient registration material. Although not required, the dentist may choose to use radiopaque material in the missing tooth area to easier visualize future implant's relationship to the existing dentition. For situations when the patient has no posterior stable occlusion or is completely edentulous occlusal bite rims or duplicated complete denture is needed. This appliance should have radiographic markers embedded at the time of 3D CBCT and sent to the laboratory for mounting on an articulator. If the duplicated denture is not available, many simple prosthodontic techniques will allow fabrication of acceptable copy. On completion of the 3D CBCT, the dentist may choose to either fabricate the guide in-office using 3D printing technology or to outsource the entire

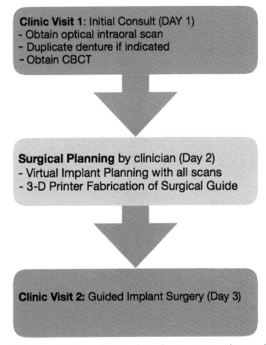

Clinic Visit 1: Initial Consult (DAY 1)
- Obtain optical intraoral scan
- Duplicate denture if indicated
- Obtain CBCT

Surgical Planning by clinician (Day 2)
- Virtual Implant Planning with all scans
- 3-D Printer Fabrication of Surgical Guide

Clinic Visit 2: Guided Implant Surgery (Day 3)

Fig. 3. Modern simplified workflow of guided implant surgery: the workflow incorporates in-office intraoral scanner, CBCT, and 3D printer into 2 clinical visits with minimal patient chair time and wait time between visits.

process. We have earlier described a protocol for surgical guide manufacturing.[8] The author prefers to obtain 3-D CBCT, impression, and plan the case virtually in the office. The fabrication of the guide is then outsourced to the outside laboratory. The second visit then is usually a surgical appointment using the fabricated guide. As discussed earlier, outsourcing the guide fabrication increases the lead time significantly but requires a less overall initial investment.

In contrast to this conventional method, in the past guides were fabricated in a multi-step process (**Fig. 4**).[9] After seeing the surgeon, the patient would have an "implant stent" fabricated by the restorative dentist. The general dentist then ideally would fabricate casts and radiopaque scanning appliance. The 3-D CBCT is then obtained with the radiographic stent in place. Casts and scans are then shared with the laboratory fabricating the guide so the laboratory may "clean up" the images and separate the teeth from bone and radiopaque scanning appliance. The "cleaned-up" image would then be reviewed by the surgeon to place the implants virtually. Finally, the completed work is shared with the laboratory, and fabrication of the guide commenced.

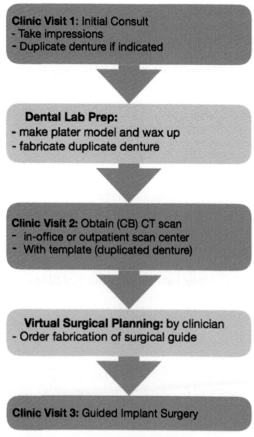

Fig. 4. Conventional workflow of guided implant surgery: does not incorporate intraoral scanner or in-office 3D printer, with optional in-office CBCT. More clinical visits and wait time to obtain CT scan and fabrication of surgical guide.

INTRAORAL SCANNERS AND BARIUM SULFATE TEMPLATE

As previously mentioned, CBCT and impressions are obtained at the initial consultation. Conventionally these impressions are poured in stone to be sent to the laboratory fabricating the final guide. If the impressions are taken in stable material, they can also be scanned directly by the laboratory. Alternatively, the practitioner may choose to use an intraoral scanner to capture the patient's dentition. A large number of scanners exist on the market, and they provide incredible benefits when compared with conventional impression techniques.[8] Image file obtained by scanners can be directly overplayed onto CBCT in separate layers for easy manipulation.[10]

When preparing for virtual implant placement, there is a need to visualize the arch in question, the opposing dentition, and the radiographic scanning appliance. Barium sulfate is a material commonly used in gastrointestinal imaging that provides excellent visualization. When used for duplicating dentures, a concentration of less than 20% will not cause noticeable scatter.[11] Another advantage of this material is that when incorporated into regular acrylic, it will not cause significant shrinkage and, therefore, will not alter denture dimensions. Once 3D CBCT with the barium sulfate duplicated denture is obtained, the images of the patient's alveolar ridge and the denture can be separated virtually for implant planning. When barium sulfate is not available, radiopaque markers can be added manually onto duplicated denture or bite rims. For this method to be successful, a minimum of 8 commercially available markers is needed.[12]

COMPUTED TOMOGRAPHY

CT scan technology is broadly classified as medical-grade (or helical) and cone-beam type.[8] Medical-grade CTs are unmatched in their precision and accuracy in maxillofacial trauma.[13] However, these studies have always been limited in outpatient dental implant surgery due to high cost, limited availability, and increased radiation. CBCT, on the other hand, has a small footprint, is comparatively inexpensive, and is widely available. The availability of 3D CBCT technology has directly increased the number of guided implant surgery cases performed.

CT data is obtained as digital imaging and communications in medicine (DICOM) files. Images are reconstructed into 4 views for proper surgical planning: cross-sectional, axial, panoramic, and 3D reconstruction (**Figs. 5–7**). Most software will initially generate axial and sagittal views. The panoramic view (automatically or manually) is then obtained from these 2 views. Many types of software provide "clean up" and scatter removal tools to provide a 3D reconstruction as an accurate volumetric representation. **Fig. 8** provides a summary of views.

VIRTUAL IMPLANT PLANNING SOFTWARE

CT capture and implant software have improved tremendously over the past decade. Notably, there is significantly less scatter in contemporary software, and hence less post-processing is required after the acquisition. A variety of virtual implant planning software currently exists on the market. Some of the software comes prepackaged with the cone-beam units, while other software must be purchased separately. Options within the software also vary significantly, as some manufacturers provide a complete suite of acquisition, interpretation, and planning, whereas others require add-ons.[14] At the minimum, the software should be able to read open DICOM files and allow for the identification of important anatomic structures. The more advanced capability of implant planning and specific fixture selection is often needed. **Fig. 9**

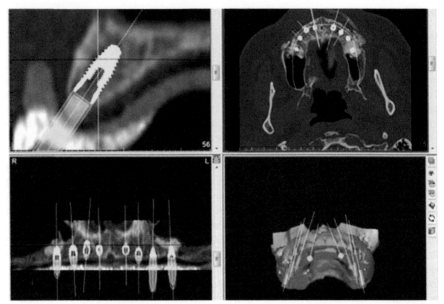

Fig. 5. Virtual implant planning: showing 4 views (cross-sectional, axial, panoramic, and 3D reconstruction). Planned for 8 maxillary implants with restorative spaces shown and barium sulfate denture template in place.

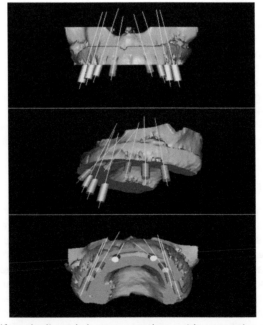

Fig. 6. Barium sulfate duplicated denture template: with restorative spaces of planned dental implants in 3D reconstruction views.

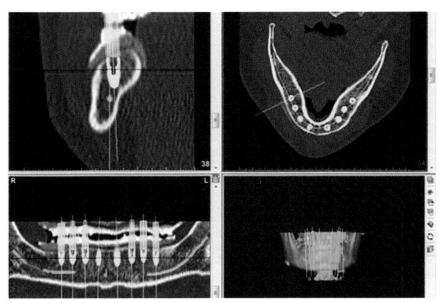

Fig. 7. Virtual implant planning: 8 mandibular implants with inferior alveolar nerve appreciated in panoramic and cross-sectional views.

shows a virtual surgical plan with specific angled implant placement. Virtual abutments can also be planned to aid in the final crown retention method.

Guided surgery is particularly important in cases planned for immediate temporization. These cases require precise final angulation, or the temporary will not fit. **Fig. 10** shows a postoperative radiograph after the placement of multiple implants using the guided technique. Guided surgery is also preferred for cases that require only axial

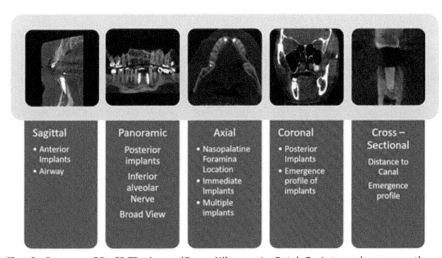

Fig. 8. Common 3D CBCT views. (*From* Nikoyan L, Patel R. Intraoral scanner, three-dimensional imaging, and three-dimensional printing in the dental office. Dent Clin North Am. 2020;64(2):366; with permission.)

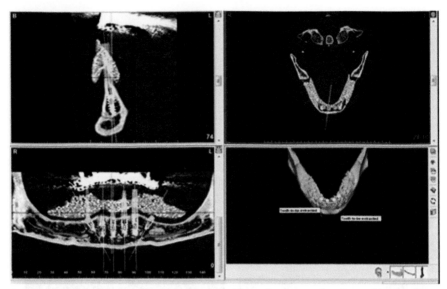

Fig. 9. Mandibular implant planning of 6 mandibular implants. The panoramic view shows angled implant placement at 45° and angled system specific multiunit abutments.

parallelism. There are other useful features of modern 3D CBCT software. These include calculation of vertical restorative space and determination of the quality of the bone among some.[15]

SELECTION AND FABRICATION OF IMPLANT SURGICAL GUIDE

The surgeon should decide if a guide is advantageous at the first consultation visit. As mentioned previously, guided surgery has many benefits over free-handed implant surgery. Even more precise are guides used in conjunction with navigation. Recently navigation implant surgery is extremely accurate with a deviation of only 0.4 mm.[16] If the surgeon wishes to use navigation during surgery, he or she must understand the inherent significant costs associated with this technology.[17,18]

Once the decision to use a guide has been made, there are several important considerations. The surgeon must evaluate the patient and decide how this guide shall be supported. If teeth are present, then the goal should be to use remaining teeth as

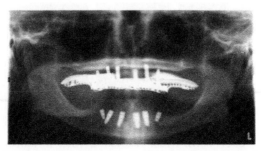

Fig. 10. Postoperative radiograph after placement of multiple implants using the guided technique.

support and fabricate tooth-supported guides. These are not only more precise but require less surgical exposure.[18] If no teeth are present or no support can be expected from the remaining teeth, then a bone-supported guide can be fabricated. These will require significantly larger surgical exposure and need fixation to the existing bone structure to be precise. The mucosa-supported guides are the least-desirable type of guides. Although these guides promise less invasive procedures, they are often not stable enough for predictable surgery. Generally, guides will either provide for progressively larger sleeves or entirely different units for each osteotomy. Some guide designs will also allow for an irrigation window to better cool the surgical site.

When the surgeon completes the planning phase and chooses the preferred type of guide, the fabrication is ready to commence. There are 3 main options for guide fabrication: dental laboratory, dental laboratory attached to a software company, and in-office/desktop stereolithographic 3D printers. Local dental laboratories can offer multiple benefits such as faster turnaround times and real-time hands-on help. Larger national laboratories generally have more experience but will require longer lead times. Laboratories that are attached to proprietary software offer the convenience of guide ordering directly within the software. These laboratories may be especially beneficial for surgeons who prefer to plan their implants themselves. Some offices may opt to fabricate the guides on their premises. After the initial expense of 3D printers, the cost per guide is significantly less when compared with the dental laboratory–made guides.[19–21] The accuracy of in-house guides increases with the surgeon's experience.[22] When in-office printed guides are used, the patient directly benefits not only from increased accuracy but decreased wait time for the implant surgery.

COMPLICATIONS OF GUIDED IMPLANT SURGERY
Sources of Error During Initial Visit

Many sources of complications must be considered when using CT-guided surgery. It is the responsibility of the surgeon to understand the possible source of errors and be prepared to make adjustments to maintain a successful implant surgery.[23] During the initial consultation, the errors can come from impressions, denture duplications, and inaccuracies of the cone-beam scan. Commonly missed error is added when the patient's bite is not registered appropriately. This inaccurate position is then used in the cone beam machine. The result will often lead to inaccurate restorative space and a nonfitting guide. In cases when denture duplication overlay is required or when stone models are scanned by the cone-beam machine, multiple 3D CBCTs will be performed. In these scenarios, to limit calibration errors, the acquisition setting should be the same.

INHERENT ERROR OF COMPUTED TOMOGRAPHY SCANS AND SURGICAL GUIDES

The surgeon should always remember that all CBCT scanners have inherent errors.[24] Although mostly very small, some of these errors can add to 0.6 mm.[25] It is critical to consider these errors when operating near vital anatomic structures. For example, if a guide is designed to avoid the maxillary sinus, it is a good practice to consider that the burr can be 1.0 mm closer than planned originally. There is also an error in the guide manufacturing process. The initial pilot burrs are usually 2.0 mm, but the cylinder or the sleeve cannot be exactly 2 mm because the burr would never fit. These access cylinders are at least 0.2 to 0.5 mm larger, and this is an additive error.[26,27]

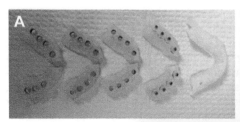
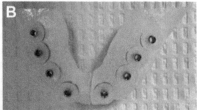
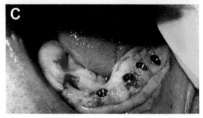

Fig. 11. (*A*) Bone-supported surgical guides with stereolithic bone model. (*B*) Bone-supported guides modified preoperative to account for change in surgical plan to quadrant implant placement while marinating guide stability. (*C*) Postoperative implant placement of lower left quadrant.

PERIOPERATIVE COMPLICATIONS AND CONSIDERATIONS

To have a predictable and safe guided surgery, it is imperative to understand possible surgical complications that can be encountered. The surgeon should review the plan ahead of the surgery and be familiar with the overall procedure. Surgical stents and drilling depth should be carefully reviewed to ensure accuracy with no manufacturing errors. If stereolithic models are provided by the laboratory, these can be compared with the current patient situation. If differences are noted then, adjustments to the guide can be made at this time. Adjustment to the existing guide should be made minimally to avoid introducing fitting errors. In some instances, it may be possible to split the guide into smaller guides that will fit and still provide precise osteotomy (**Fig. 11**).

Some errors just cannot be corrected. If the guide continues not to fit even after significant adjustment, it probably will not be of any surgical use. Guides are usually produced for a specific surgical system and are not interchangeable. Last, if the guide on the stereolithic model is vastly different from the virtual plan, then it should not be used. When faced with a nonfitting guide or improper guide, the surgeon must decide whether to abort the procedure or continue without the guide. It is imperative that the surgeon is familiar with the procedure and can effectively complete it without a guide.

SUMMARY

CT-guided implant surgery offers many benefits compared with free-handed surgery. Cost and access to specialized technology was always a barrier to the mainstream use of guides in dentistry. The recent decrease in the cost of 3D image acquisition and interpretation has paved the way for the increase in guided surgery utilization. The fabrication technology has also improved, further driving the cost down. Performing implant surgery with the help of guides is now widely taught and accepted throughout the dental implant fields. As this technology pushes the limits of implant dentistry, it should, however, be viewed with caution. Practitioners that were not comfortable performing implant surgery before suddenly find themselves lured by apparent ease and predictability of the procedure. Complications happen even when guides are used, and the surgeon must anticipate and be capable of correcting them.

CLINICS CARE POINTS

- Guided implant surgery is more accurate and precise than free-handed implant surgery.
- Possible complications of CT-guided implant surgery include wax-up, radiographic tem- plate, the accuracy of CT scan, the accuracy of surgical guides, and the overheating of bone.
- CT-guided implant surgery has become a mainstay in successful implant surgery, with in- office cone-beam CT, intraoral scanners, and 3D-printers reducing clinical visits and maintain accuracy.

DISCLOSURE

The authors have nothing to disclose.

REFERENCES

1. Carter JB, Stone JD, Clark RS, et al. Applications of cone-beam computed tomography in oral and maxillofacial surgery: an overview of published indications and clinical usage in United States academic centers and oral and maxillofacial surgery practices. J Oral Maxillofac Surg 2016;74(4):668–79.
2. Mora MA, Chenin DL, Arce RM. Software tools and surgical guides in dental-implant-guided surgery. Dent Clin North Am 2014;58:597626.
3. Schneider D, Marquardt P, Zwahlen M, et al. A systematic review on the accuracy and the clinical outcome of computer-guided template-based implant dentistry. Clin Oral Implants Res 2009;20(Suppl 4):73–86.
4. Scherer U, Stoetzer M, Ruecker M, et al. Template-guided vs. non-guided drilling in site preparation of dental implants. Clin Oral Investig 2015;19(6):1339–46.
5. Block MS, Emery RW, Cullum DR, et al. Implant placement is more accurate using dynamic navigation. J Oral Maxillofac Surg 2017;75:1377–86.
6. Jung RE, Schneider D, Ganeles J, et al. Computer technology applications in surgical implant dentistry: A systemic review. Int J Oral Maxillofac Implants 2009; 24(suppl):92–109.
7. Block MS, Emery RW. Static or dynamic navigation for implant placement—choosing the method of guidance. J Oral Maxillofac Surg 2016;74:269–77.
8. Nikoyan L, Patel R. Intraoral scanner, three-dimensional imaging, and three-dimensional printing in the dental office. Dent Clin North Am 2020;64(2):365–78.
9. Flugge TV, Nelson K, Schmelzeisen R, et al. Three-dimensional plotting and printing of an implant drilling guide: simplifying guided implant surgery. J Oral Maxillofac Surg 2013;71:1340–6.
10. Mangano F, Gandolfi A, Luongo G, et al. Intraoral scanners in dentistry: a review of the current literature. BMC Oral Health 2017;17:149.
11. Basten CH, Kois JC. The use of barium sulfate for implant templates. J Prosthet Dent 1996;76(4):451–4.
12. Zahran MH, Fenton A. A radiopaque implant template for partially edentulous patients. J Prosthet Dent 2010;103:390–2.
13. Steinbacher DM. Three-dimensional analysis and surgical planning in craniomaxillofacial surgery. J Oral Maxillofac Surg 2015;73:S40–56.

14. Vannier MW, Marsh JL. Three-dimensional imaging, surgical planning, and image-guided therapy. Radiol Clin North Am 1996;34:545.
15. Ganz SD. Three-dimensional imaging and guided surgery for dental implants. Dent Clin North Am 2015;59:265–90.
16. Nardy C, Wexler A, Persky N, et al. Navigation surgery for dental implants: assessment of accuracy of the image guided implantology system. J Oral Maxillofac Surg 2004;62:116–9.
17. Farley NE, Kennedy K, McGlumphy EA, et al. Split-mouth comparison of the accuracy of computer-generated and conventional surgical guides. Int J Oral Maxillofac Implants 2013;28:563–72.
18. Widmann G, Bale RJ. Accuracy in computer-aided implant surgery—a review. Int J Oral Maxillofac Implants 2006;21:305.
19. Deeb GR, Allen RK, Hall VP, et al. How accurate are implant surgical guides produced with desktop stereolithographic 3-dimensional printers? J Oral Maxillofac Surg 2017;75:2559.e1-e8.
20. Lal K, White G, Morea D, et al. Use of stereolithographic templates for surgical and prosthodontic implant planning and placement. Part I. The concept. J Prosthodont 2006;15:51.
21. Ozan O, Turkyilmaz I, Ersoy AE, et al. Clinical accuracy of 3 different types of computed tomography-derived stereolitho- graphic surgical guides in implant placement. J Oral Maxillofac Surg 2009;67:394.
22. Vercruyssen M, Cox C, Coucke W, et al. A randomized clinical trial comparing guided implant surgery (bone- or mucosa-supported) with mental navigation or the use of a pilot-drill template. J Clin Periodontol 2014;41:717–23.
23. Block MS, Chandler C. Computed tomography–guided surgery: complications associated with scanning, processing, surgery, and prosthetics. J Oral Maxillofac Surg 2009;67:13–22.
24. Kobayashi K, Shimoda S, Nakagawa Y, et al. Accuracy in measurement of distance using limited cone-beam computed tomography. Int J Oral Maxillofac Implants 2004;19:228.
25. Hiroyuki T, Eiichi H, Tooru K, et al. Study of clinical validity on helical CT and limited cone-beam CT (3DX CT) for tooth length measurement. J Orthod Waves 2004;63:78.
26. Van Assche N, Van Steenberghe D, Guerrero ME, et al. Accuracy of implant placement based on pre-surgical planning of three-dimensional cone-beam images: a pilot study. J Clin Periodontol 2007;34:816.
27. Scarano A, Carinci F, Quaranta A, et al. Effects of bur wear during implant site preparation: an in vitro study. Int J Immunopathol Pharmacol 2007;20:23.

Implant Material Sciences

Allen Glied, DDS[a],*, Junaid Mundiya, DMD[b]

KEYWORDS

- Alloy • Dental implant • Titanium • Zirconium • Metal

KEY POINTS

- While selecting a dental implant, the microstructure of the implant, its surface composition, characteristics, design, toughness, strength, corrosion, wear, and fracture resistance should be considered.
- Current dental implant used are Titanium- Zirconium Alloy, Zirconia, Titanium, Titanium Alloy, Aluminum, Titanium, Zirconium oxides, Ceramic, Metal alloys, Cobalt, chromium alloy, and Iron chromium nickel-based alloy.
- Features of dental implants are shape, threads, surface texture, length, and diameter.

INTRODUCTION

In the past, the only way to replace missing teeth was to have a removable appliance. However, these days, dental implants are commonly being used to replace missing teeth. The dental implants are improving as a result of new technological and scientific advances.[1]

Different materials have been used in the past for dental implants such as lead, stainless steel, and gold. Currently, the focus is on using Roxolid, surface-modified titanium implants, and zirconia. These materials have superior esthetic and functional characteristics for dental implants.[2]

Many factors come into play when selecting a dental implant: the microstructure of the implant, its surface composition, characteristics, design factor, toughness, strength, corrosion, wear, and fracture resistance.[3]

HISTORY

Dental implants can be traced back to the 1800s. In the early 1800s, Maggiolo used gold in the shape of a tooth root. Then toward the turn of the century, Harris used teeth made out of porcelain. The post of these teeth was coated with lead-coated platinum. Zemenski then used porcelain, gutta-percha, and rubber as implantation techniques.

In the early 1900s, Lambotte implants were fabricated using aluminum, brass, copper, gold, magnesium, and soft steel plated with gold and nickel. Then in

[a] Department of Dentistry, St. Barnabas Hospital, 4422 Third Avenue, Bronx, NY 10457, USA;
[b] Department of Oral and Maxillofacial Surgery, The Brooklyn Hospital Center, 121 Dekalb Avenue, Brooklyn, NY 11201, USA
* Corresponding author.
E-mail address: allenglied@gmail.com

Dent Clin N Am 65 (2021) 81–88
https://doi.org/10.1016/j.cden.2020.09.006
0011-8532/21/© 2020 Elsevier Inc. All rights reserved.

Pennsylvania, Sholl used porcelain teeth implant having a corrugated porcelain root. The concept of submerged implant and healing tissue and dental implant immobility was introduced by E.J. Greenfield. The modern era encompasses using synthetic polymers, metal alloys, and ceramic for dental implants.[4]

DEFINITION

There are few properties of material science that need a review to understand the material sciences of dental implants.[5]

An implant should have a high compressive and tensile strength to improve its functional stability and to prevent fractures. When an implant is able to transfer stress from the implant to bone it is reported as interfacial shear strength. This causes low stresses on the implant. During cyclic loading, the implant can have brittle fractures. Therefore, there should be high yield strength and fatigue strength. The modulus of elasticity of bone is 18 GPa. Therefore, the goal is to have an implant material that has a comparable modulus of elasticity. This will cause a more uniform distribution of stress at implant and minimize the relative movement at the implant-bone interface. The ductility of the dental implant is necessary for contouring and shaping of the implant. The ADA recommends a minimum ductility of 8%. Increasing the toughness of an implant prevents fracture of the implant. Increasing the hardness of the implant decreases the incidence of wear of implant material.[5]

Implant surfaces influence its response to tissue and cells. By increasing the surface area of an implant, it improves cell attachment to the bone. Implant surface has been divided into surface roughness as minimally rough (0.5–1 m), intermediately rough (1–2 m), and rough (2–3 m). The texture of implants can vary as well, such as concave or convex. The concave texture is by being treated with hydroxyapatite coating and titanium plasma spraying. The convex texture is treating the implant surface by subtractive treatment such as etching and blasting. Furthermore, the implant surface is classified based on the orientation of surface irregularities such as anisotropic and isotropic surface irregularity. Anisotropic surfaces have clear directionality and vary considerably in roughness. Isotropic surface irregularity has similar topography independent of measuring direction.[6]

Any implant material should show favorable biocompatibility. Materials are defined by their corrosion property to be biocompatible. Corrosion can result in the weakening of the restoration, roughening its surface, or releasing elements from the alloy or metal. Corrosion can be attributed to electrochemical, galvanic, pitting, or crevice reaction. Electrochemical corrosion can be defined as anodic oxidation and cathodic reduction resulting in metal deterioration and charge transfer. This reaction occurs due to electrons, and it can be prevented by the presence of a passive oxide layer on the metal surface. Galvanic corrosion reaction is due to the difference in electrical gradients. If there is leakage of saliva between implant and superstructure such as abutment or crown, it can lead to nickel or chrome ions to pass to periimplant tissue. Galvanic corrosion can lead to bone reabsorption. This bone loss will eventually lead to loss of implant stability and will lead to a failure of the implant. Pitting corrosion is when the metal ions from the implant combine with chloride ions. Pitting corrosion is due to small surface pits of an implant. The formation of these surface pits leads to roughening of implant surfaces. Crevice corrosion is due to metallic ions creating a positive charge environment when they dissolve. This usually occurs at narrow interfaces such as implant screw and bone interfaces.[7–9]

DISCUSSION

This section focuses on introducing different implant materials used currently and then looking back on what was used in the past.

Titanium-Zirconium Alloy

Titanium-zirconium alloy has better fatigue strength and increased elongation compared with pure titanium. Monophasic structures of titanium-zirconium alloy are sandblasted and acid-etched for it to be topographically identical to the pure titanium implant. Because titanium-zirconium alloy has better mechanical properties and good biocompatibility, it can be used for thin implants and implant components that can be subjected to high strains. This leads to the growth of osteoblasts, which are essential for osseointegration. Titanium-zirconium alloy is used by Straumann Roxolid implant, and it has 50% stronger than pure titanium.[10]

Zirconia

Ceramic implants were introduced as an alternative to titanium implants due to their properties of less plaque build-up, aesthetic consideration, and it being kind to soft tissue.[11] Zirconia structures are characterized in 3 crystal forms: monoclinic, cubic, and tetragonal. At room temperature, Zirconia is in its monoclinic structure and changes into the tetragonal structure at 1170 C. This structure changes into a cubic phase at 2370 C. As these structures are called, they are unstable and break into pieces. The cubic phase of Zirconia is stabilized by adding CaO, MgO, and Y2O3 (Yttrium). This structure is called partially stabilized zirconia combining monoclinic, cubic, and tetragonal phases in order of importance. The tetragonal zirconia polycrystals only contain the tetragonal phase. This phase is obtained by adding Y2O3 (Yttrium) at room temperature. The properties that make tetragonal zirconia polycrystal a suitable biomedical material are low porosity, high bending, high density, and compression strength.[12]

Titanium

Titanium is most commonly used for dental implants. Titanium is biocompatible due to the formation of a stable oxide layer on its surface. Pure commercial titanium is classified into 4 different grades based on their oxygen content. Grade 1 has the least oxygen content (0.18%) and grade 4 has the most (0.4%). Different materials are added to commercially pure titanium to further enhance its properties. Vanadium is added due to its ability to act as an aluminum scavenger to prevent corrosion. Aluminum is added to increase strength and decrease density. Iron is added for corrosion resistance. Titanium is a dimorphic metal. It exists as a hexagonal closed packed crystal lattice, alpha-phase less than 883 C. When higher than 883 C, it transforms into a body-centered cubic lattice, beta-phase. Titanium is the material of choice for dental implants due to its high passivity, rapid formation, controlled thickness, resistance to chemical attack, catalytic activity for several chemical reactions, and modulus of elasticity compatible with bone. The major disadvantage of titanium is its color. The gray color titanium is not esthetically appealing when soft tissue is not optimal or if there is thin mucosa.[13–17]

Titanium Alloys

Titanium alloy exists in alpha, beta, and alpha-beta forms. When titanium is heated and combined with either element such as Al and Va and then cooled it results in titanium alloy. Alpha-phase titanium is combined with aluminum as a stabilizer. This results in increased strength and decreased weight of the titanium-aluminum alloy. The beta-phase is combined with vanadium as a stabilizer. The alpha to beta transformation occurs at a range of temperatures as Al or Va is added to titanium. The alloys most commonly used for dental implants are the 6% Al and 4% Va alpha-beta variety.[18]

Aluminum, Titanium, Zirconium Oxides

High ceramics from aluminum, titanium, and zirconium oxides are used to form endosteal plate, root form, and pin type dental implants. These alloy oxides have a high modulus of elasticity, compressive, tensile, and bending strength greater than compact bone. This results in specialized design requirements for this class of biomaterial.[6]

Ceramic

Ceramic is rarely used as a surgical implant due to low ductility and brittleness. However, it does have positive properties such as good strength, inert behavior, and minimum thermal and electrical conductivity. The use of ceramic is limited to implant dentistry.[19]

Metal Alloys

Metals such as gold, stainless steel, cobalt-chromium biomechanical properties made them an implant material of choice. These metals have a good finish, they are easy to process, and are able to be sterilized. These metals are still used in prosthetic components of implants for superstructures, bars, and crowns. However, the success and advancement of titanium-based implants and alloy have made them obsolete.[19]

Cobalt-Chromium Alloy

Cobalt, chromium, and molybdenum are the major elements in the composition of this alloy. Cobalt provides a continuous phase for basic properties. Chromium provides corrosion resistance. Molybdenum provides strength and bulk corrosion resistance. The ductility of this alloy is enhanced by controlling the carbon and nickel biocorrosion products. The alloy can be used to manufacture customized subperiosteal implant frames.[20,21]

Iron-Chromium Nickel-Based Alloy

Iron-based alloys were used in ramus blade, stabilizer pin, and mucosal inserts. These implants are not commonly used anymore. If a patient is allergic to any of the material, the use of this implant is not advised. This alloy has a high galvanic potential and corrosion resistance. It is also prone to pitting corrosion. If titanium, cobalt, zirconium, or carbon implant are used in combination with iron chromium-nickel alloy, it can lead to galvanic coupling and biocorrosion.[6]

FEATURES OF DENTAL IMPLANTS
Shape

Dental implants are commonly available in tapered or parallel types. The tapered type of dental implants is known to have better primary stability compared with a parallel type.[22] The increase in primary stability of tapered implants is due to their lateral compression of the bone and increased stiffness of the interfacial bone.[23] Tapered implants can be used in softer bones such as posterior maxilla for greater stability. They are helpful in avoiding damaging roots of adjacent teeth that may be in close proximity to a site of interest.[24] Tapered implants require a higher insertion torque compared with parallel implants.[25] Both parallel and tapered implants can be used for immediate or delayed implant placement; however, because of higher primary stability of tapered implants, they are preferred.[24,26]

Threads of Implant

There are 3 different types of thread implants that are commonly used in implant dentistry. These are V-shaped, reverse buttress, and square-shaped.[27,28] Studies have shown that the square thread design of a dental implant shows more bone to implant contact and greater reverse torque measurement compared with reserve buttress and V-shaped thread.[29]

The threads of dental implants can be further characterized by pretaping and self-tapping implants. Pretapping implants have lower primary stability compared with self-taping implants.

The osteotomy for pretaping implants needs to be prepared using a tapered drill. These threads prepared from the taping drills are used to accommodate the pretaper implants. Pretapping implants are recommended for dense bones such as anterior and posterior mandible. Self-tapping implants make their own threads into the osteotomy site as they are being inserted at desired locations. Self-tapping implants can be used for the anterior and posterior maxilla.[30,31]

Surface Texture

The surface texture of dental implants can either be smooth or rough. Rough-surfaced implants have a larger surface area compared with smooth surface implants. As the surface area increases it encourages bone healing and periimplant soft tissue.[32] The greater the surface area the greater distribution of forces to which implant is exposed. Rough surface implants also have higher primary stability compared with smooth surface implants.[33] Research also shows that rough dental implants have greater bone apposition[34] and higher removal torque values.[35] The implant surface is roughened by either blasting or acid etching or adding biocompatible material such as hydroxyapatite.[35–37] If rough dental implants are exposed to the oral cavity, they have a tendency to accumulate plaque and bacteria, leading to periimplantitis.[38]

Implant Length

The length of a dental implant is governed by the bone available, adjacent anatomic structures, width, and quality of bone. Generally speaking, the longer the implant the greater the surface contact hence higher primary stability. This is not a linear relationship. For example, a 10 mm implant has 30% more surface area compared with a 7-mm implant, whereas, a 13-mm implant only has 20% more surface area compared with a 10 mm implant.[39] There has been a movement to use shorter implants if there is a limit in available bony or proximity of vital structures such as maxillary sinus or neurovascular bundle. Research shows the survival rate after 2 years for 5-mm implants is 93.1% compared with 9.5 mm implants at 98.6%.[40] Therefore, shorter implants may fail in 4 to 6 years compared with standard implants that may fail in 6 to 8 years.[41]

Implant Diameter

When choosing a dental implant to replace a tooth, the diameter of implants plays a major role in its success and implants the ability to withstand the occlusal load.[42] As an increase in length is associated with the increased surface, the same goes for implant diameter. Increasing the diameter in a 3-mm implant by 1 mm increases the surface area by 35% over the same length.[43] As the surface area of the implant increases, it lessens the stress to the crestal bone area and reduces both crestal bone loss and early loading implant failure.[43] In instances where there is not enough bone, and augmentation is not possible, short and wide implants can be used. They can also be used when the bone bed is not optimal.[44] Wide implants are used to increase the stability of the implant and improve stress distribution.[41,45] Wide implants are also used in immediate implant placement after tooth extraction.[46]

SUMMARY

Implant dentistry is the current phase of dentistry. With advances in technology, biomedical science, surgical technique, and success rate implant, dentistry is a hot topic. However, implant material science is not talked about as often as it should. The study of material science along with biomechanical sciences will provide optimization of design and material concepts for surgical implants.[47]

CLINICS CARE POINTS

- Dental Implants should have high compressive and tensile strength to improve its functional stability and prevent fractures.
- Increasing implant surface area, will improve cell attachment to the bone.
- Titanium-zirconium alloy has better mechanical properties and good biocompatibility. It is used for thin implants, and implant components.
- Diameter of Implant plays a role it its success. A wider implant will increase its ability to withstand occlusal load.

DISCLOSURE

The authors have nothing to disclose.

REFERENCES

1. Hulbert SF, Bennett JT. State of the art in dental implants. J Dent Res 1975; 54(Spec No B):B153–7.
2. Saini M, Singh Y, Arora P, et al. Implant biomaterials: A comprehensive review. World J Clin Cases 2015;3(1):52–7.
3. Parr GR, Gardner LK, Toth RW. Titanium: The mystery metal of implant dentistry. Dental materials aspect. J Prosthet Dent 1985;54:410–4.
4. Block MS, Kent JN, Guerra LR. Implants in dentistry. Philadelphia: W.B. Saunders company; 1997. p. 4.
5. Muddugangadhar BC, Amarnath GS, Tripathi S, et al. Biomaterials for Dental Implants: An Overview. Int J Oral Implantol Clin Res 2011;2:13–24.
6. Wennerberg A, Albrektsson T. On implant surfaces: a review of current knowledge and opinions. Int J Oral Maxillofac Implants 2010;25:63–74.
7. Manivasagam G, Dhinasekaran D, Rajamanickam A. Biomedical implants: corrosion and its prevention - A Review. Recent Patents on Corrosion Science. vol. 2. Bentham Open; 2010. p. 40–54.
8. Adya N, Alam M, Ravindranath T, et al. Corrosion in titanium dental implants: literature review. J Indian Prosthodont Soc 2005;5:126–31.
9. Chaturvedi TP. An overview of the corrosion aspect of dental implants (titanium and its alloys). Indian J Dent Res 2009;20:91–8.
10. Chiapasco M, Casentini P, Zaniboni M, et al. Titanium-zirconium alloy narrow-diameter implants (Straumann Roxolid(®)) for the rehabilitation of horizontally deficient edentulous ridges: prospective study on 18 consecutive patients. Clin Oral Implants Res 2012;23:1136–41.
11. Özkurt Z, Kazazoğlu E. Zirconia dental implants: a literature review. J Oral Implantol 2011;37:367–76.

12. Adatia ND, Bayne SC, Cooper LF, et al. Fracture resistance of yttria-stabilized zirconia dental implant abutments. J Prosthodont 2009;18:17–22.
13. Cranin AN, Silverbrand H, Sher J, et al. The requirements and clinical performance of dental implants. In, Smith DC, Williams DF, editors. Biocompatibility of dental materials. vol. 4. Bona Raton: CRC Press; 1982. p. 197-229.
14. Tschernitschek H, Borchers L, Geurtsen W. Nonalloyed titanium as a bioinert metal–a review. Quintessence Int 2005;36:523–30.
15. Wennerberg A, Albrektsson T, Andersson B. Bone tissue response to commercially pure titanium implants blasted with fine and coarse particles of aluminum oxide. Int J Oral Maxillofac Implants 1996;11:38–45.
16. Meffert RM, Langer B, Fritz ME. Dental implants: a review. J Periodontol 1992;63: 859–70.
17. Williams DF. Implants in dental and maxillofacial surgery. Biomaterials 1981;2: 133–46.
18. Ravnholt G. Corrosion current and pH rise around titanium coupled to dental alloys. Scand J Dent Res 1988;96:466–72.
19. Sykaras N, Iacopino AM, Marker VA, et al. Implant materials, designs, and surface topographies: their effect on osseointegration. A literature review. Int J Oral Maxillofac Implants 2000;15:675–90.
20. Arvidson K, Cottler-Fox M, Hammarlund E, et al. Cytotoxic effects of cobalt-chromium alloys on fibroblasts derived from human gingiva. Scand J Dent Res 1987;95:356–63.
21. Phillips RW. Skinner's science of dental materials. 8th edition. Philadelphia: WB Saunders; 1982.
22. Romanos GE, Basha-Hijazi A, Gupta B, et al. Role of clinician's experience and implant design on implant stability. An ex vivo study in artificial soft bones. Clin Implant Dent Relat Res 2014;16:166–71.
23. Sennerby L, Ericson LE, Thomsen P, et al. Structure of the bone-titanium interface in retrieved clinical oral implants. Clin Oral Implants Res 1991;2:103–11.
24. Alves CC, Neves M. Tapered implants: from indications to advantages. J Periodont Rest Dent 2009;29:161–7.
25. Menicucci G, Pachie E, Lorenzetti M, et al. Comparison of primary stability of straight-walled and tapered implants using an insertion torque device. Int J Prosthodont 2012;25:465–71.
26. Jacobs SH, O'Connell BC. Dental implant restoration: principles and procedures. 1st edition. New Malden (United Kingdom): Quintessence Publishing; 2001.
27. Misch CE. Contemporary implant dentistry. 2nd edition. St Louis (MO): Elsevier; 2008.
28. Warreth A, McAleese E, McDonnell P, et al. Dental implants and single implant-supported restorations. J Ir Dent Assoc 2013;59:32–43.
29. Steigenga J, Al-Shammari K, Misch C, et al. Effects of implant thread geometry on percentage of osseointegration and resistance to reverse torque in the tibia of rabbits. J Periodontol 2004;75:1233–41.
30. Rabel A, Köhler SG, Schmidt-Westhausen AM. Clinical study on the primary stability of two dental implant systems with resonance frequency analysis. Clin Oral Investig 2007;11:257–65.
31. Yoon HG, Heo SJ, Koak JY, et al. Effect of bone quality and implant surgical technique on implant stability quotient (ISQ) value. J Adv Prosthodont 2011;3:10–5.
32. Cochran DL. A comparison of endosseous dental implant surfaces. J Periodontol 1999;70:1523–39.

33. Oue H, Doi K, Oki Y, et al. Influence of implant surface topography on primary stability in a standardized osteoporosis rabbit model study. J Funct Biomater 2015;6:143–52.
34. Novaes AB Jr, Souza SL, de Oliveria PT, et al. Histomorphometric analysis of the bone-implant contact obtained with 4 different implant surface treatments placed side by side in the dog mandible. Int J Oral Maxillofac Implants 2002;17:377–83.
35. Klokkevold PR, Johnson P, Dadgostari S, et al. Early endosseous integration enhanced by dual acid etching of titanium: a torque removal study in the rabbit femur. Clin Oral Implants Res 2001;12:350–7.
36. Wong M, Eulenberger J, Schenk R, et al. Effects of surface topology on the osseointegration of implant in trabecular bone. J Biomed Mater Res 1995;29: 1567–75.
37. Le Guehennec L, Goyenvalle E, LopezHeredia MA, et al. Histomorphometric analysis of the osseointegration of four different implant surfaces in the femoral epiphyses of rabbits. Clin Oral Implants Res 2008;19:1103–10.
38. Renvert S, Roos-Jansåker AM, Claffey N. Nonsurgical treatment of peri-implant mucositis and peri-implantitis: a literature review. J Clin Periodontol 2008;35(8 Suppl):305–15.
39. Misch CE. Short dental implants: a literature review and rationale for use. Dent Today 2005;24:64–8.
40. Jokstad A. The evidence for endorsing the use of short dental implants remains inconclusive. Evid Based Dent 2011;12:99–101.
41. Monje A, Chan HL, Fu JH, et al. Are short dental implants (<10 mm) effective? A meta-analysis on prospective clinical trials. J Periodontol 2013;84:895–904.
42. Allum SR, Tomlinson RA, Joshi R. The impact of loads on standard diameter, small diameter and mini implants: a comparative laboratory study. Clin Oral Implants Res 2008;19:553–9.
43. Misch CE, Qu M, Bidez MW. Mechanical properties of trabecular bone in the human mandible: implications for dental implant treatment planning and surgical placement. J Oral Maxillofac Surg 1999;57:700–6.
44. Renouard F, Nisand D. Impact of implant length and diameter on survival rates. Clin Oral Implants Res 2006;17(Suppl 2):35–51.
45. Ivanoff CJ, Sennerby L, Johansson C, et al. Influence of implant diameters on the integration of screw implants. An experimental study in rabbits. Int J Oral Maxillofac Surg 1997;26:141–8.
46. Langer B, Langer L, Herrmann I, et al. The wide fixture: a solution for special bone situations and a rescue for the compromised implant. Part 1. Int J Oral Maxillofac Implants 1993;8(4):400–8.
47. Smith DC. Dental implants: materials and design considerations. Int J Prosthodont 1993;6:106–17.

Immediate Implants

Raymond Fan, DDS[a,b,*], Harvey A. Quinton, DDS[c],
Marvin B. Golberg, DDS, BS[d], Jason E. Portnof, DMD, MD, FICD[b]

KEYWORDS

- Immediate implant • Implant provisional • Atraumatic extraction

KEY POINTS

- By reducing treatment time and number of surgical procedures, immediate implants have become a valuable alternative to tooth replacement.
- Meticulous surgical and restorative considerations can provide the ideal situation for an immediate implant placement.
- The steps described allow for fabrication of both the provisional and the final implant restoration.

The patient that is a candidate for immediate endosseous dental implant placement must meet high scrutiny. Careful planning and meticulous surgical and restorative considerations are paramount in ensuring the success of the immediate dental implant.

Before any implant evaluation, a review of medical history is important to identify any conditions that could affect surgical implant placement or healing. Systemic diseases are important to consider, as these conditions could affect implant healing. When evaluating a patient's past medical history, the practitioner should take into account systemic diseases, such as diabetes and osteoporosis, and local insults, such as tobacco use and smoking.

Although these are only some of the systemic conditions that can raise red flags in a patient's medical history, they are some of the most important to heed caution. These conditions may be relative contraindications for traditional 2-stage implant placement and make for a much less ideal candidate in the setting of immediate implant

[a] Department of Oral and Maxillofacial Surgery, Nova Southeastern University, College of Dental Medicine, 3103 Southwest 76th Avenue, Fort Lauderdale, FL 33314, USA; [b] Surgical Arts of Boca Raton, 9980 N Central Park Blvd #113, Boca Raton, FL 33428, USA; [c] Department of Cariology and Restorative Dentistry, Nova Southeastern University, College of Dental Medicine, 3103 Southwest 76th Avenue, Fort Lauderdale, FL 33314, USA; [d] Department of Prosthodontics, Nova Southeastern University, College of Dental Medicine, 3103 Southwest 76th Avenue, Fort Lauderdale, FL 33314, USA
* Corresponding author. Surgical Arts of Boca Raton, 9980 N Central Park Blvd #113, Boca Raton, FL 33428, USA
E-mail address: rayfan.e@gmail.com

Dent Clin N Am 65 (2021) 89–102
https://doi.org/10.1016/j.cden.2020.09.007
0011-8532/21/© 2020 Elsevier Inc. All rights reserved.

placement. A comprehensive informed consent process that includes a thorough review of all risks, benefits, alternatives, and complications is necessary.

Immediate implant placement is the sequence of placing an implant into a freshly extracted tooth site. There are many advantages to placing an implant immediately after extraction when compared with the more traditional delayed surgery. There are fewer surgeries required along with providing the option to place an immediate temporary restoration to avoid any esthetic compromises.

One of the key elements required in immediate implant placement is bone. There must be enough good-quality bone to engage the implant to facilitate stability for osseointegration. As a result, atraumatic extraction technique is paramount for immediate implant success. The use of periotomes and sectioning of teeth allow for well-preserved alveolar bone. Periotomes are used to expand and separate the gingival attachments from the tooth and periodontium. Atraumatic movements with careful luxation to prevent alveolar bone fracture is critical to maintain enough bone for implant placement. Multiroot teeth are commonly sectioned into their individual roots to allow for a less traumatic extraction.

More recently, piezosurgery units have been used for atraumatic extractions. Piezosurgery uses ultrasound frequencies in the range of 22,000 to 35,000 Hz to cut through bone. In addition, piezosurgical cutting allows for creation of a bone window if exposure is needed for an extraction. This bone window can later be used as an autogenous bone graft.

Preservation of bone, more specifically, preservation of the walls of the tooth socket will allow for a more predictable immediate implant. Not only is preservation of the walls of the tooth socket important but also maintenance of the furcal bone through atraumatic extraction is essential for immediate implant placement. Furcal bone can be used to help engage the immediate implant and obtain primary stability. In the anterior region, preservation of the buccal bone is essential in maintaining soft tissue contour.

A freshly extracted tooth socket will have up to 5 walls. Ideally, the buccal, lingual, mesial, distal, and apical walls remain intact after removal of the tooth structure. If all the walls are present after extraction, the site is known as a 5-walled defect. A 5-walled defect will provide the ideal environment for implant placement. A 4-walled defect, an extraction site missing one of the above, will usually require bone grafting at the time of implant placement. Although not ideal, it usually still allows for a suitable site for immediate implant placement. A 3-walled defect will likely need bone grafting before implant placement and is usually not amenable to immediate placement because of the lack of bone structure.[1] There must be enough bone for the implant to engage and achieve primary stability for osseointegration.

Primary stability is determined by the amount of bone and quality of bone engaged to the implant. Primary stability can be determined through multiple methods. Some common methods of determining primary stability are through insertion torque or resonance analysis. Insertion torque values are measured in newton per centimeters (N/cm) and are commonly measured with the implant motor. Although there are many protocols available for insertion torque values in regards to implant placement, 30 N/cm is a commonly accepted insertion torque value to predict primary stability. At this time, there is no definitive value to predict for success in different loading concepts.[2] Other quantitative measures include resonance frequency analysis. Resonance frequency analysis determines implant stability by sending a magnetic pulse through the implant, which is interpreted to a numerical value called the implant stability quotient (ISQ). The ISQ value measures the stiffness of the implant-bone interface.[3]

Insertion torque values and bone volume have been positively correlated with resonance frequency analysis/ISQ values.[4] Quality of bone can be defined by the amount of cortical bone and medullary bone available, or location in the jaw. The hard tissue evaluation incorporates the quality and shape of bone, the Lekholm and Zarb classification.[5] This classification quantifies bone in 4 categories based on the amount of cortical and trabecular bone. Type 1 bone is large homogenous cortical bone. It is described as very dense with little blood supply compared with the other types of bone. Type I bone is found in the anterior mandible where there is mostly cortical bone. Type 2 bone is composed of a thick cortical layer surrounding a dense medullar bone. Type 2 bone can be found in the posterior mandible. Type 3 bone consists of a thin cortical layer surrounding a dense medullar bone. Type 3 bone can be found in the anterior maxilla. Type 4 bone consists of a thin cortical layer surrounding a sparse medullar bone. Type 4 bone is generally found in the posterior maxilla. This bone is considered to be very "soft" and can lead to higher failure rates.[6]

Studies have shown the mandible (type 1 and type 2 bone) to have higher survival of implants when compared with the maxilla (**Table 1**). The maxilla being type 3 and 4 bone has less cortical bone and more medullary bone. As a result, implants have less bone resistance/interface to stabilize.[7] ISQ values of implants placed in the mandible have been found to be more stable than the maxilla. Achieving primary stability in immediate implants is critical to their success. Without obtaining primary stability, more traditional 2-stage techniques are more favorable.

Knowing the implant divergence or convergence is a critical part of the virtual plan, particularly for immediate implant placement. The trajectory of implant placement is not only determined by the amount of residual bone left after extraction but also determined by the position of the planned final restoration. For example, in the anterior esthetic zone, implants are ideally positioned just palatal to the incisal edge of the proposed restoration in an axial direction. Palatal positioning allows for screw access to be just palatal to the facial surface. An implant placed too facially will create a host of problems, including an unideal access position for the final restoration as well as possible bone loss and soft tissue recession. An implant placed too palatally can create a ridge lapped restoration leading to a hygienic problem. After placement of the implant, there will be a gap between the implant and the facial wall known as the labial gap. Studies have shown that grafting of the labial gap allows for improved preservation of the labial wall (**Fig. 1**).[8] The 3-dimensional position of the implant needs to be considered when deciding to place an immediate implant.

Preservation of the facial wall is crucial to obtaining an esthetic result. The facial wall has 3 sources of blood supply: the endosseous bone marrow, periosteum, and periodontal ligament. The periodontal ligament is lost after extraction of the tooth. If a flap is raised, there will be loss of periosteal blood supply to the bone, leaving only the endosseous marrow as the remaining blood supply to the bone. Atraumatic extraction without flap elevation will provide the best chance for maintenance of the

Table 1 Classification of bone quality		
Classification	**Composition**	**Location**
Type 1	Dense cortical bone, little medullary bone	Anterior mandible
Type 2	Thick cortical bone and dense medullary core	Posterior mandible
Type 3	Thin cortical bone with a dense medullary core	Anterior maxilla
Type 4	Thin cortical bone with little medullary bone	Posterior maxilla

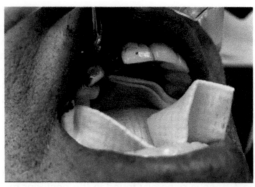

Fig. 1. Intraoperative immediate implant tooth number 7 with particulate bone grafting and platelet rich plasma.

facial bony wall.[8] Immediate implant placement with bone grafting of the labial gap and placement of a well-contoured provisional that secures the graft and blood clot allows for minimal loss of facial bone.[9] Atraumatic extraction, palatal placement of the implant, gap grafting, and provisional restoration placement for stabilization of blood clot and graft materials will provide an environment for the smallest amount of facial plate resorption and ultimately the best chance for an esthetic result.

Treatment planning of the potential implant site begins with both the clinical and the radiographic examination. The clinical examination involves both evaluation of the soft and hard tissue within the mouth. The smile line, gingival show, and gingival type will all factor into the decision making of implant placement in the anterior esthetic zone. The thick biotype resists gingival recession and causes minimal changes when surgically manipulated. Thin biotype gingiva has more recession when manipulated surgically and is more unforgiving to work with. Thin scalloped biotypes will be more prone to recession and cause more black triangular spaces in between teeth, a consideration critical when planning an immediate implant in the esthetic zone.

A greater amount of keratinized tissue allows for a more implant-friendly environment. The abundance of keratinized tissue provides a seal or cuff around implants that promotes an environment that is much more easily cleansed.

Radiographic assessment should be evaluated in combination with a panoramic radiograph and computed tomographic (CT) image. Panoramic radiographs provide a broad view of the overall hard tissue of the mouth. Some of the limitations of panoramic radiographs are that they have magnification of up to 25% to 30% so measurements should be taken with the knowledge of this magnification. Furthermore, the image is 2 dimensional. CT imaging allows for the operator to view the hard tissue in a 3-dimensional view. There are programs that allow for virtual implant placement incorporated into the CT viewing system so implant position, angle, and orientation can be visualized before placement (**Fig. 2**).

Implant site assessment should include clinical measurements of mesial and distal, occlusal plane to ridge, and buccal lingual lengths of the edentulous site. In the posterior, there should be a minimum of 5 to 7 mm from the crest of bone to the occlusal plane. The implant should be placed 2 to 3 mm apical to the clinical cementoenamel junction. An implant placed too high will result in a sharp transition into the gingiva, causing an esthetic and cleansing problem. An implant placed too deep will result in a deep pocket associated with the crown. In the anterior zone, 2 mm of bone buccally and lingually from the implant will provide enough support to prevent

A

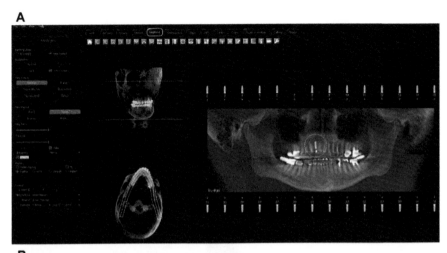

B

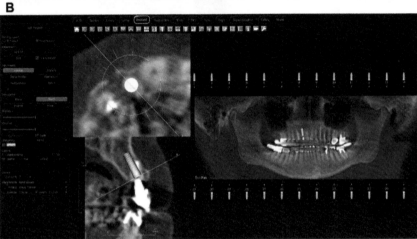

Fig. 2. Virtual workup for immediate implant placement for tooth number 7.j. (*A*) Panoramic view of virtual implant placement in tooth site #7. (*B*) Axial, sagittal, and panoramic view of virtual implant placement in tooth site #7.

recession and bone loss. Given the esthetic concerns with the anterior, 2 mm is preferred, whereas, in the posterior, 1 mm of bone on the buccal and lingual aspects will be sufficient. Lingual concavities should be taken into consideration when placing an implant into the mandible. These lingual concavities can cause lingual fenestrations, which can lead to dehiscence of the soft tissue or even infection. In the maxilla, plate perforations can occur in the anterior labial plate.

Evaluation of anatomic sites are critical in the treatment planning process. The inferior alveolar nerve and implant should have a minimum of 2 mm of separation. The implant to mental foramen distance should be 5 mm. Implants should be placed 3 mm apart from each other to facilitate enough blood supply to allow for proper bone formation and osseointegration. Implants to natural dentition should be 1.5 mm apart (**Fig. 3**).

The difference between implant to adjacent implant and implant to adjacent natural dentition is the periodontal ligament. Natural dentition has a periodontal ligament that

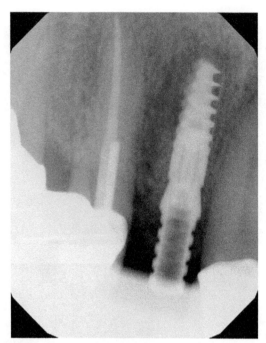

Fig. 3. Postoperative radiograph of immediate implant placement number 7.

contributes to additional blood flow and supply to the alveolar bone, whereas an implant does not have a periodontal ligament. As a result, 3 mm is necessary to facilitate enough blood supply to the bone in the implant-implant interface. If implants are placed too close to each other (<3 mm), break down of the interdental bone will occur.[9] Without underlying bone support, the soft tissue will recede, causing black triangles. Interdental papillae are supported by underlying bone levels. The smaller the distance from interdental alveolar bone to the contact point between adjacent teeth correlates to the presence of the papilla (**Table 2**).[10]

Immediate implants have become an appealing option for patients. They decrease both treatment time and number of surgical procedures. By following the parameters considered, immediate implants can be an appropriate and predictable alternative for tooth replacement.

The fabrication of a digitally created esthetic and functional provisional restoration brings your patient 1 step closer to completion of their implant procedure (**Fig. 4**). The permanent restoration is, of course, the ultimate goal of implant placement. The techniques as described accomplishes that goal, and interestingly, almost all the

Table 2	
Relationship of crestal bone to presence of papilla	
Distance from Contact Point to Interdental Crestal Bone	**Percentage of Time the Papilla Is Present**
5 mm	100
6 mm	56
≥7 mm	27

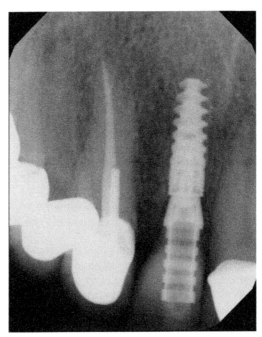

Fig. 4. Two months postoperative radiograph of tooth number 7 immediate implant with temporary restoration.

steps used to fabricate the provisional restoration are used in the fabrication of the permanent crown. The digitally stored files need only minor correction between the provisional (resin material) and permanent (IPS e.max CAD) restoration.

The scanning system used in this discussion is the Sirona Omnicam with 4.5.2 software. An on-site milling machine is used in this example. The other milling option is to send the scanned file to an off-site laboratory.

ADMINISTRATION

Once the computer software is launched, one must complete the administration, directing the program through a sequence of screens to define required parameters. First, enter the patient's name, chart ID, and dentist's name. You may scan the software program with any of these entries to locate a case. Next, choose the type of restoration from a list of options. We are selecting a screw-retained crown for the restoration type, followed by the design mode (biogenetic individual), and the manufacturer and material (Telio CAD Ivoclar Vivadent Abutment, milling), Next, select the implant company and platform size followed by TiBase, which is our ScanBody type. You must select a ScanPost option if the implant is placed too deep under the gingiva. This will raise the TiBase 2 mm. The final step in Administration is to select the implant site.

ACQUISITION

This process begins by removing the implant healing cap and securing the ScanPost or TiBase and ScanBody in the proper orientation. The notch on the TiBase must face mesial or distal so that the sprue emerges buccal or lingual. The ScanBody only seats in 1 position; this will allow you to accurately align and seat the completed provisional restoration. Confirm full seating with a radiograph. It is imperative to capture the gingival contour immediately once the healing abutment is removed. To do this, the placement of the ScanPost and ScanBody should be completed as quickly and safely as possible so that the gingival tissue does not rebound.

SCANNING SEQUENCE

Scan 1: All surfaces surrounding the ScanBody must be captured along with the soft tissue. A 360° acquisition is required.

Scan 2: Remove the ScanBody to scan the uncovered TiBase to the midline of the arch. It is necessary to capture the proximal surfaces of the adjacent teeth.

Scan 3: Scan the opposing arch, capturing 2 teeth on either side of the corresponding implant tooth.

Scan 4: Buccal bite with TiBase in place if possible. If the TiBase interferes when the patient occludes for the scan, remove the TiBase and put the healing cap back in place.

Once all scans have been captured, place the implant arch model image in line with the crosshairs at the midline. Click OK after setting this alignment. Select the model icon on the tool bar and then align the buccal cusp tips to the curve of Spee. Next, line up the upper model so it is parallel to the long axis of the tooth, which is the curve of Wilson. These 2 settings will correctly position the model for proper occlusion.

Complete the following steps in this order:

- Modify the emergence profile from the gingival view to display a proper crown proposal.
- Contour the surfaces of the crown with provided icons to physiologically contour to the adjacent teeth, for example, marginal ridge heights, buccal and lingual contours, occlusion, and emergence profile.
- Display the opposing jaw to adjust the occlusion with icons for buccal and lingual cusp interdigitation.
- Check the mesial and distal contacts by making the lower jaw transparent. Adjust the contacts to a light green color.
- From the apical view, remove crown bulkiness so gingival tissue is not displaced.
- Smooth out crown proposal so it does not collect food.

There are various other icons that are available at different stages of scanning and design that the operator may become familiar with for finite modifications.

The proposed provisional implant crown is now ready for milling.

After the provisional crown is milled in the Omnican (Sirona Dentsply), which takes approximately 12 minutes, it is ready for polishing, characterization, and glazing. Before cementation on the TiBase, the mesial and distal contacts and occlusion are adjusted, if needed, intraorally. The provisional crown is then cemented on the TiBase extraorally, which allows extraneous cement to be easily identified and removed. The benefit of this procedure is that no cement remains subgingival to cause failure of the implant. Follow the directions provided by the manufacturer of the cement for this extraoral step. After the provisional crown is screwed into place, the access hole is filled with sterilized Teflon tape and a direct composite restoration. Confirm final seating with a radiograph.

For the final restoration, after osteointegration, merely change the milling block composition under the Administration title on the toolbar. Minor digital adjustments may be made to produce a final restoration that has proper contours, contacts, thickness, and so forth before milling (**Figs. 5–9**).

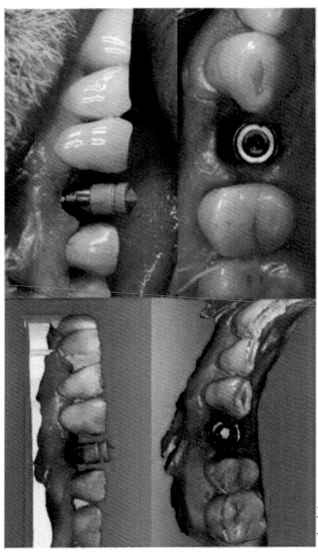

Fig. 5. Scan with scan body/post.

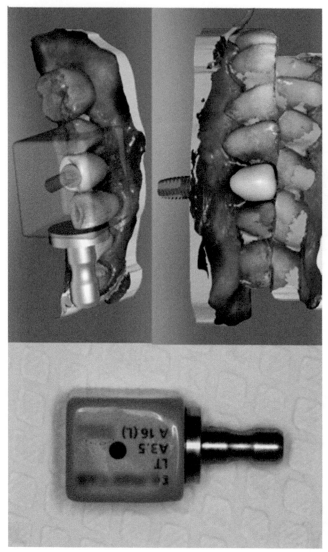

Fig. 6. Hybrid crown design.

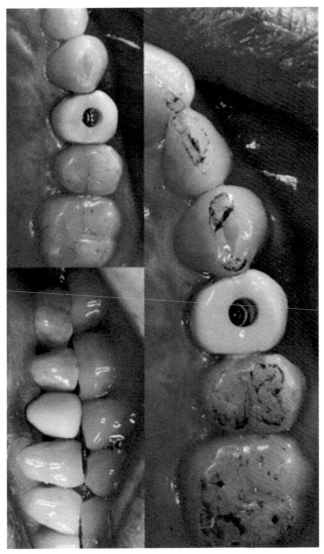

Fig. 7. Clinical try-in.

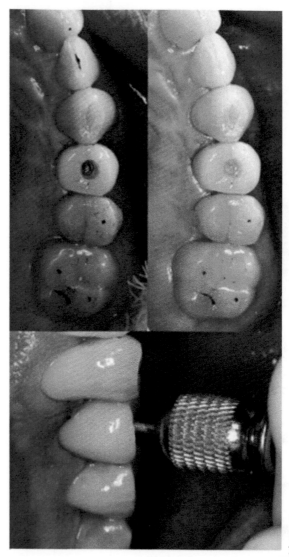

Fig. 8. Seating hybrid crown.

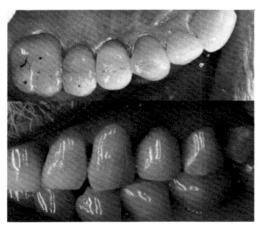

Fig. 9. Completed case.

The ease and joy of experiencing an aesthetic and accurate final restoration digitally is our future.

CLINICS CARE POINTS

- Indications and contraindications for immediate implant placement
- Atraumatic extraction
- Restoratively driven implant placement
- Implant scanning and restoration work flow

DISCLOSURE

The authors have nothing to disclose.

REFERENCES

1. Barber HD, Spivey J. Implant placement immediately following tooth extraction. In: Fonseca RJ, editor. Oral and maxillofacial surgery: 3-volume set. Saunders; 2017. p. 541–2.

2. Placement of implants - Torque. (n.d.). Available at: https://www.for.org/en/treat/treatment-guidelines/edentulous/treatment-procedures/surgical/surgical-protocols-general/placement-implants-torque. Accessed April 20, 2020.

3. Trisi P, Carlesi T, Colagiovanni M, et al. Implant Stability Quotient (ISQ) vs Direct in Vitro Measurement of Primary Stability (Micromotion): Effect of Bone Density and Insertion Torque. Journal of Osteology and Biomaterial 2010;1(3).

4. Makary C, Alberto R, Gilberto S, et al. Implant primary stability determined by resonance frequency analysis. Implant Dent 2012;21(6):474–80.

5. Lekholm U, Zarb GA. Patient selection and preparation. Tissue integrated prostheses: osseointegration in clinical dentistry. Chicago: Quintessence Publishing Company; 1985. p. 199–209.

6. Goiato MC, dos Santos DM, Santiago JF Jr, et al. Longevity of dental implants in type IV bone: a systematic review. Int J Oral Maxillofac Surg 2014;43(9): 1108–16.

7. Shiffler K, David L, Mark R, et al. Effect of length, diameter, intraoral location on implant stability. Oral Surg Oral Med Oral Pathol Oral Radiol 2016;122(6):e193–8.

8. Tarnow D, Chu S, Salama M, et al. Flapless postextraction socket implant placement in the esthetic zone: part 1. The effect of bone grafting and/or provisional restoration on facial-palatal ridge dimensional change—a retrospective cohort study. Int J Periodontics Restorative Dent 2014;34(3):323–31.

9. Tarnow DP, Cho SC, Wallace SS. The effect of inter-implant distance on the height of inter-implant bone crest. J Periodontol 2000;71(4):546–9.

10. Tarnow DP, Magner AW, Fletcher P. The effect of the distance from the contact point to the crest of bone on the presence or absence of the interproximal dental papilla. J Periodontol 1992;63(12):995–6.

Vertical and Horizontal Augmentation of Deficient Maxilla and Mandible for Implant Placement

Amanda Andre, DDS[a],*, Orrett E. Ogle, DDS[b,c]

KEYWORDS

- Alveolar bone loss • Horizontal bone augmentation • Vertical bone augmentation
- Bone grafting

KEY POINTS

- The ideal position of a dental implant should not be compromised in the setting of a deficient maxillary or mandibular alveolar ridge. Overall, bone augmentation techniques can be highly predictable and can provide significant horizontal and vertical gain.
- Since there is currently no true consensus in the literature on which bone grafting technique or material is strictly indicated for each clinical scenario, dental professionals can benefit from gaining an understanding on the various methods to achieve horizontal and vertical augmentation of the deficient alveolar ridge.
- The surgical techniques presented in this article for the augmentation of the deficient alveolar ridge can vary from simple to advanced and require proper training for successful outcomes and minimizing complications.

INTRODUCTION

The loss of alveolar bone is a common phenomenon linked to various systemic and local factors. Systemic factors include age, nutrition, osteoporosis, and other skeletal disturbances, and local factors include the premature loss of teeth, trauma, pathology, and periodontal disease. In the United States, partial edentulism affects the majority of the population and the number of partially edentulous individuals is expected to increase to more than 200 million in the next 8 years.[1] The increased focus in preventative dental care over the past years has positively impacted tooth retention and thus a decrease in fully edentulous individuals is expected. Interestingly, the premature loss

[a] The Brooklyn Hospital Center, 121 Dekalb Avenue, Brooklyn, NY 11201, USA; [b] Mona Dental Program, Faculty of Medicine, Univ. of the West Indies, Kingston 6, Jamaica; [c] Oral and Maxillofacial Surgery, Woodhull Hospital, Brooklyn, NY 11206, USA
* Corresponding author.
E-mail address: aafernandez@tbh.org

Dent Clin N Am 65 (2021) 103–123
https://doi.org/10.1016/j.cden.2020.09.009
0011-8532/21/© 2020 Elsevier Inc. All rights reserved.

of permanent teeth remains correlated with an increase in age. The growth of a more socially active and more esthetically demanding aging population in the United States has increased the demand for more comfortable, functional, and esthetic dental prosthetic solutions. The placement of dental implants broadens the treatment options for these individuals. Prosthetically driven implant restorations may not only significantly improve the patient's treatment outcomes by improving the esthetics, occlusion, phonetics, retention, and stability of the prosthesis, but also preserve the remaining alveolar bone. The atrophy of the maxillary and mandibular alveolar arches is a common occurrence that can pose many challenges for the rehabilitation of these patients, both surgically and restoratively. In contemporary implant dentistry, a practitioner may choose between the use or augmentation of the remaining bone based on the clinical and radiographic presentation. In this article, we discuss the various indications and techniques for the vertical and horizontal augmentation of the deficient maxilla and mandible for endosseous implant placement. Ridge preservation and socket augmentation procedures are beyond the scope of this article.

PATTERNS OF BONE LOSS

The classic study by Cawood and Howell[2] demonstrated there are predictable patterns of progressive horizontal and vertical anatomic changes following the loss of teeth (**Box 1**). The loss of teeth induces the progressive loss of alveolar bone until completely resorbed.[2,3] In addition, the loss of basal bone from ill-fitting dentures or occlusal overloading can further contribute to the atrophy of the ridge. Identifying the various patterns of bone loss can facilitate the treatment planning and increase the predictability of the rehabilitation of atrophic ridges.

When teeth are lost prematurely, it can lead to a decrease in the alveolar ridge's volume owing to the lack of functional stimulus necessary to preserve its vertical and horizontal dimensions. Function influences the delicate balance that exists at the cellular level between bone resorption and bone formation.[4] When permanent teeth are loss prematurely, the loss of stimulus from the forces of mastication in the area lead to a shift to bone resorption.

Generally, the loss of teeth in the maxilla tends to occur before the loss of teeth in the mandible and mandibular anterior teeth are commonly the last teeth remaining in the mouth.[5] However, the rate of resorption of the alveolar crest of the mandible is 4 times the average rate of resorption of the maxilla. The rate of resorption occurs more rapidly within the first 6 months after the loss of teeth.[3] Combination syndrome is a well-documented condition seen in patients with a completely edentulous maxilla and a partially edentulous mandible with preserved anterior teeth. This syndrome leads to a classical pattern of severe resorption of the anterior maxilla and posterior mandible, overgrowth of the maxillary tuberosities, papillary hyperplasia of the hard plate, and extrusion of the lower anterior teeth.[6] The treatment for combination syndrome with dental implants

Box 1 Cawood and Howell Classification of Edentulous Jaws	
I	Dentate
II	Immediately after extraction
III	Well-rounded ridge form, adequate in height and width
IV	Knife-edge ridge form, adequate in height and inadequate in width
V	Flat ridge form, inadequate in height and width
VI	Depressed ridge form, with some basilar loss evident

has made it possible for the rehabilitation of posterior occlusion, the redistribution of the forces of mastication, and the prevention of further bone loss.

The loss of teeth can also be attributed to the body's response to the presence of bacterial biofilm in the oral cavity or trauma from occlusal forces. Periodontal disease can lead to the permanent destruction of supportive periodontal structures, alveolar bone, and ultimately the teeth involved. Without treatment, the resulting inflammatory reaction leads to an average bone loss per year of approximately 0.2 mm for facial surfaces and 0.3 mm for proximal surfaces, with a radius of 1.5 to 2.5 mm from the site of bacterial biofilm formation.[4] In addition, bone destruction caused by persistent occlusal trauma results in a widening of the periodontal ligament and resorption of adjacent bone. These changes to the adjacent bone can lead to tooth mobility and when paired with inflammatory reactions to the bacterial biofilm can result in vertical bone loss or unusual bone loss patterns.[4] The most prevalent form of bone loss caused by periodontal disease is horizontal bone loss, whereas vertical or angular bone loss tends to occur in areas of greater bone volume.

Vertical bone loss was classified by Goldman and Cohen on the basis of the number of osseous walls present in the defect (**Fig. 1**). Consequently, various defect patterns can arise after dental extractions. Furthermore, Misch and Dietsh[7] classified the resulting extraction socket defects based on the amount of remaining bony walls and provided recommendations on the appropriate graft materials and techniques to be used for the restoration of such defects (**Fig. 2**). The 5-wall defect results from extraction sockets or cystic cavities. Bone grafting is optional in these defects owing to the tendency of 5-wall defects to fill in with bone without additional surgical interventions. For this reason, the use of inexpensive materials is recommended when considering socket preservation procedures. The 4-wall defect typically consists of missing labial and occlusal walls, whereas the 2- and 3- wall defects present a larger area for bone augmentation and require the use of autogenous bone. Moreover, the 1-walll defect is the most challenging to augment and, thus, block grafts are usually recommended for the restoration of the ridge's volume.

Deteriorating changes to the quality of the soft tissue architecture can also occur owing to the loss of alveolar bone. The alveolus is typically protected by a strong layer of keratinized attached gingiva. Upon the loss of alveolar bone, the soft tissue can be replaced with a less keratinized oral mucosa, allowing for the area to be more easily traumatized upon normal function.[5] The loss of keratinized mucosa can add to the challenges in placing dental implants in the esthetic zone.

HORIZONTAL AND VERTICAL REQUIREMENTS FOR IMPLANT PLACEMENT

A successful treatment outcome in relation to dental implants depends the restoration of the patient's function, comfort, speech, and esthetics. Alveolar bone atrophy in the vertical or horizontal dimensions may obstruct the surgeon's ability to place endosseous implants in the desired position for the prosthetic rehabilitation of the arch. The development of advanced techniques has allowed for the achievement of these outcomes despite the patient's level of maxillary or mandibular atrophy. Owing to the predictability of bone augmentation procedures, the practitioner should avoid compromising the ideal position of the implant when adequate bone width and height are not available. Nonetheless, the fact remains that the greater the loss of teeth and bone volume, the more challenging the process of achieving a functional and esthetic outcome. Careful treatment planning must take into account the 3-dimensional position of the implant in the bone and the horizontal and vertical requirements for implant placement.

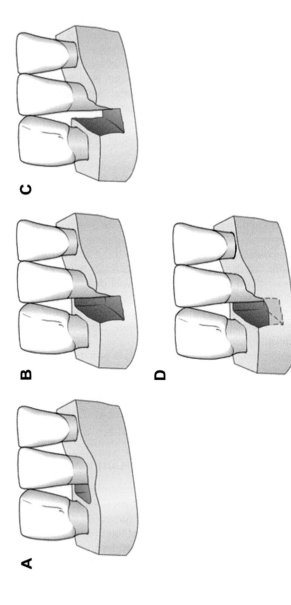

Fig. 1. Representation of vertical defects of the right lateral incisor. (*A*) Three-wall defect: distal, lingual, and facial. (*B*) Two-wall defect: distal and lingual. (*C*) One-wall defect: distal. (*D*) Combined osseous defect with 3 walls in its apical half and 2 in the occlusal half. (*From* Camargo PM, Takei HH, Carranza FA. Bone loss and patterns of bone destruction. In: Newman MG, Takei HH, Klokkevold PR, Carranza FA, editors. Newman and Carranza's clinical periodontology. 13th edition. Philadelphia: Elsevier; 2019. p. 323–5; with permission.)

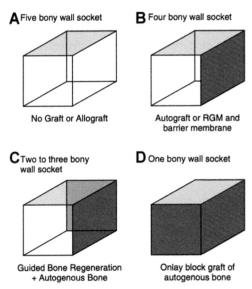

A Five bony wall socket

No Graft or Allograft

B Four bony wall socket

Autograft or RGM and
barrier membrane

C Two to three bony
wall socket

Guided Bone Regeneration
+ Autogenous Bone

D One bony wall socket

Onlay block graft of
autogenous bone

Fig. 2. Classification of wall defects. (*A*) A 5-wall defect usually results from tooth extraction sockets or cystic cavities. (*B*) Four-wall defect. (*C*) Three-wall defect and 2-wall defect. (*D*) A 1-wall defect usually has the lingual/palatal wall present. RGM, resorbable graft material. (*From* Resnik RR, Suzuki JB. Atraumatic tooth extraction and socket grafting. In: Resnik RR, editor. Misch's contemporary implant dentistry. 4th ed. Elsevier; 2020. p. 900; with permission.)

A cone beam computed tomography scan offers the most accurate measure for the available bone structure in the mesiodistal, buccolingual, and apicoronal planes. To minimize damage to adjacent teeth, the ideal distance from the implant to adjacent tooth should be at least 1.5 mm. However, to achieve soft tissue health, the distance between the neck of the implant and the crown of the adjacent tooth should be increased to at least 2.0 mm. In addition, if the coronal distance between the implant and the tooth exceeds 4.0 mm, the cantilever effect would lead to bone loss, magnified occlusal forces, and ultimately possible restoration and/or implant failure. After implant placement, the width of the remaining bone should be at least 2.0 mm on the facial aspect and 1.0 mm or more on the lingual or palatal aspect to prevent bone recession owing to a lack of blood supply. It is widely accepted that, to determine the horizontal dimension required for implant placement, the practitioner must follow the formula: Implant diameter + 2.0 mm facial bone + 1.0 mm lingual bone.[8] Therefore, the horizontal dimension of the available bone should be at least 3.00 mm or greater than the diameter of the implant.

As opposed to calculated measurements, the vertical dimension requirements depend on soft tissue height, prosthetic needs, and proximity to vital structures. The ideal depth of placement of a dental implant is 2.0 to 4.0 mm apical to the adjacent cemento–enamel junction or free gingival margin to allow for adequate prosthetic crown soft tissue emergency profile. The fabrication material of the final prosthesis should be taken into account.[8] Typically, a space of 15 mm is suggested from the crest of the alveolar ridge to the incisal edge of the prosthesis. The specific crown height space (CHS) requirements depend on the selected material for the final restoration. If the interocclusal space is deemed insufficient or excessive, it can be detrimental to the survival of the prosthesis and additional procedures should be considered.[9] Vital structures should be identified in the treatment planning phase with the assistance of 3-dimensional imaging studies or computer-generated models. To prevent traumatic injury to the nerve, implants should be positioned at least 2.0 mm away from the inferior alveolar nerve canal or mental foramen. Moreover, bleeding and other iatrogenic complications can result from the penetration of the dental implant through the inferior border of the mandible or border of the maxillary sinus and nasal cavity and, thus, great care should be taken to avoid these structures (**Box 2**).[8]

There is no consensus in the literature in regard to strict guidelines on which technique or material is indicated for each bone deficiency or clinical scenario.[8,10] Rather, the decision should be made after careful consideration and treatment planning. The combination of different techniques and materials is encouraged to achieve optimal treatment outcomes.

HORIZONTAL AUGMENTATION

Advanced horizontal bone augmentation procedures are indicated when the bone volume available in the proposed implant site is deemed to be insufficient for the prosthetically ideal placement of the dental implant. The final decision on which bone augmentation technique is adequate for each clinical scenario remains the responsibility of the clinician because there are no clear set protocols in the literature.[10] Clinicians should be familiar with the various options for restoring the deficient alveolar ridge (**Table 1**). Some of the most predictable surgical techniques available are:

- Tunnel technique using particulate bone

Box 2
Implant Placement Considerations

Mesiodistal	
Implant–tooth (apical)	>1.5 mm
Implant–tooth (coronal)	>2.0 mm, <4.0 mm
Implant–implant	>3.0 mm
Buccolingual/faciopalatal	
Facial/buccal thickness	>2.0 mm
Lingual/palatal thickness	>1.0 mm
Apicocoronal	
Implant platform-cemento–enamel junction/free gingival margin	2–4 mm
Distance from vital structures	
Inferior alveolar nerve canal or mental foramen	>2 mm
Inferior border of the mandible	Avoid cortical bone perforation
Nasal cavity	Avoid cortical bone perforation
Inferior border of maxillary sinus	Without bone grafting, can penetrate approximately 1–2 mm into the sinus
Interocclusal/CHS	
Alveolar ridge–incisal edge of prosthesis	<15 mm

Data from Resnik RR, Misch CE. Ideal implant positioning. In: Resnik RR, editor. Misch's contemporary implant dentistry. 4th ed. Elsevier; 2020. p. 670–705.

Table 1
Summary of horizontal bone augmentation techniques

Technique	Indication	Potential Bone Gain	Recommended Time to Implant Placement
Tunnel technique	2-wall defect Satisfactory vertical height <4 mm ridge width A ridge that widens as it approaches the basal bone	1–4 mm	4 mo
GBR	2-wall defect, 3-wall defect, 4-wall defect	3–6 mm	9–12 mo
Onlay bone grafting	1-wall defect <3 mm ridge width	4 mm Ramus 3–4 mm Symphysis 4–6 mm	4–6 mo
Ridge Split/Expansion	3–4 mm ridge width	2–3 mm	Immediate or 4 mo
Distraction Osteogenesis	>5 mm horizontal deficiency	Not reported	3–4 mo

- Guided bone regeneration (GBR)
- Onlay block grafting
- Ridge splitting or expansion technique
- Distraction osteogenesis

Tunnel Technique Using Particulate Bone

The placement of particulate bone under the periosteum using a tunneling technique for space maintenance has shown to successfully increase the width of the alveolar ridge. This technique is minimally invasive, simple, and can be more cost effective than other augmentation procedures. In an article by Block,[11] the reported indications for the procedure are (1) satisfactory vertical height, (2) a lack of at least 4.0 mm of bone width, and (3) widening of the ridge as it approaches the basal bone. The ideal defect type for this procedure is the 2-wall defect.

The technique described starts with a crestal incision on the superior aspect mesial to the site of the defect running inferior in a vertical fashion. The blunt end of a periosteal elevator is used to create a subperiosteal tunnel posterior to the incision site. At the crest of the ridge, the periosteum is elevated over the ridge. Excessive lingual dissection should be avoided. Using a TB-type syringe, the particulate material is deposited in a posterior to anterior direction, directly against bone and removed at an angle to create a bevel. Digital pressure is then used to mold the graft until the desired shape is achieved. The incision is then closed using interrupted resorbable sutures. The recommended bone grafting particle sizes range from 350 to 500 μm and the volume from 0.5 mL to 1.5 mL. A healing period of at least 4 months is recommended before implant placement.[11] Overall, the use of allogenic or xenogeneic grafting materials seems to result in a higher potential for horizontal gain, compared with the use of synthetic materials.[12] The potential bone gain of this technique has not been widely reported in systematic reviews, however, case studies show a 2.0- to 4.0-mm augmentation after 4 months of healing time.[11]

A retrospective cohort study by Deeb and colleagues[13] compared the treatment outcomes between 21 patients treated by the tunnel technique and 31 treated with the open technique. After a 6-month healing period, their data showed no significant difference between the outcomes of the tunnel technique versus GBR using a titanium-reinforced polytetrafluoroethylene membrane for the augmentation of horizontal ridge augmentation. The tunnel technique provides a minimally invasive option for patients for the rehabilitation of the deficient alveolar ridge.

Guided Bone Regeneration

GBR is one of the most common and predictable methods for the treatment of horizontal bone defects. Space maintenance can be provided by nonresorbable and resorbable membranes preventing the migration of undesired soft tissue and guiding the growth of bone into the grafted site. There is evidence to support the use of GBR for horizontal augmentation at the time of implant placement for ridges measuring approximately 4 mm or as a staged procedure in preparation for implant placement for residual crests measuring less than 3 mm.[10] Nonresorbable membranes include titanium mesh, expanded polytetrafluoroethylene, and titanium-reinforced expanded polytetrafluoroethylene membrane. Resorbable membranes include collagen, polylactic acid, amniotic membrane, pericardial membrane, and dura mater.[14] The barrier material seems to have little effect on horizontal ridge augmentation and although there are more complications reported with the use of titanium meshes (ie, dehiscence), the conclusion on recent systematic reviews has not shown the data to be statistically significant (**Figs. 3–5**).[12]

Karmon and colleagues[15] described a novel technique combining GBR and the tunnel technique with the use a subperiosteal bag for horizontal bone augmentation. The authors created a "bag" by perforating, folding and suturing a Bio-Gide bilayer resorbable collagen membrane. The bag was then filled with Bio-Oss bovine-derived xenograft bone substitute. A vertical incision was made and a subperiosteal tunnel created distal to the site. The bag was inserted inside the tunnel with the perforated side facing the alveolar ridge and the nonperforated side of the bag facing the flap. Primary closure was then achieved with resorbable sutures. The time recommended from grafting procedure to implant placement in this study was 6 months.

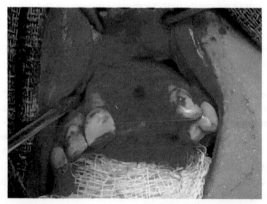

Fig. 3. Exposed severe defect of the anterior maxilla owing to mechanical trauma.

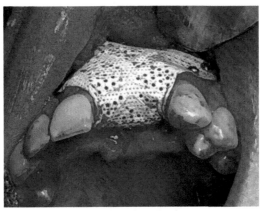

Fig. 4. Placement of reinforced polytetrafluoroethylene mesh for GBR and augmentation of the deficient anterior maxilla, secured with membrane tent screws.

Onlay block bone grafting

Autogenous bone remains the gold standard for alveolar bone augmentation owing to its osteogenic, osteoinductive, and osteoconductive properties. When indicated, the donor site is typically selected depending on the size of the required bone block and type of defect. Block grafts are the procedure of choice for the effective augmentation of 1-wall defects. A recent systematic review by Milinkovic and Cordaro[10] reported a mean linear horizontal bone gain of 4.3 mm after an average healing period of 5.2 months when bone block grafts were used. Correspondingly, another recent systematic review by Troeltzsch and colleagues[12] that analyzed 184 studies, reported an overall weighted mean of a 4.5 mm increase in horizontal gain. In accordance, the calculated mean gain of horizontal bone thickness using autogenous block grafts in a review of 42 cases by Von Arx and Buser[16] was 4.6 mm with a range between 2 and 7 mm.

Intraoral sites such as the mandibular symphysis, ramus, maxillary tuberosity, and bony exostoses can be harvested for augmentation of small size (<5.0 mm) defects. The harvesting of these sites can often be performed under local anesthesia and have minimal morbidity. In contrast, when greater amounts of bone (>5.0 mm) are required, donor sites such as the tibia, anterior iliac crest, posterior iliac crest, and calvarium can provide substantial amounts of cancellous, corticocancellous, or cortical bone (**Fig. 6**). Although the harvesting of these distal sites can be done safely, it is recommended for the procedure to be performed under general anesthesia by trained oral surgeons, to minimize more significant complications.[17]

Ridge Split or Expansion Technique

The literature supports alveolar ridge split/expansion osteotomies for the augmentation of alveolar ridges between 3.0 and 4.0 mm to gain 2.0 and 3.0 mm of alveolar bone (**Fig. 7**). Milinkovic and Cordaro[10] reported a mean bone gain of 2.95 mm among 6 studies with an average healing time of 4.5 months.[10] A technique described by Dym and colleagues[17] recommends the use of different size osteotomes increasing in size to force the direction of the split buccally, grafting of the site, and closure by primary intention or by the covering of the graft with a membrane before closing with sutures. Another described variation to this technique is the island flap osteotomy, which allow for simultaneous vertical and horizontal augmentation. In the island flap osteotomy

A

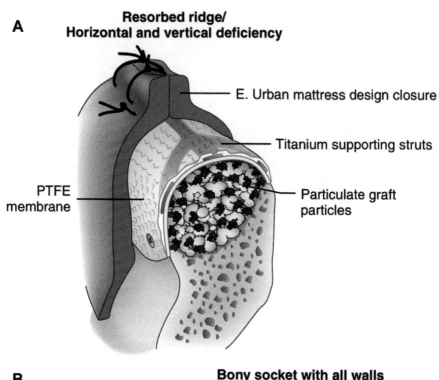

**Resorbed ridge/
Horizontal and vertical deficiency**

E. Urban mattress design closure

Titanium supporting struts

PTFE
membrane

Particulate graft
particles

B

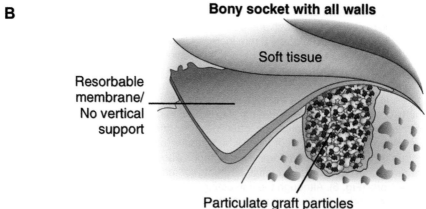

Bony socket with all walls

Soft tissue

Resorbable
membrane/
No vertical
support

Particulate graft particles

Fig. 5. Use of resorbable (A) and nonresorbable (B) membranes to protect the regenerative space fill and prevent soft tissue ingrowth. Nonresorbable membranes (A) such as polytetrafluoroethylene (PTFE) membranes provide structural support, which prevents the collapse of the soft tissue into the grafted site. (*From* Caldwell CS. Particulate membrane grafting/guided bone regeneration. In: Resnik RR, editor. Misch's contemporary implant dentistry. 4th ed. Elsevier; 2020. p. 962; with permission.)

technique, the buccal plate is intentionally fractured to create a segment of bone attached to the buccal periosteum. The use of Piezo surgery as an adjunct simplifies the technique and increases the safety of the procedure by decreasing the potential risk for soft tissue damage and thermal necrosis.[18]

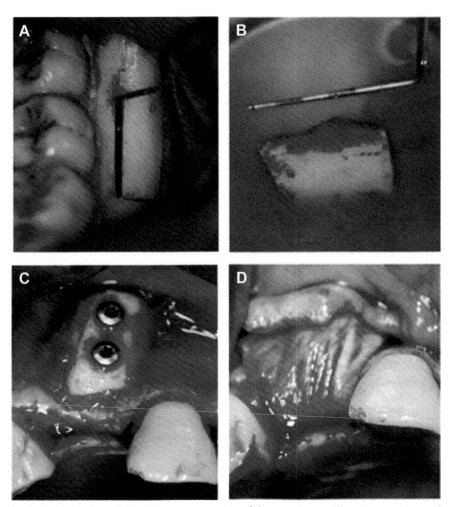

Fig. 6. Onlay block graft for ridge augmentation of the anterior maxilla using corticocancellous onlay mandibular block graft. (*A*) Bone osteotomy in mandibular molar area. (*B*) Corticocancellous bone graft. (*C*) Onlay graft fixation with miniscrews. (*D*) Covering the graft with a collagen membrane. (*From* Mansour A, Al-Hamed FS, Torres J, et al. Alveolar bone grafting: Rationale and clinical applications. In: Alghamdi H, Jansen J, editors. Dental implants and bone grafts. Cambridge, MA: Woodhead Publishing; 2020. p. 62; with permission.)

Distraction Osteogenesis

Distraction osteogenesis is a technique used for severe defects requiring more than 5.0 mm of expansion. The general alveolar distraction timeline consists of the surgical placement of the distractor followed by a latency period of 5 to 7 days. The distraction period involves adjustments of 0.5 mm to 1.0 mm daily. A consolidation period of 8 to 12 weeks follows, the distractor device is removed and implant placement can take place.[19] Although distraction osteogenesis is more commonly used for vertical ridge augmentation, it has also been reported for the augmentation of the narrow alveolar

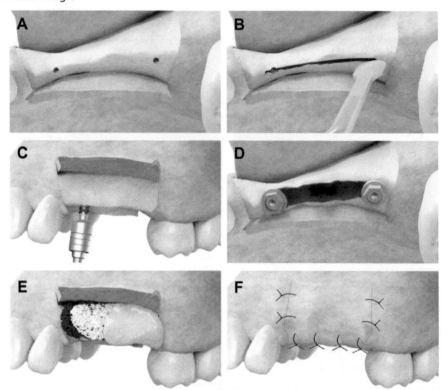

Fig. 7. Diagram showing the ridge splitting technique for the augmentation of the deficient alveolar ridge. (*A*) Implant marks. (*B*) Sagittal osteotomy connecting marked implant sites. (*C*) Use of motorized bone expander. (*D*) Dental implants placed. (*E*) Bone graft placed into osteotomy site. (*F*) Flap repositioned and sutured. (*From* Anitua E, Alkhraisat MH. Is alveolar ridge split a risk factor for implant survival? J Oral Maxillofac Surg. 2016;74(11):2183; with permission.)

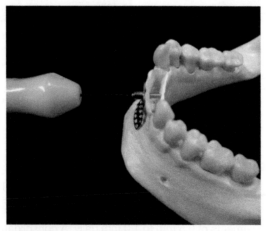

Fig. 8. Horizontal alveolar distraction device placed on a model. (*From* Funaki K, Takahashi T, Yamuchi K. Horizontal alveolar ridge augmentation using distraction osteogenesis: comparison with a bone-splitting method in a dog model. Oral Surg Oral Med Oral Pathol Oral Radiol Endod. 2009;107(3):351; with permission.)

ridge (**Fig. 8**).[20] The surgical technique was described in a case study by Garcia-Garcia and colleagues.[20] An incision is made in the mucosa along the crest of the alveolar ridge without a release. A tunnel is created between the vestibular mucosa and bone to the level of the base of the transport segment. The vestibular and lateral osteotomies are made using a ridge-splitting osteotome. The distractor screw is placed through the freed transport segment in a vestibular–lingual direction. The slow tension forces between the basal bone and transport device allow for the gradual growth of bone and soft tissue.

VERTICAL AUGMENTATION

It is generally accepted that the minimum bone height for successful placement of dental implants in ideal bone density is 10 mm (plus a margin of 2 mm from vital landmarks such as the inferior alveolar canal, floor of nose or maxillary sinus). Alveolar bone height less than 10 mm will require vertical augmentation to improve functional biomechanics and reduce excessive stresses on the implant. The consensus panel of the International Congress of Oral Implantologists recommended that vertical bone height for fixed prosthesis should be based on the excessive CHS[9] rather than an absolute number. According to the consensus panel, excessive CHS conditions relate to a CHS that is more than 15 mm. (The definition of CHS is from the bone to the occlusal plane.) An increased CHS of more than 15 mm is usually a result of the vertical loss of alveolar bone from long-standing edentulism. Vertical augmentation should aim to decrease the CHS to less than 15 mm. The ideal space for a cement-retained prosthesis is 9 mm to 10 mm in the posterior and 10 mm to 12 mm in a maxillary central. This dimension allows an ideal 3 mm of soft tissue, 2 mm of occlusal or porcelain thickness, and a 5-mm height for the abutment.[21] Prosthesis design is, therefore, an important consideration before surgical decisions are made. Overgrafting may produce a very short CHS, which would be unacceptable for prosthetic rehabilitation. An implant-retained removable prosthesis, in contrast, hand needs at least 15 mm to 17 mm of CHS. Overgrafting would also be deleterious in this reconstruction.

The issue of excessive CHS should be addressed before implant placement. Surgical augmentation of the residual ridge height will reduce the CHS and improve implant biomechanics. Surgical techniques available to remedy the problem are:

- Onlay block bone grafts
- Interpositional bone grafts
- GBR
- Distraction osteogenesis
- Particulate bone grafts with titanium mesh or barrier membranes.

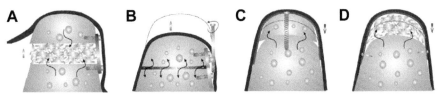

Fig. 9. Techniques for vertical ridge augmentation. (*A*) Interpositional graft. (*B*) Distraction osteogenesis. (*C*) Onlay bone graft. (*D*) GBR. (*From* Sheikh Z, Sima C, Glogauer M. Bone replacement materials and techniques used for achieving vertical alveolar bone augmentation. Materials. 2015;8(6):2953–93.)

A staged approach to reconstruction of the jaws is often preferred to simultaneous implant placement, especially when large volume gains are required (**Fig. 9**).[9]

Onlay Block Grafting

Onlay block bone grafting is when a block of transplanted bone tissue is placed directly unto the recipient bone at the intended implant site. Most often in the outpatient setting, the bone is harvested from the mandibular symphysis (which offers the greatest bone volume), external oblique ridge (lower morbidity compared with symphysis grafts), and rarely from coronoid process. These sites are readily available and will provide good bone quality and quantity with few postoperative complications. Allogenic grafts and anorganic bovine bone are other options with predictable success. Bone substitutes have not been shown to be reliable for vertical augmentation of the dentoalveolar process.

A conservative corticotomy is first performed at the recipient site to encourage blood clot formation and bone marrow osteoblast precursor migration into the graft. The bone block is next harvested from the selected donor site, contoured, and is laid over the prepared recipient site devoid of soft tissues, where it is fixated with osteosynthesis titanium screws as an onlay graft to achieve the desired vertical augmentation of the alveolar ridge. Placement of the bone graft should be guided by an augmentation template.[22] Close contact and good initial stabilization of the block graft to the recipient bed is critical to achieving a successful clinical result. Tension-free closure of the overlying soft tissue is required.

Interpositional Bone Grafts

The concept of interpositional or "sandwich" grafting is based on the theory that a bone graft placed between 2 pieces of pedicled bone with internal cancellous bone will undergo rapid and complete healing and graft incorporation.[23] The main advantage of this technique is the preservation of the attached gingiva. The bone pedicles are achieved through a vascularized segmental osteotomy performed on the alveolar bone. Success of the technique depends on maintaining the vascularization of the bone pedicles from the overlying periosteum. The free vascularized osteoperiosteal flap, in combination with the bone graft in the gap, raises the superior/inferior flap to the desired position to achieve vertical ridge augmentation. The incision is made in the free mucosa at least 10 mm lateral to the mucogingival junction to allow for closure. A vertical releasing incision is placed about 5 mm anteriorly to the planned graft site. If the graft site is close to the mental foramen, a mucosa-only dissection should be performed to isolate the branches of the mental nerve. The nerve branches may be retracted atraumatically with vessel loops.

The periosteum is incised 3 to 5 mm inferiorly to the planned osteotomy site and is elevated inferiorly only, maintaining the periosteal attachments to the superior aspect of the ridge. The lingual mucosa should not be elevated. The horizontal osteotomy is made above the inferior alveolar canal. The vertical bone cuts are made with minimal elevation of the periosteum. The osteotomy cuts should be made through the lingual cortical plate. A finger should be placed over the lingual mucosa to feel the cutting blade exit the bone but not the lingual mucosa. The alveolar ridge segment is mobilized passively and elevated to the extent of the soft tissue attachments.

Fixation is achieved with an X-shaped miniplate (1.2-mm screws) The plate should be attached first to the superior mobilized segment of the crest. After the plate is secured to the mobilized segment, it is raised to the desired height, oriented to minimize sharp edges on the lingual mucosa, and the final screws placed in the inferior intact bone. The space is then grafted. Cancellous/particulate marrow, autogenous block grafts, or a freeze-dried mineralized allograft may be used. The allograft has the advantage in that there is no donor site surgery. After the graft is placed, the incision should be closed without tension. Endosteal implants should be placed at 3 months after grafting.

Guided Bone Regeneration

GBR is a surgical procedure that uses barrier membranes to direct the growth of new bone. It may be achieved with or without particulate bone grafts and/or bone substitutes. Osseous regeneration by GBR depends on the migration of pluripotential and osteogenic cells (eg, osteoblasts derived from the periosteum and/or adjacent bone and/or bone marrow) to the bone defect site and exclusion of cells impeding bone formation (eg, epithelial cells and fibroblasts).[24] To ensure successful GBR, 4 principles need to be met: exclusion of epithelium and connective tissue, space maintenance, stability of the fibrin clot, and primary wound closure.[25] GBR is often considered to be the preferred technique for vertical ridge augmentation because it is highly predictable and has a low complication rate.

The surgical procedure for GBR depends on the size of the defect and on the prosthetic plan. For small defects, GBR and implant placement can be done at the same time if the osseous defect around the implant is small and good primary stabilization of the implant can be achieved. To increase the alveolar height and improve the ridge shape in larger defects, the GBR should be done before implant placement. For small defects in which GBR and implant placement is being done simultaneously, the use of an allograft material is recommended. For ridges with severe vertical bone loss, an autogenous graft combined with a xenograft should be used.

For small defects, a trapezoid flap can be used to expose the crest, followed by implant placement. The implant should be placed above the height of the atrophic ridge and covered by the graft material. The membrane is placed and secured. The wound is closed tension free.

In moderate to severe vertical edentulous bone loss, the goal is to replace the original bone crest of the edentulous area. The same incision that is used for the interpositional graft is used. If a large vertical bone loss area is to be grafted, a greater number of releasing incisions will be needed for tension-free flap closure because failure often occurs because of wound dehiscence. A full-thickness mucoperiosteal flap is elevated to adequately expose the edentulous area. Small bur holes are drilled through the cortex or a corticotomy is performed. The bone graft material is placed and molded to form and covered with a membrane, which is stabilized with titanium bone tacks. In the posterior maxillary, a vertical GBR procedure and maxillary sinus grafting using the lateral window approach could be done simultaneously. Treatment of complex vertical defects requires a stable and stiff membrane, usually made of titanium or metal-reinforced polytetrafluoroethylene.[26]

Distraction Osteogenesis

Distraction osteogenesis is a technique used to generate new bone after an osteotomy and gradual distraction. It is based on the biological principle of bone callus mechanical elongation through slow and progressive separation under tension of the 2 bone fragments surrounded by the callus to achieve new bone formation at the distraction gap.[27] In the edentulous alveolar ridge, small distraction devices are used to simultaneously gradually lengthen the bone and expand the soft tissue.

A horizontal mucoperiosteal incision is made following the mucogingival junction extending the extent of the defect to be elevated. The mucoperiosteal flap is elevated to about 5 mm beyond the planned osteotomy site. At the ends of the defect to be elevated, vertical tunneling is done toward the alveolar crest to facilitate vertical osteotomies. After adequate exposure, the distraction device should be adapted to the buccal cortex and the osteotomy line scored. In a long alveolar defect, 2 distraction devices are recommended to better control the vector of elongation at both bone edges. The horizontal and vertical osteotomies can be performed with a 701 fissure bur under copious irrigation with sterile water, taking care not to injure the medial mucosa and to preserve the blood supply to the bone from the medial periosteum. After completion of the osteotomies the alveolar segment is immobilized and the distractor is replaced. The distractor should be activated and the transport segment elevated about 5 mm to check for vertical movement without bony interferences. It is then brought back to the original position and the wound closed in layers—periosteal closure and mucosal closure.

The distraction phase should be started in 5 to 7 days to allow for the formation of a callus and healing of the soft tissue. The time period for distraction depends on the amount of augmentation that is required. The segment should be moved 0.5 mm twice daily to achieve a rate of 1 mm/d (**Fig. 10**). After distraction, a consolidation period of about 2 months should be maintained to allow the stretched callus to mature with the support of the device. It is important to keep the callus stable in the stretched position. We use a consolidation period of 1 week for each 1 mm of distraction and to wait for 1 month after removal of the distractor before implants are placed.

The procedure to be used for vertical augmentation is based on the amount of elevation that is, required from the residual alveolar crest for standard length crowns. The necessary bone elevation required can be divided as follows: small 3 to 5 mm, medium 6 to 9 mm, and large 10 mm.

- Small augmentations: onlay bone grafts, staged GBR
- Medium augmentations: GBR, onlay bone grafts, interpositional grafts with or without membranes
- Large augmentations: GBR, distraction osteogenesis, onlay graft (unpredictable)

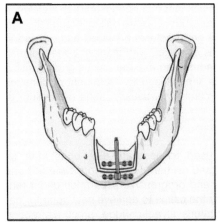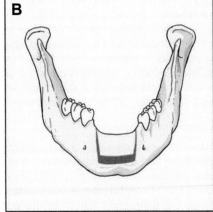

Fig. 10. Vertical distraction of deficient alveolar bone. (*From* Hariri F, Chin SY, Rengarajoo J, et al. Distraction osteogenesis in oral and craniomaxillofacial reconstructive surgery, osteogenesis and bone regeneration. In: Yang H, editor. Osteogenesis and bone regeneration. https://doi.org/10.5772/intechopen.81055).

Table 2 Complications by method of augmentation	
Method of Augmentation	**Complications**
Onlay graft	More complications in the vertical than in the horizontal bone grafts. Wound dehiscence Premature exposure of graft Mobility of the graft with fibrosis of the interface Resorption of graft before implant placement Screw loosening or fracture Infection
GBR	Wound dehiscence Premature exposure of the membrane Failure of the regeneration Additional graft needed at time of implant placement, to obtain sufficient implant stability
Distraction osteogenesis	Flap damage Inability to mobilize the transport fragment Tipping of transport segment Improper vector at one of the ends Lingual inclination of the transport segment in the mandible. Interference of the distractor with occlusion Fracture of the distractor Perforation of the mucosa by the transport segment Dehiscence of incision Resorption of the transport segment Infection
Ridge split	Only for vertically sufficient but horizontally insufficient alveolar ridges Flap damage Bad split Fracture of the buccal plate Complete loss of buccal bone Wound dehiscence Deficiency of the buccal volume at time of implant placement Buccal bone fracture at time of implant surgery Infection
Inlay bone graft	Only corrects vertical defects, not horizontal defects Flap damage Wound dehiscence Necrosis of alveolar segment Loss of graft Inadequate vertical augmentation for crown height.

COMPLICATIONS

Complications related to ridge augmentation can occur at the time of surgery, in the early postoperative stages, or late in the postoperative phase. Complications at the time of surgery include hemorrhage, soft tissue flap injury, injury of nerves, bone fracture, and an inability to obtain a tension-free closure (there is a relationship between flap tension and early wound dehiscence). Early complications include hematoma,

Box 3	
Complications related to bone augmentation procedures	
GBR	
Soft tissue dehiscence	1.7%
Membrane exposure	6.6%
Infection	2%
Insufficient augmentation	2%
Onlay bone grafts	
Soft tissue dehiscence	
Horizontal augmentation	25.9%
Vertical augmentation	18.2%
Infection	
Horizontal augmentation	11%
Vertical augmentation	9%
Insufficient augmentation	
Horizontal augmentation	37%
Vertical augmentation	9%
Distraction osteogenesis	
Wound dehiscence	4.7%
Displacement of the transport segment	41.6%
Lack of device activation	5.4%
Fracture of transport segment	1.8%
Infection	14.5%
Fracture of device	1.5%
Perforation of mucosa during distraction	1.7%
Ridge Split Technique	
Fracture of buccal plate in a 2-step procedure	6.7%
With immediate implant placement	23%

wound dehiscence, membrane and graft exposure, and infection. Late complications include significant graft resorption, shifting of the graft, fibrous union of the grafted bone, bony defects, and poor esthetics.

It should be noted that ridge augmentation in the vertical dimension has a higher complication rate and implant failure rate when compared with horizontal augmentations or sinus lift procedures (**Table 2**).[28]

An Internet literature search of articles listing bone grafting complications were selected and analyzed. The quality of the reports was not evaluated. The only criterion was that the article listed percentages for any complication related to alveolar ridge

Box 4
Generalizations
• The survival rates of implants placed into grafted areas are comparable with survival rates of implants placed into pristine bone.[33]
• Survival rates of implants placed in horizontally and vertically augmented alveolar ridges are high.[28]
• Augmentation of vertical alveolar ridge defects exhibit higher complication rates than those for horizontal defects.[34]
• Complications are higher in smokers.[35]

augmentation. The numbers shown in **Box 3** were selected from several Internet sources and averaged when more than one report was available. It must be emphasized that this search did not meet the standards of a review article nor was meta-analysis possible.

OUTCOMES

Advanced alveolar bone loss will always pose a problem for prosthetic rehabilitation for the individual. Retention and function of dentures are usually not satisfactory. The majority of these patients will not have sufficient bone in either vertical or horizontal dimensions for implants placement and will require ridge reconstruction before implant insertion. Augmentation of the residual alveolar bone will allow for the placement of dental implants with prosthetic rehabilitation which will be comfortable and very functional. Ridge augmentation has proven successful over a number of years with high implant survival rates. Implants placed in grafted maxillomandibular regions, displayed a success rate of 95.17%.[29] In a systematic review of 23 retrospective studies during a 5-year period, Albrektsson and Donos[30] reported a success rate of 97.7%.

In a more recent study that looked at 1222 patients with 2729 implants placed in pure native bone compared with those placed after a separate bone graft procedure from 1985 to 2012, the cumulative survival rates at 5 and 10 years were 92% and 87% for implants placed in native bone and 90% and 79% for implants placed in grafted bone, respectively.[31] The results from multivariate analysis (Cox regression) indicated no significant difference in survival between the 2 groups in this study. There was no difference in the dental implant survival rate when implants were placed in native bone or bone-grafted sites. Smoking and lack of professional maintenance were significantly related to increased implant loss.

In a systematic review of onlay grafts by Clementini and colleagues,[32] they observed a success rate of implants in areas of autogenous graft, ranging from 72.8% to 97%, in most of the reviewed studies (**Box 4**).

SUMMARY

Ridge augmentation for implant procedures has been shown to be very successful. There are several techniques available to the dentist but they require some degree of surgical expertise and experience. No particular technique has been shown to be superior. This article has presented the indications, techniques, and complications of the various procedures for alveolar ridge augmentation. This information will educate the general dental practitioner of the techniques available and provide information on the surgical procedures that could be used to discuss with patients when they are being referred to a specialist.

CLINICS CARE POINTS

- The greater the loss of teeth and consequently bone volume, the more challenging the process of achieving a functional and esthetic outcome becomes. A combination of surgical techniques may be required in order to achieve successful outcomes.
- The horizontal dimension of the available bone for implant placement should be 3 mm or greater than the diameter of the proposed implant.

- The vertical dimension requirements depend on tissue height, prosthetic needs and the proximity of the implant to vital structures.

DISCLOSURE

The authors have nothing to disclose.

REFERENCES

1. Dye BA, Thornton-Evans G, Li X, et al. Dental caries and tooth loss in adults in the United States. Hyattsville: U.S. Department of Health and Human Services, CDC, NCHS; 2015.
2. Cawood JI, Howell RA. A classification of edentulous jaws. Int J Oral Maxillofac Surg 1998;17:232–6.
3. Atwood DA, Coy WA. Clinical, cephalometric, and densitometric study of reduction of residual ridges. J Prosthet Dent 1971;26(3):280–95.
4. Camargo PM, Takei HH, Carranza FA. Bone Loss and Patterns of Bone Destruction. In: Newman and Carranza's clinical periodontology. 13th edition. St. Louis: Elsevier, Inc.; 2019. p. 316–27.
5. Carr AB, Brown DT. Partially, edentulous, epidemiology, physiology, and terminology. In: McCracken's removable partial Prosthodontics. 13th edition. St. Louis: Elsevier, Inc.; 2016. p. 2–7.
6. Tolstunov L. Combination syndrome: classification and case report. J Oral Implantol 2007;33(3):139–51.
7. Misch CE, Dietsh F. Bone-grafting materials in implant dentistry. Implant Dent 1993;2(3):158–67.
8. Resnik RR, Misch CE. Misch's contemporary implant dentistry. 4th edition. Canada: Elsevier; 2020.
9. Misch CE, Goodacre CJ, Finley JM, et al. Consensus conference panel report: crown-height space guidelines for implant dentistry—Part 1. Implant Dent 2005;14(4):312–21.
10. Milinkovic I, Cordaro L. Are there specific indications for the different alveolar bone augmentation procedures for implant placement? A systematic review. Int J Oral Maxillofac Surg 2014;43(5):606–25.
11. Block MS. Horizontal ridge augmentation using particulate bone. Atlas Oral Maxillofac Surg Clin North Am 2006;14(1):27–38.
12. Troeltzsch M, Troeltzsch M, Kauffmann P, et al. Clinical efficacy of grafting materials in alveolar ridge augmentation: a systematic review. J Craniomaxillofac Surg 2016;44(10):1618–29.
13. Deeb GR, Wilson GH, Carrico CK, et al. Is the tunnel technique more effective than open augmentation with a titanium-reinforced polytetrafluoroethylene membrane for horizontal ridge augmentation? J Oral Maxillofac Surg 2016;74(9):1752–6.
14. Haggerty CJ, Vogel CT, Fisher GR. Simple Bone Augmentation for Alveolar Ridge Defects. Oral Maxillofac Surg Clin North Am 2015;27(2):203–26.
15. Karmon B, Tavelli L, Rasperini G. Tunnel Technique with a Subperiosteal Bag for Horizontal Ridge Augmentation. Int J Periodontics Restorative Dent 2020;40(2):223–30.
16. Von Arx T, Buser D. Horizontal ridge augmentation using autogenous block grafts and the guided bone regeneration technique with collagen membranes: a clinical study with 42 patients. Clin Oral Implants Res 2006;17(4):359–66.

17. Dym H, Huang D, Stern A. Alveolar bone grafting and reconstruction procedures prior to implant placement. Dent Clin North Am 2012;56(1):209–18.
18. Kirpalani T, Dym H. Role of Piezo surgery and lasers in the oral surgery office. Dent Clin North Am 2020;64(2):351–63.
19. Vega LG, Bilbao A. Alveolar distraction osteogenesis for dental implant preparation: an update. Oral Maxillofac Surg Clin North Am 2010;22(3):369–85.
20. Garcia-Garcia A, Somoza-Martin M, Gandara-Vila P, et al. Horizontal alveolar distraction: a surgical technique with the transport segment pedicled to the mucoperiosteum. J Oral Maxillofac Surg 2004;62(11):1408–12.
21. Kendrick S, Wong D. Vertical and horizontal dimensions of implant dentistry: numbers every dentist should know. Inside Dent 2009;4287:2–5.
22. Essig H, Rücker M, Tavassol F, et al. Intraoperative Navigation und computerassistierte Chirurgie in der MKG-Chirurgie–Onkologische Chirurgie und rekonstruktive Tumorchirurgie. OP-JOURNAL 2011;27(02):130–7.
23. Frame JW, Browne RM, Brady CL. Biologic basis for interpositional autogenous bone grafts to the mandible. J Oral Maxillofac Surg 1982;40(7):407–11.
24. Liu J, Kerns DG. Suppl 1: mechanisms of guided bone regeneration: a review. Open Dent J 2014;8:56.
25. Wang H-L, Boyapati L. "PASS" principles for predictable bone regeneration. Implant Dent 2006;15(1):8–17.
26. Matilinna K. Barrier membranes for tissue regeneration and bone augmentation techniques in dentistry. Singapore: Pan Stanford Publishing; 2014.
27. Chiapasco M, Consolo U, Bianchi A, et al. Alveolar distraction osteogenesis for the correction of vertically deficient edentulous ridges: a multicenter prospective study on humans. Int J Oral Maxillofac Implants 2004;19(3):399–407.
28. Jensen SS, Terheyden H. Bone augmentation procedures in localized defects in the alveolar ridge: clinical results with different bone grafts and bone-substitute materials. Int J Oral Maxillofac Implants 2009;24(Suppl):218–36.
29. Salmen FS, Oliveira MR, Gabrielli MAC, et al. Bone grafting for alveolar ridge reconstruction. Review of 166 cases. Rev Col Bras Cir 2017;44(1):33–40.
30. Albrektsson T, Donos N. Implant survival and complications. The Third EAO consensus conference 2012. Clin Oral Implants Res 2012;23(Suppl 6):63–5.
31. Tran DT, Gay IC, Diaz-Rodriguez J, et al. Survival of dental implants placed in grafted and nongrafted bone: a retrospective study in a university setting. Int J Oral Maxillofac Implants 2016;31(2):310–7.
32. Clementini M, Morlupi A, Agrestini C, et al. Success rate of dental implants inserted in autologous bone graft regenerated areas: a systematic review. Oral Implantol (Rome) 2011;4(3–4):3–10.
33. Klein MO, Al-Nawas B. For which clinical indications in dental implantology is the use of bone substitute materials scientifically substantiated? Eur J Oral Implantol 2010;4:11–29.
34. Rocchietta I, Fontana F, Simion M. Clinical outcomes of vertical bone augmentation to enable dental implant placement: a systematic review. J Clin Periodontol 2008;35(8 Suppl):203–15.
35. Widmark G, Andersson B, Carlsson GE, et al. Rehabilitation of patients with severely resorbed maxillae by means of implants with or without bone grafts: a 3- to 5-year follow-up clinical report. Int J Oral Maxillofac Implants 2001;16(1):73–9.

Implant Surgery Update for the General Practitioner
Dealing with Common Postimplant Surgery Complications

Rinil Patel, DDS*, Earl Clarkson, DDS

KEYWORDS

- Implant complications • Nerve injury • Infection • Antibiotics • Sinusitis
- Membrane perforation • Edema

KEY POINTS

- Postimplant surgery complications are common.
- Nerve injuries should be identified and diagnosed based on degree of injury.
- Routine implants do not need antibiotics unless patient returns with an infection.
- Sinusitis first-line antibiotic is amoxicillin with or without clavulanate.
- Ibuprofen and dexamethasone can reduce postoperative edema and discomfort.

INTRODUCTION

The introduction of implants has revolutionized restorative and surgical dentistry. With the evolution of technology, implants have become more affordable, become smaller, and come with different surface types and shapes. However, even with these technological advances, knowledge of the anatomy, surgical skill, and management of common complications are of upmost importance. Postimplant placement complications can be separated into 2 categories: early failure or late failure. Early failure usually is within the first 6 months or before osseointegration, whereas late failures are after the first 6 months or during the restorative phase.[1,2] Primary predictors of implant failure include poor bone quality, chronic periodontitis, systemic diseases, smoking, advanced age, implant location, parafunctional habits, loss of implant integration, and inappropriate prosthesis.[3] This article discusses common postimplant surgery failures and management of these complications.

NYC Health + Hospitals/Woodhull, 760 Broadway, Room 2C-320, Brooklyn, NY 11206, USA
* Corresponding author.
E-mail address: rinilpateldds@gmail.com

Dent Clin N Am 65 (2021) 125–134
https://doi.org/10.1016/j.cden.2020.09.010
0011-8532/21/Published by Elsevier Inc.

dental.theclinics.com

NEUROSENSORY DISTURBANCES AND NERVE INJURY

Neurosensory disturbances throughout the maxillofacial region can occur because of trauma, neoplasms, infections, or secondary to a surgical procedure. Two common neurosensory injury classification systems are Seddon and Sunderland. The classifications systems are explained in **Table 1**.

A review of published literature reveals studies investigating the incidence of injury are inconsistent.[4] Published articles of nerve injury from implant placement range between 0% and 13% with some reporting incidence rates as high as 40%.[5,6] These inconsistencies are primarily due to interchangeable definitions of nerve injury and evaluation. Neurosensory disturbances can be permanent or transient. Patients usually suffer varying degrees of the following symptoms: numbness to teeth, chin, cheeks, and lips, speech impediments, problems with speech and mastication, inability to control food and liquid with unintended drooling, and occasionally, chronic pain.[7]

Nerve damage is more likely to occur when placing dental implants in the mandible. As bone resorption occurs in the mandible, the distance from the alveolar crest to the inferior alveolar nerve and mental nerve decreases, consequently increasing the chance of accidental nerve injury. Nerve damage after implant surgery is mainly caused by direct or indirect injury from osteotomy drilling or implant placement, stretching of the nerve caused by excess traction of the flap, or direct needle injury.[8] Postoperative edema can be another cause of paresthesia; however, this usually will resolve once the edema subsides.[9] The most common areas to be affected are the lower lip and chin region; although unlikely, but still possible, are the tongue, palate, and localized tissues.

In order to avoid nerve injuries, the practitioner should always refer to radiographic imaging before implant placement. If 3-dimensional imaging is available, this is far

Table 1
Classification of nerve injuries and associated findings

Injury Type	Extent of Injury	Recovery Time	Surgical Treatment
Sunderland 1st degree (Seddon neuropraxia)	Transient ischemia, anoxia, ± segmental demyelination, intrafascicular edema causing block of conduction	Fast: hours to weeks	None indicated
Sunderland 2nd degree (Seddon axonotmesis)	Axon and myelin interruption (intact endoneurium, perineurium, and epineurium)	Slow: weeks Regeneration rate 1–3 mm/d	None indicated
Sunderland 3rd degree	Injury involves endoneurium (intact perineurium and epineurium)	Slow: weeks to months	Nerve exploration can be considered
Sunderland 4th degree	Injury involves endoneurium and perineurium (intact epineurium)	Spontaneous recovery not likely	Microneurosurgery
Sunderland 5th degree (Seddon neurotmesis)	Complete nerve transection, continuity disruption	Spontaneous recovery not possible	Microneurosurgery

Adapted from Miloro M, Kolokythas A. Traumatic injuries of the trigeminal nerve. In: Fonseca RJ, Walker RV, Barber HD, et al, editors. Oral and maxillofacial trauma, 4th edition. St. Louis: Elsevier Saunders; 2013. p. 662; with permission

superior to traditional 2-dimensional imaging. If only 2-dimensional imaging is available, using a radiographic marker will help calibrate any digital measurements and reduce the margin of error for inaccuracies. Using available software to map and highlight the nerve will always help plan for accurate placement as well as using implant planning software. Another important factor to consider is the length of each implant drills. Traditionally, implant drills have measurement markings to denote the depth within the bone. However, the start and stop point of these measurements may vary from manufacturer to manufacturer. There can be an additional 0.5 to 2 mm at the tip of the drill from the indicator line. It is crucial to read your implant manufacturer's catalog or contact the representative to understand the exact length and where the depth measurements are taken from. Another way to ensure proper depth management is by taking intraoperative radiographs. These radiographs will help the clinician know where he or she is within the bone. Another way to avoid nerve damage is to control flap retraction. Overreflection of a flap, especially in the area of the mental nerve, can cause stretching and transient neurosensory disturbances, and always place retractors on bone, not the soft tissue.

If a postoperative patient is noted to have a neurosensory injury, the first important step is early identification and diagnosis of the degree of injury. Subsequently, management is based upon mechanism, location, and degree of injury. An injury from overretraction of a flap (Seddon neuropraxia, Sunderland first degree) could completely resolve on its own or with adjunctive pharmacologic therapy. If a crush injury is suspected directly from an implant, similar to **Fig. 1**, then the implant should be backed out immediately or removed completely.[5] In addition, pharmacologic

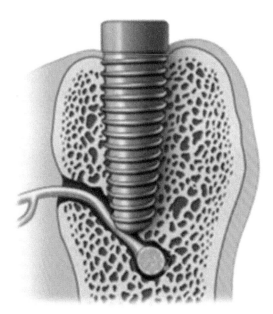

Fig. 1. Implant-related nerve injury that can occur when the implant is in proximity to the closed canal with possible bleeding, edema, and development of a compartment syndrome that causes deleterious effects on the nerve, even in the short term. (*From* Miloro M, Kolokythas A. Traumatic injuries of the trigeminal nerve. In: Fonseca RJ, Walker RV, Barber HD, et al, editors. Oral and maxillofacial trauma, 4th edition. St. Louis: Elsevier Saunders; 2013. p. 666; with permission.)

therapy should also be initiated with close monitoring of the patient. Subjective findings the patient may share should be documented, but objective findings should also be noted. Baseline testing should include testing for touch with von Frey hairs, 2-point discrimination with a Boley gauge or similar, temperature, and taste (if involvement of lingual nerve is suspected). Evaluations should be completed every 3 weeks postoperatively to assess for changes in the patient's condition. If the patient has persistent anesthesia at 6 to 9 weeks, microneurosurgery should be considered, and appropriate referrals given to the patient in a timely fashion.[10]

PREOPERATIVE ANTIBIOTICS AND POSTOPERATIVE INFECTIONS

The routine use of prophylactic antibiotics in implant dentistry seems to be widespread. However, the use of preoperative, perioperative, and postoperative antibiotics in dental implant surgery remains controversial. A search of the literature can show postoperative infections as high as 5.9% to 11.5% with antibiotics and as low as 7.0% without antibiotics.[11] According to Mazzocchi and colleagues,[12] apart from individuals suffering from systemic diseases, most patients undergoing dental implant surgery are healthy individuals who do need antibiotics for small surgical wounds. A study published in the *Journal of Hospital Infection* reported there was some evidence that 2 g of amoxicillin given 1 hour preoperatively reduced early failures of dental implants, although further research was needed to confirm the findings.[13]

The 2 most common types of dental implant-associated infections are peri-implant mucositis and peri-implantitis. Peri-implant mucositis is inflammation confined to the soft tissues surrounding an implant without signs of bone loss following normal bone remodeling. Peri-implantitis is an inflammatory process that affects both the soft tissue and the bone surrounding an implant beyond what is biologically expected (**Fig. 2**).[14] **Table 2** outlines the distinctions between the two.

The main problems when determining frequency of peri-implant mucositis and peri-implantitis are the lack of a common definition, study populations, and implant structures. Presently, there is no reliable evidence for treating perimucositis and peri-implantitis. Although some clinicians advise systemic antibiotics and oral agents to clean the surface of implants, there has yet to be a double-blind, randomized,

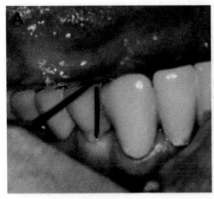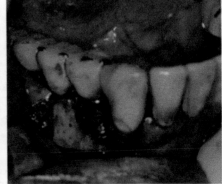

Fig. 2. Peri-implantitis in the right mandible. Probing with exudate, probing depth ≥4 mm, bone loss. (*From* Misch CE. An implant is not a tooth: a comparison of periodontal indices. In: Misch CE, editor. Dental implant prosthetics. St. Louis: Elsevier Mosby; 2015. p. 63; with permission.)

Table 2			
Diagnostic comparison of peri-implantitis versus peri-implant mucositis			
	BOP ± Exudate	**Probing Depth ≥4 mm**	**Radiographic Bone Loss**
Peri-implant mucositis	+	+	−
Peri-implantitis	+	+	+

Abbreviation: BOP, bleeding on probing
  From Robertson K, Shahbazian T, MacLeod S. Treatment of peri-implantitis and the failing implant. Dent Clin North Am. 2015;59(2):331; with permission.

placebo-controlled trial to prove this.[13] Because of this, treatment goals should incorporate preventing further bone loss, functionality of the implant, esthetics, and ultimately, loss of the implant itself.[4] In order to do so, the treatment modalities can include mechanical debridement, pharmacologic treatment (ie, chlorhexidine irrigation, local antibiotics, systemic antibiotics), surgical debridement, and correct anatomic conditions that impair plaque control.[13] Further treatment options are explained in "An Update on the Treatment of Peri-Implantitis" by Raza Hussan and Michael Miloro in this issue.

Following implant surgery, if a patient returns with tissue erythema, pain, or other signs of an active infection, the clinician must differentiate between normal postoperative symptoms versus active infection. If a patient returns with abscess formation, an incision and drainage should be completed and the patient should be started on antibiotic therapy.[2] During incision and drainage, any purulent drainage should be cultured and submitted for bacterial sensitivity. If a fistula is noted and the clinician is unsure of the infection source, a gutta percha cone can be inserted into the fistula and along with radiographic imaging to trace the source. If an implant is removed, it is important to understand the survival rate of subsequent implant placement decreases. Agari and colleagues[15] noted over a 7-year study with placement of 5532 implants that the survival rate for initial implants was 95%. However, the survival rate at first reimplantation was 77%; survival rate at second reimplantation was 73%, and by the third reimplantation, survival rate was 50%.

SINUSITIS AND SINUS MEMBRANE PERFORATIONS

Of the paranasal sinuses, the maxillary sinus is the largest, approximately 15 mL in volume, and tends to increase with the loss of the maxillary premolars and molars. Sinus augmentation is indicated when a patient presents with an edentulous and atrophic maxillary alveolus that cannot support an implant. When inserting dental implants in the posterior maxilla, the clinician should always be aware of the location to the maxillary sinus, the Schneiderian membrane, and the possible complications that can arise. When a dental implant becomes infected, sinusitis can easily occur because of the local spread of inflammation.[16] Sinusitis is one of the most commonly diagnosed diseases in the United States. It refers to inflammation within the maxillary sinus and is characterized as acute when lasting less than 4 weeks, subacute when lasting 4 to 8 weeks, and chronic when lasting longer than 8 weeks.[17] When dealing with sinusitis, it is important to understand the bacterial species that can cause an acute infection. The usual pathogens in an acute bacterial sinusitis include *Streptococcus pneumoniae*, *Haemophilus influenzae*, and *Moraxella catarrhalis*, while anaerobes, other Streptococci, Staphylococci, and Neisseria are also frequently isolated in sinus aspirate cultures.[18,19]

According to the literature, maxillary sinusitis secondary to sinus augmentation ranges between 0% and 20%, whereas perforation of the sinus membrane ranges between 10% and 55%.[20,21] In this setting, maxillary sinusitis can be explained by obliteration or blockage of the ostium (because of edema, hematoma, or dislodged graft), impaired mucus production, or impaired ciliary function (**Fig. 3**). Perforations are usually due to operator error, anatomic variations within the sinus, thin membranes, sinus pathologic condition, bony septa, second sinus surgery, or excess placement of graft material.[20] It is prudent not to overpack the bone graft material, as this can also lead to blockage of the ostium, leading to inflammation and then infection of the maxillary sinus.

With the introduction of newer instruments to facilitate the operator during sinus augmentation procedures, the incidence of perforations, in theory, should decrease. Examples of these instruments include Piezosurgery (Mectron s.p.a., Italy) or Dentium Advanced Sinus Kit (Dentium USA, Cypress, California), which use either ultrasonic transduction or diamond-coated burs to help prevent membrane perforations when accessing the maxillary sinus. When initially performing a lateral window, the operator should ensure the access is large and above the alveolus, as this will facilitate lifting the membrane in subsequent steps. Another trick that can help, if a small portion of the membrane is noted to be "stuck" along the floor or wall, opening a wet 4 × 4 gauze and carefully and continually feeding the gauze into an area where the membrane is already lifted can sometimes help free the adhered segment.

Amoxicillin with or without clavulanate is considered to be the first-line antibiotic choice of acute sinusitis. For those penicillin-allergic, either doxycycline, a respiratory fluoroquinolone (levofloxacin or moxifloxacin), or a combination therapy of clindamycin plus a third-generation oral cephalosporin (cefixime or cefpodoxime) is recommended.[22] Oral cephalosporins are no longer recommended for the empiric monotherapy as well as trimethoprim-sulfamethoxazole and macrolides (azithromycin and

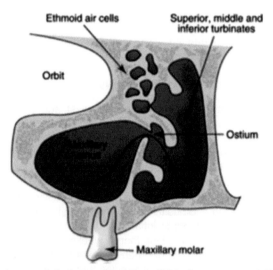

Fig. 3. Maxillary sinus and drainage via ostium. If blockage occurs at the ostium due to edema, hematoma, or dislodged graft, then the sinus would be unable to drain, leading to sinusitis. (*From* Treadway AL, Bankston SA. Dental implant prosthetic rehabilitation: sinus grafting. In: Bagheri SC, Bell RB, Khan HA, editors. Current therapy in oral and maxillofacial surgery. 1st edition. St Louis (MO): Elsevier Saunders; 2012. p. 168; with permission.)

clarithromycin) owing to unacceptably high rates of resistance to *S pneumoniae* and *M catarrhalis*.[19] Concurrently with antibiotics, other adjunctive therapies should include adequate hydration (6–8 glasses of water daily), sleep, nutrition, systemic or nasal decongestants, nasal saline sprays, and pain control, while minimizing irritants such as smoking.[5,19]

Box 1
Classification of sinus perforations with options for repair: Vlassis and Fugazatto

Class I
   Perforation is adjacent to the osteotomy site. Class I perforations are often "sealed off" as a result of the membrane folding on itself following completion of elevation.
   Repair Options: If membrane has folded over itself, no further treatment needed. If the perforation is small and isolated, collage tape is placed over the area with 3-mm overlap onto unaffected membrane and place graft material at the borders of the collagen tape. Margins of intact membrane can be sutured over perforations or suture a medial-free margin to periosteum lateral to osteotomy with resorbable suture.

Class II
   Perforation is located in the midsuperior aspect of the osteotomy, extending mesiodistally for two-thirds of the dimension of total osteotomy site. This occurs most with an infrastructure design of the osteotomy, rather than removing a bony window.
   Repair options: same as class I perforation. Note, suturing may be more difficult in this scenario.

Class III
   Perforation is located at the inferior border of the osteotomy at its mesial or distal sixth. This is the **most common perforation** and is almost always the result of inadequacy of osteotomy or improper execution of membrane reflection. Conversion of ostetomy design from a square to a rounded edge will dramatically decrease instance.
   Repair options: completion of membrane reflection rarely results in covering a class III perforation. If the membrane may be elevated around the perforation, thus allowing sufficient movement of both margins of the tear, then suturing may be an option, with subsequent covering with a lamellar bone sheet. If margins cannot be elevated, the ostetomy site should be extended to include the perforated area, begin elevating at a new site, and lead toward the perforation, then suture the perforation. Last option would be to use a large lamellar bone sheet and produce a pouch over the perforated region.

Class IV
   Perforation is located in the central two-thirds of the inferior border of the osteotomy site. Such a perforation is rare and is almost always caused by lack of care when preparing the osteotomy site. A tear in this area is also seen with improper septal elevation. Such a tear also enlarges dramatically as management is attempted and represents a considerable clinical challenge.
   Repair options: repair options are similar to those of class III, except rather than extending the ostetomy site, a new ostetomy site should be prepared.

Class V
   Perforation is a preexisting area of exposure of the sinus membrane, due to combination of extensive antral pneumatization and severe ridge resorption. Prior oral-antral fistula may also be a contributing factor.
   Repair options: an ostetomy is performed, which results in the creation of 2 free-floating semiluna areas around the class V perforation. These "islands" are positioned over each other and sutured, and the area is covered with resorbable tape. Once such closure is accomplished, a conventional ostetomy site is then prepared lateral to the perforation.

From Vlassis JM, Fugazzotto PA. A classification system for sinus membrane perforations during augmentation procedures with options for repair. *J Periodont.* 1999;70(6):692–9; with permission.

Sinus membrane perforations and tears are frequently caused by forceful elevation. In 1999, Vlassis and Fugazatto[23] published a classification system with options for repair (**Box 1**).

POSTOPERATIVE EDEMA

Postoperative edema is characterized by accumulation of fluid in interstitial tissue. The amount of edema is proportional to the amount of tissue injury, and more edema is likely with more loose connective tissue at the surgical site.[24] Postoperative swellings can have a negative impact on the surgical site and a patient's clinical condition. The main mediators of the inflammation in the postoperative stage are cyclooxygenase (COX) and prostaglandins. When tissue is manipulated or injured, phospholipids are converted to arachidonic acid, which then produces prostaglandins and thromboxane A_2 (collectively known as prostanoids) via COX enzymes.[25] It is important to be able to distinguish normal postoperative edema versus an acute infection (**Fig. 4**).

Postoperative edema can be minimized with shorter surgical times, flapless surgeries, practitioner experience, elevation, ice, and pharmacologic management. Generally, postoperative edema will begin shortly after surgery and will increase for 48 hours, peaking at about 72 hours.[26] The use of nonsteroidal anti-inflammatory drugs (NSAIDs) provides analgesia and anti-inflammatory effects by inhibiting the synthesis of prostaglandins from arachidonic acid, while glucocorticoids alter the connective tissue response to injury by inhibiting phospholipase A_2, thereby reducing arachidonic acid release.[25]

Prescribing 600 mg ibuprofen 1 hour before surgery and 600 mg 6 hours after the first dose or 4 mg dexamethasone 1 hour before surgery and 4 mg 6 hours after the first dose significantly reduced pain up to 3 days after surgery, reducing discomfort 2 days after surgery.[27] The author of this article supports prescribing 600 mg ibuprofen 1 hour before and every 6 hours thereafter for up to 3 to 5 days as needed for pain, supplemented with 1000 mg acetaminophen as needed for breakthrough pain (not to exceed 4000 mg in 24 hours), and 4 mg dexamethasone 1 hour before surgery and 4 mg 6 hours after the first dose. Alternatively, a methylprednisolone tapering dose pack may be prescribed. When prescribing steroids, close postoperative

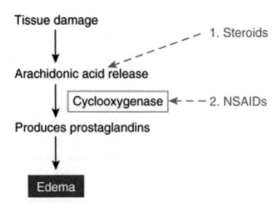

Fig. 4. Pathophysiology of edema and inhibitor mechanism of glucocorticoids and NSAID medications. (*From* Resnik RR. Pharmacology in implant dentistry. In: Resnik RR, editor. Misch's contemporary implant dentistry. 4th ed. Elsevier; 2020. p. 366; with permission.)

management is recommended, although most patients will not have any adverse outcomes.

CLINICS CARE POINTS

- Obtaining adequate imaging before implant placements can avoid neurosensory disturbances.
- Early identification and treatment of neurosensory disturbances are key for successful recovery.
- Recurrent infections from peri-implantitis or perimucositis decrease chances of implant survival.
- After removal of an infected dental implant, odds of successful osteointegration of the subsequent implant decrease.
- The use of diamond-coated rotary instruments will help decrease membrane perforation when creating a bony window for sinus augmentation,
- Postoperative edema can be decreased by starting the patient on preoperative steroids.

DISCLOSURE

The authors have nothing to disclose.

REFERENCES

1. Froum SJ. Dental implant complications etiology, prevention, and treatment. Hoboken: Wiley-Blackwell; 2010.
2. Singh P, Cranin AN. Atlas of oral implantology. Maryland Heights: Mosby; 2010.
3. Manor Y, Oubaid S, Mardinger O, et al. Characteristics of early versus late implant failure: a retrospective study. J Oral Maxillofac Surg 2009;67(12): 2649–52.
4. Khoury F, Keeve P, Ramanauskaite A, et al. "Surgical treatment of peri-implantitis - Consensus Report of Working Group 4." International Dental Journal, U.S. National Library of Medicine. 2019. Available at: www.ncbi.nlm.nih.gov/pubmed/ 31478576. Accessed April 20, 2020.
5. Dym H. Implant procedures for the general dentist. Philadelphia: Elsevier; 2015.
6. Fonseca RJ. Oral & maxillofacial trauma. St. Louis: Elsevier; 2013.
7. Libersa P, Savignat M, Tonnel A. Neurosensory disturbances of the inferior alveolar nerve: a retrospective study of complaints in a 10-year period. J Oral Maxillofac Surg 2007;65(8):1486–9.
8. Park YT, Kin SG, Moon SY. Indirect compressive injury to the inferior alveolar nerve caused by dental implant placement. J Oral Maxillofac Surg 2012;70(4): e258–9.
9. Garg AK. Implant dentistry a practical approach. Maryland Heights: Elsevier; 2010.
10. Park C, Indresano T. Nerve evaluation protocol 2014. Oakland: California Association of Oral and Maxillofacial Surgeons; 2014.
11. Figueiredo R, Camps-Font O, Valmaseda-Castellon E, et al. Risk factors for postoperative infections after dental implant placement: a case-control study. J Oral Maxillofac Surg 2015;73(12):2312–8.
12. Mazzocchi A, Passi L, Moretti R. Retrospective analysis of 736 implants inserted without antibiotic therapy. J Oral Maxillofac Surg 2007;65(11):2321–3.

13. Pye AD, Lockhart DEA, Dawson MP, et al. A review of dental implants and infection. J Hosp Infect 2009;72(2):104–10.
14. Rosen P, Clem D, Cochran D, et al. Academy report: peri-implant mucositis and peri-implantitis: a current understanding of their diagnoses and clinical implications. J Periodontol 2013;84(4):436–43.
15. Agari KM, Le B. Re-implantation of dental implants in sites of previous failure. J Oral Maxillofac Surg 2018;76(10). https://doi.org/10.1016/j.joms.2018.06.124.
16. Ueda M, Kaneda T. Maxillary sinusitis caused by dental implants: report of two cases. J Oral Maxillofac Surg 1992;50(3):285–7.
17. Salvin R, Spector S, Bernstein I. The diagnosis and management of sinusitis: a practice parameter update. J Allergy Clin Immunol 2005;116(6):S13–47.
18. Cook HE, Haber J. Bacteriology of the maxillary sinus. J Oral Maxillofac Surg 1987;45(12):1011–4.
19. Hupp JR, Ferneini EM. Head, neck, and orofacial infections: an interdisciplinary approach. St. Louis: Elsevier; 2016.
20. Timmenga NM, Raghoebar GM, Boering G, et al. Maxillary sinus function after sinus lifts for the insertion of dental implants. J Oral Maxillofac Surg 1997;55(9):936–9.
21. Nolan P, Freeman K, Kraut R. Correlation between Schneiderian membrane perforation and sinus lift graft outcome: a retrospective evaluation of 359 augmented sinus. J Oral Maxillofac Surg 2014;72(1):47–52.
22. Rosenfeld R, Piccirillo J, Chandrasekhar S, et al. Clinical practice guideline (update): adult sinusitis. Otolaryngol Head Neck Surg 2015;152(2_suppl):S1–39.
23. Vlassis JM, Fugazzotto PA. A classification system for sinus membrane perforations during augmentation procedures with options for repair. J Periodontol 1999;70(6):692–9.
24. Resnik RR, Misch CE. Misch's avoiding complications in oral implantology. St. Louis: Elsevier; 2018.
25. Ricciotti E, Fitzgerald GA. Prostaglandins and inflammation. Arterioscler Thromb Vasc Biol 2011;31(5):986–1000.
26. Niamtu J. Cosmetic facial surgery. Elsevier; 2018.
27. Bahammam M, Kayal R, Alasmari D, et al. Comparison between dexamethasone and ibuprofen for postoperative pain prevention and control after surgical implant placement: a double-masked, parallel-group, placebo-controlled randomized clinical trial. J Periodontol 2017;88(1):69–77.

Prosthodontic Principles in Dental Implantology

Adjustments in a Coronavirus Disease-19 Pandemic-Battered Economy

Ricardo A. Boyce, DDS, FICD[a,b,*]

KEYWORDS

- Personal protective equipment (PPE) • Implant-protective occlusion (IPO)
- Patient-reported outcome measures (PROM) • Quality of life (QOL)
- Oral rehabilitation/reconstruction • Fixed dental prostheses (FDP)
- Implant overdentures (IOD)
- Implant-supported fixed complete dental prostheses (IFCDPs)

KEY POINTS

- Since the coronavirus disease 2019 pandemic, several businesses have closed and many people have been left jobless.
- The current recession will have a negative impact on dentists and dental offices in the United States and worldwide.
- The modern-day dentist will need to be conservative and may need to implement payment plans as means to encourage patients to invest in implant treatment.
- Long spanned and/or complex implant cases should have mandatory occlusal-protected appointments.
- The general practitioner is challenged on a daily basis to make clinical decisions based off of the patient's anatomy, needs, and wishes, in order, to select the best prostheses.

More than 5 million dental implants are placed annually by dentists in the United States, according to the American Dental Association. Oral health enhances a patients' quality of life.[1] Pjetursson and colleagues[2,3] reported that "the survival rates of implant-supported single crowns and fixed dental prostheses (FDPs) range between 89% and 94% at 10 years.

The current pandemic of coronavirus disease 2019 (COVID-19) has caused >1 million deaths worldwide and >230,000 deaths in the United States, and these numbers are growing every day. On a brighter note, more than 30 million people have recovered worldwide. Coronaviruses are a group of viruses that can cause a

[a] The Brooklyn Hospital Center, 121 Dekalb Avenue, Box 187, Brooklyn, NY 11201, USA; [b] New York University, College of Dentistry, New York, NY, USA
* The Brooklyn Hospital Center, 121 Dekalb Avenue, Box 187, Brooklyn, NY 11201.
E-mail addresses: raboycedds@yahoo.com; rboyce@tbh.org

Dent Clin N Am 65 (2021) 135–165
https://doi.org/10.1016/j.cden.2020.09.011
0011-8532/21/© 2020 Elsevier Inc. All rights reserved.

variety of respiratory illnesses (ie, pneumonia) that can lead to respiratory failure. SARS-CoV-2 (severe acute respiratory syndrome coronavirus 2) was renamed COVID-19 (coronavirus disease 2019). Current medical/ dental literature on the COVID-19 pandemic suggests that dentists, oral surgeons, and otolaryngologists–head and neck surgeons are at high risk of contagion owing to the exposure to saliva, blood, aerosol, and droplets.[4,5] This crisis has resulted in people being quarantined in their homes (in attempts to contain the spread of the virus), schools closing, restaurants closing, businesses cutting staff or closing themselves, and ultimately leading to millions of people losing their jobs (income). More than 30 million people in the United States have claimed themselves jobless (unemployed) at the end of April, 2020. The recession in the United States will eventually rebound in a positive direction with time. At the beginning of the pandemic, the effect on dentists and staff were challenging owing to some office closings and the temporary hold on all elective procedures (recommended by state governors), while only focusing on dental emergencies. The dental implant market in the United States and globally will take a hit financially during the pandemic. There will be patients who were able to afford implants (before the pandemic) who will be unaffected, there may be another working class who (once were able) may not be in a position to afford or consider implants as a necessity. The modern-day dentist should be understanding, may have to be more conservative with their patients' treatment plan, and suggest to them ways of investing in an implant 1 or 2 at a time. The dental office may need to implement down payments or payment plans (before treatment) as a way of encouraging implant care. This consideration can be extended by the doctor that has a heart for providing quality dentistry for their fellow man or woman, that is, the patient. The modern-day dentist or general practitioner (GP) should implement reproducible treatment protocols, which will propel more successful outcomes.[6] The 5 concepts for dental implant success include (1) past medical history, (2) examination and occlusion, (3) dental imaging, (4) fixed verses removable prosthodontics, and (5) surgery, and are reviewed in this article (**Fig 1**).[7] The goal is to bring forth proven contributions of evidence based dentistry in the complex discipline of dental implantology in a format that will strengthen the decision making process of the GP in the clinical setting. At the end of this article, the reader will be able to make efficient, intelligent, and methodical treatments based off current scientific research (systemic reviews, randomized controlled trials, meta-analysis, and retrospective studies) and the foundation of textbooks on dental implantology. The objective during this challenging time in our profession is to make dental implants affordable for the patient, enhance their ability to function, improve their aesthetics, and improve their overall quality of life. Pictures (from cases) have been included to describe certain topics discussed, is in no way to lead or influence the GP to use a particular treatment. The pictures are to be used as visual aids to bring light to the literature being discussed. Because there are so many variables mentioned in this article, the reader should always consider whatever works for them or more conservative approaches when it comes to their case(s).

The first discussion will be on the use of personal protective equipment (PPE) for the safety of the doctor(s), dental hygienist, and staff. The Centers for Disease Control and Prevention and other state and local health department have continued to instruct and respond to the outbreak of the COVID-19 respiratory disease. All patients should be triaged over the phone, queried about any recent travel histories, if they have tested positive for COVID-19 (or awaiting test results), if they have a fever (>100.4°F), chills, shaking, body aches, headache, itchy throat, dry throat, dry cough, shortness of breath, or loss of smell or taste. They should also be asked if their family members or loved ones (having contact) have had the virus. The patients should be instructed

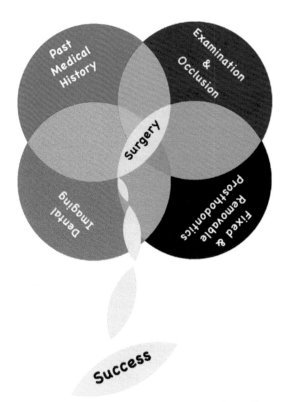

Fig. 1. The 5 concepts for dental implant success. (*Courtesy of* Ricardo A. Boyce, DDS, FICD. © 2015.)

to wear some sort of mask or face covering to protect themselves and others before their office visit. Please note that the questions mentioned should be followed up on arrival to the dental clinic. All members of the health care team (dentists, dental hygienists, dental assistants, and receptionist) should be wearing masks and washing their hands throughout the day and be prepared to triage all patients (before any treatment). The temperature should be taken with a contact-free forehead thermometer. Patients should have a review of systems and their vitals (temperature) checked before treatment. Those patients that present to the office (or queried over the phone) with a fever (>100.4°F) and any of the other symptoms mentioned should not be treated and given another appointment at least 2 weeks from the date (or until the patient is cleared from the virus/disease).[8,9] The dentist can prescribe acetaminophen (if the patient does not have in their possession or at home) should any fever exist and be instructed to contact their physicians and/or specialists for medical advice (a medical consult can be written). If the patient presents with symptoms of new confusion, dyspnea, severe dysphagia, airway compromise, bluish lips (or face), persistent pain or pressure in the chest, and fever, then emergency medical services should called immediately. Until more is learned about this virus, appointments should be booked to allow social distancing in the reception area and every patient should be treated as if they were COVID-19 positive. The use of air purifiers or air scrubbers (with HEPA filters and UVC light disinfection) can be considered for each treatment room. The rooms to be allowed to be aired out (or with the windows open) in between cases. Dental procedures can be performed if there is absence of contacts and/or symptoms.[5] High-speed handpieces and ultrasonic devices should be minimized; the use of rubber dams are highly recommended.[8,9]

When patients arrive they should be given level 1 masks (if they do not present with one) to wear in waiting room. The goal of the office staff should be to protect all patients and staff. When the procedures are about to start, all staff (in the surgical room) should be should be wearing N-95 or KN95 or level 3 (depending on the procedure) masks or masks with a face shield or goggles and/or a separate face shield; in addition, a full-length gown should also be worn. The clinician can review a list of guidelines and recommendations from the Centers for Disease Control and Prevention's website (https://www.cdc.gov/coronavirus/2019-ncov/hcp/dental-settings.html). Good judgment for PPE should be used for the type of procedure, because it can be adjusted for minor follow-up procedures. The dental staff should perform hand hygiene using alcohol-based hand sanitizer and alcohol hand rubs before and after all patient contact, contact with potentially infectious material, and before putting on and upon removal of PPE, including gloves. The recommendation is to wash hands with soap and water for at least 20 seconds. If hands are visibly soiled, use soap and water before returning to alcohol-based hand sanitizer.

The donning (putting on) and doffing (taking off) should be done by those health care workers who are treating and in direct contact with patients. Those dental professionals who work in a hospital or have to consult COVID-19–infected patients (on the floors) may feel more comfortable using a P 100 or N 100 mask instead of an N-95 mask. Any clinician who will be performing implant procedures in the hospital operating room will be practicing surgical scrubbing, gowning, and gloving, and others can obtain a more detailed description of donning and doffing on the Centers for Disease Control and Prevention's website (https://www.cdc.gov/hai/pdfs/ppe/ppe-sequence.pdf).

Good oral health is a shared responsibility between the patient and the dental provider. Patients must be informed and motivated to perform their daily home care duties until their next visit (or recall). Prudent safety recommendations for the GP providing care for implants in the ambulatory setting/dental office include but are not limited to (1) placing the patient in an upright position (whenever possible), (2) placement of a 4 × 4 gauze in the area of the oropharynx to protect objects falling (if the office does not have them, a 2 × 2 will be suffice, unfolding it will be even better), and (3) attach dental floss to Hex tools (**Fig. 2**). In the unlikely case an implant part should accidently be swallowed by the patient, they will need to be directed to the nearest hospital for a chest radiograph.

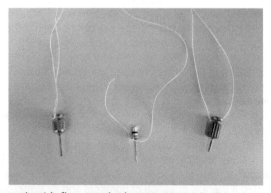

Fig. 2. Restorative tools with floss attached to prevent aspiration.

The GP often instructs the patient how to maintain their dentition, as well as, having the following extended responsibilities: (1) obtain a good medical history, (2) request a medical consult with the patient's physician or specialist (when necessary), (3) obtain necessary laboratory tests based on the patient's past medical history (ie, complete blood count with differential, hemoglobin A1c, international normalized ratio, etc), and (4) inform the patient of their risk factors associated with dental implant placement. An updated list of medical conditions with risk factors for failure or potential complications of implant placement are provided in **Box 1**.[7]

There are several documented literatures on the cluster phenomenon[10–12] and parafunctional habits associated with implant failure.[13] Rose and colleagues[14] stated that "meticulous screening and patient selection can help reduce the risk of failure or potential complications during implant treatment." Potential complications in the risk factor category include to discomfort, pain, and purulence. Patients with multiple comorbidities and taking multiple medications may be potential risks for implant failure. Systematic reviews and meta-analysis have proved that there is a statistically significant increased implant failure rate with patients on selective serotonin reuptake inhibitors and proton pump inhibitors.[15] If the patient (symptomatic or asymptomatic) asks for the implant to be removed owing to any of the aforementioned reasons (included in **Box 1**), the implant is considered to have failed.

Individual risk assessments are necessary before implant surgery.[16] In light of COVID-19, geriatric patients with serious chronic diseases (ie, pulmonary, cardiac, etc) may be at increased risk of sudden death; therefore, medical consults should be sent to physicians and specialist before implant surgery (now more than ever). As for these older patients, it may be safe and wise to provide alternative prosthodontic treatment in the form of conventional partial dentures and/or complete dentures.

The GP should be skilled enough to handle the implant case and if not then refer the patient to a dental specialist who can execute surgical strategies for the various hard and soft tissue deficiencies, such as (1) anatomic preconditions, (2) lack of keratinized mucosa, (3) local diseases affecting the teeth and implants, (4) mechanical overload, (5) tissue morphology and phenotype, (6) expansion of the floor of the sinus, (7) extraction(s), (8) trauma to orofacial structures, (9) migration of teeth and malpositioning of implants, and (10) iatrogenic factors.[17]

Chiapasco and colleagues[18] listed 5 main methods to augment the local bone volume at deficient sites as follows: (a) osteoinduction by the use of growth factors; (b) osteoconduction where a grafting material serves as a scaffold; (c) distraction osteogenesis, by which a fracture is surgically induced and then pulled apart; (d) guided bone regeneration, which allows spaces maintained by barrier membranes to be filled with bone; and (e) revascularized bone grafts, where vital bone segment is transferred to its recipient bed with its vascular pedicle. There are different regenerative

---

Box 1
Risk factors for implant placement

Moderate to severe neutropenia	Atypical odontalgia or atypical facial pain
Patients on corticosteroids	Radiation therapy to the head and neck
Cancer chemotherapy	Myocardial infarction within 6 mo
Patients on IV bisphosphonates	Gravid patient
Poorly controlled diabetics	Heavy smoking habits
Malignancy/terminal illness	Cluster phenomenon
Psychological instability	Parafunctional habits
Selective serotonin reuptake inhibitors	Proton Pump Inhibitors

techniques that can be implemented to reconstruct deficient alveolar ridges, namely, lateral, vertical, or combined bone augmentation.[19] The approaches to achieve this reconstruction is by the use of bone blocks, particulated grafts, and/or barrier membranes. There are a variety of biomaterials that can be applied, including autogenous, allogenic, xenogenic, and synthetic bone substitute (resorbable and nonresorbable).[20] The goal is to achieve primary stability of the implant and avoid any micro movement, which could lead to poor revascularization of the graft site.

There are no well-documented series of scientific studies that show the superiority of an implant company over another. The most important biological event (of osteointegration) is in the clinical healing phase of the dental implant is cell adhesion at the interface between it and the host tissue.[21] A meta-analysis and systematic reviews have showed that rough-surfaced implants demonstrated favorable results compared with machined implants.[6] Ogle[21] also stated that "the success and failure is more dependent on patient related, procedural, and prosthetic parameters than implant shape."

Clinicians interested in short implants ($\leq$6 mm) should be mindful that studies have shown higher rates of prosthetic complications (microrotation and rocking).[22,23] The complications and rotational movements seem to decrease when the prostheses were splinted. Meta-analysis of randomized clinical trials reported that long implants show a higher survival rate than extrashort implants (after a 5-year timeframe).[24]

Chen and Buser[25] published a list of protocols for implant placement after extractions: (a) type 1 (immediate implant placement): the implants are placed on the same day as the extraction; (b) type 2 (early implant placement): the implants are placed 1 to 2 months after the extraction; (c) type 3 (delayed implant placement): the implants are placed 3 to 4 months after the extraction; and (d) type 4 (late or conventional placement): 4 to 6 months or greater after implant placement. The patient who presents with infection in the bone may benefit from the delayed or late/conventional to improve the chances of success. In cases where there is difficulty in achieving primary stability (and challenges to stabilize the implant), good clinical judgment would be to consider a conventional loading approach to avoid micromovements to increase the survival rate, which directly impacts the affect the esthetic outcome. Canellas and colleagues[26] showed a statistically significant difference in favor of delayed implant placement in their meta-analysis. Gallucci and colleagues[27] created a comprehensive protocol combining implant placement and loading (**Fig. 3**, highlighting the well documented and insufficiently documented cases):

- Type 1A: immediate placement and immediate restoration/loading
- Type 1B: immediate placement and early restoration/loading
- Type 1C: immediate placement and conventional restoration/loading
- Type 2A: early placement with soft tissue healing and immediate restoration/loading
- Type 2B: early placement with soft tissue healing and early restoration/loading
- Type 2C: early placement with soft tissue healing and conventional restoration/loading
- Type 3A: early placement with partial bone healing and immediate restoration/loading
- Type 3B: early placement with partial bone healing and early restoration/loading
- Type 3C: early placement with partial bone healing and conventional restoration/loading
- Type 4A: late placement and immediate restoration/loading
- Type 4B: late placement and early restoration/loading
- Type 4C: late placement and conventional restoration/loading

	Loading Protocol		
	Immediate restoration/loading (type A)	Early loading (type B)	Conventional loading (type C)
Implant placement protocol			
Immediate placement (Type 1)	Type 1A CD	Type 1B CD	Type 1C SCV
Early placement (Type 2-3)	Type 2-3A CID	Type 2-3B CID	Type 2-3C SCV
Late placement (Type 4)	Type 4A CD	Type 4B SCV	Type 4C SCV

Note. Type 1A: Immediate Placement + Immediate Restoration/Loading; Type 1B: Immediate Placement + Early Loading; Type 1C: Immediate Placement + Conventional Loading; Type 2-3A: Early Placement + Immediate Restoration/Loading; Type 2-3B: Early placement + Early Loading; Type 2-3C: Early Placement + Conventional Loading; Type 4A: Late Placement + Immediate Loading; Type 4B: Late Placement + Early Loading; Type 4C: Late Placement + Conventional Loading.
CD (yellow): clinically documented; CID (red): clinically insufficiently documented (includes loading protocols that are not documented); CWD (green): clinically well documented; SCV: scientifically and clinically validated.

Fig. 3. Classification according to implant placement and healing protocol. (*From* Gallucci GO, Hamilton A, Zhou W, et al. Implant placement and loading protocols in partially edentulous patients: A systemic review. Clin Oral Implants Res. 2018;29(Suppl 16):126; with permission.)

Gallucci and colleagues[27] stated that type 1C is the most scientifically and clinically validated approach. The most documented approach, type 4C, is the standard of care when treatment modifiers such as bone augmentation, low insertion torque, reduced diameter implants, and patient local and systemic factors are present. The Group 2 ITI Consensus Report reviewed these new implant protocols for descriptive analysis: (a) immediate implant placement, same day as the extraction(s); (b) early implant placement: (soft tissue healing) 4 to 8 weeks or (partial bone healing) 12 to 16 weeks after the tooth extraction(s); and (c) late implant placement: placed after complete bone healing, more than 6 months after tooth extraction.[28] The implant loading protocols defined as follows: (a) immediate loading: dental implants are connected to a prosthesis in occlusion with the opposing arch within 1 week subsequent to implant placement; (b) immediate restoration: dental implants are connected to a prosthesis, held out of occlusion with the opposing arch within 1 week subsequent to implant placement; (c) early loading: dental implants are connected to the prosthesis between 1 week and 2 months after implant placement; and (d) conventional loading: dental implants are allowed a healing period of more than 2 months after implant placement with no connection of the prosthesis.[28]

Morton and colleagues[28] showed the percentage of the survival rates for the new set of protocols (types 1A–4C; see **Fig. 3**). Their consensus statement on this topic revealed a 98% survival rate with type 1A (yellow); a 98% survival rate with type 1B (yellow); a 96% survival rate with type 1C (green); types 2A and 2B both have clinically insufficient documentation (red); a 96% survival rate with type 2C (green); a 98% survival rate with type 4A (yellow); a 98% survival rate with 4B(green); and a 98% survival rate with type 4C(green). The reader should be mindful there is no gold standard for implant placement after extraction(s); however, the implant placement and loading protocol should be planned before surgery.[28]

Establishing proper occlusion can dictate the success of each case. Occlusal treatment at the time of delivery and at follow-up visits cannot be overemphasized. Several studies[29,30] have proven that most reported complications (prosthetic or bony) are associated with occlusion. In dental implantology, another form of dental implant complication(s) refer to "a problem with any of the replaceable components of the implant system."[31] Misch stated that "most common complications of the implant prostheses relate to biomechanical factors, such as porcelain fracture, unretained prostheses (cement or screw), abutment screw loosening, early implant failure after loading, and implant component fracture.[32–34] The GP is encouraged to implement an occlusal plan to provide an implant-protective occlusion to decrease biomechanical complications and improve clinical longevity.[32–35] It has been documented that the implant system handles the stress of mastication and occlusal interferences poorly.[32] If occlusal treatment visits are not properly provided for the patient it can result in implant(s) failure. The benefits of implant-protective occlusion are as follows: (1) no premature occlusal contacts or interferences, (2) mutually protected articulation, (3) implant body angle to occlusal load, (4) cusp angle of crowns, (5) cantilever or offset loads, (6) crown height (vertical height), (7) implant crown contour, (8) occlusal contact position, (9) timing of occlusal contacts, and (10) protect the weakest component.[32] The screw could fracture as a result of occlusal overload or torqueing beyond the manufacturer's recommendation. The sequence of internal mechanical complications of the screw that can lead to failure are as follows: the screw loosening leading → screw bending; the screw bending leading → screw fracturing; and screw fracturing leading → fracturing of the platform of the implant, which could ultimately lead to failure of the implant. It is recommended that all bent screws be replaced by new ones before retorqueing, owing to the high risk of breakage (this can be requested by the manufacturer or the dental laboratory). It is important to note that, after the implant placement, the cover screw, healing cap, and temporary crown should be hand torqued until delivery of the final restoration(s) or prostheses when it will be torqued according to the manufacturer's recommendation. There are a few times when skillful clinicians may be fortunate enough to remove a broken screw embedded within the implant. If not possible, the implant may have to be buried (leaving it nonfunctional) or be removed (trephination) or a cast post/core and crown be cemented. If a problem like one of these described occur in the office then referral to a specialist would be recommended.

Papaspyridakos and colleagues[35] revealed in their systematic review that "wears" are the most common minor complication and "fracture of the prosthetic material" are the major complication with implant-supported fixed complete dental prostheses for the edentulous patients. They went further to recommend for patients to wear nightguards to prevent any complications of the prostheses. A more current retrospective study (with 1–12 years of follow-up) of implant-supported fixed complete dental prostheses detailed (the annual rate in percentage) of minor complications as (1) wear of the prosthetic material (9.8%), (2) decementation of cement retained implant-supported fixed complete dental prostheses (2.9%), and (3) loss of the screw access filling material (2.7%).[36] The annual rate of major complications from this same study are as follows: (1) fracture of prosthetic material (1.9%), (2) fracture of the occlusal screw (0.3%), and (3) fracture of the framework (0.3%).[36] Moreover, to avoid repairs, remakes, and wasted chair time, a nightguard as a part of the final delivery is recommended.[36] The use of nightguards and orthodontic retainers have been recommended in the partially dentate patient (with implants) to prevent interproximal contact loss, which could lead to peri-implantitis.[37] There are a number of clinical complications published in the literature that may compromise the successful outcome of dental implants (ie, biologic, technical/mechanical, esthetic, or phonetic).[38,39] Heitz-Mayfield and colleagues[16] stated that "Bleeding on probing (BOP) has a positive predictive value (7% to 58%) for the diagnosis of peri-implantitis." Peri-implant mucositis characteristically includes BOP, and/or suppuration, probing depths of less than 4 mm with no evidence of bone loss (is reversible), is considered a precursor to peri-implantitis.[40] A diagnosis of peri-implantitis involves evidence of inflammation, infection, and progressive bone loss (classified as mild, moderate, or severe), if not treated can lead to failure of the implant.

Over the past 2 decades, cone beam computed tomography has proved to become a valuable armamentarium in dental implantology treatment planning (**Fig. 4**).[41,42] This 3-dimensional imaging modality allows the clinicians the ability to access bone density before implant placement, measure the bone height, and width to properly predict the placement of the implant more accurately.[43] This allows the GP (along with the help of the dental laboratory) the ability to develop a more "prosthetically driven" process, to allow the patient the option of receiving a prosthesis on the day of surgery. Moreover, this outcome should never be promised to the patient because of the possibility of complications that can occur somewhere in the case (ie, unsatisfactory aesthetics). It is imperative that the surgeon use cone beam computed tomography scans to assess vital structures in the image of the maxilla and/or mandible. An awareness and knowledge of surgical anatomy is important to the success of the case. Aziz

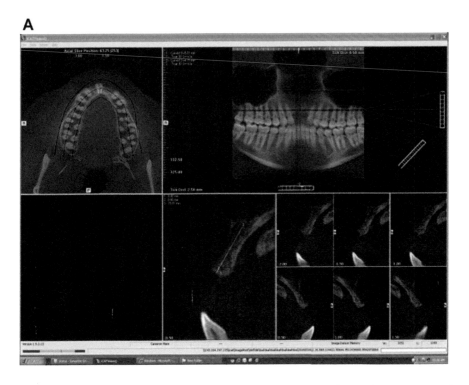

Fig. 4. (*A*) Cone beam computed tomography. (*B*) Axial view of cone beam computed tomography.

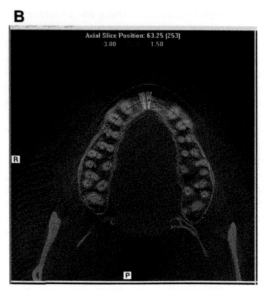

Fig. 4. (*continued*).

affirmed that "prevention of an inferior alveolar nerve (IAN) injury is directly related to proper and thorough preoperative implant planning. He also stated, "The etiology of IAN injury is usually associated with inadequate planning or overzealous implant placement (ie, miscalculation).[44] This miscalculation can also occur in the area of the maxillary sinuses, the mental foramen, nasopalatine canal, and the lingual concavity of the mandible. There are a variety of virtual systems (**Figs. 5** and **6**) on the market for the clinician to choose from to plan for the placement of implant(s). The modern-day GP can use software to select the implant company, choose the length of the implant, platform size, draw the nerve (if needed), choose virtual teeth (and abutment), and position (move and rotate) the implant to prevent any perforations and fenestrations (**Fig 6**).

In this particular case, we used the virtual company Simplant from a cast and the scanned image(s) to a computer-milled template or tooth supported stereolithographic surgical guide was made to fit the patient (**Figs. 7–11**). Note that the amount of bone loss (loss of interdental papilla) in the area of #8 and #9 from a history of trauma, bilateral posterior crossbite, anterior open bite, and overjet (appreciated in picture with paralleling pins, in **Figs. 11–13**).

In this case, the decision was made to restore at a later date owing to the degree of overjet, which would alter the aesthetics (see **Fig. 12**). The final placement of implant #8 is shown in **Fig. 14**. Implants #8 and #9, completed with postoperative radiograph, are shown in **Fig. 15**. The patient's preexisting flipper (**Fig. 16**) was reamed out on the intaglio surface and a soft reline material was placed so that it would not place heavy pressure on the implants #8 and #9. Subsequently, the flipper was taken out of occlusion. Gold custom (UCLA) abutments were milled (**Fig.17A**), cotton pellets placed in the vents to protect the screws (see **Fig.17B**). The occlusion was adjusted, then the connected permanent crowns were cemented (**Fig. 18**).

The discussion of dental implants are at the forefront of most treatment plans involving any missing tooth or teeth. Today, more patients are requesting edentulous spaces to be restored with FDPs; however, owing to financial constraints (from the current economic recession) it may lead the patient to gradually invest in the fixed

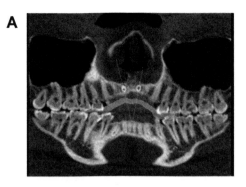

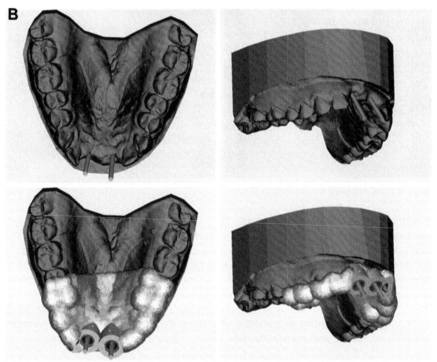

Fig. 5. (*A*) Shows a cone beam computed tomography with a virtual image of paralleling pins. (*B*) Virtual image of paralleling pins in the cast and with surgical guide.

partial dentures at a later date. Nonetheless, the GP will need to provide this group of patients with evidenced based knowledge, goals, and treatment to satisfy their needs and expectations.

Many patients may not be ready to lose their periodontally compromised dentition; however, some will eventually transition from removable partial dentures to a complete denture or complete overdentures or implant-supported fixed complete dental prostheses. An early start of implant placement may turn out to be a wise investment for the patient (**Fig. 19**). Wittneben and colleagues[45] stated "in partially edentulous patients demanding a fixed rehabilitation, the choice between tooth- or implant-supported fixed dental (FDP's) needs to be made." Nonetheless, the patient should

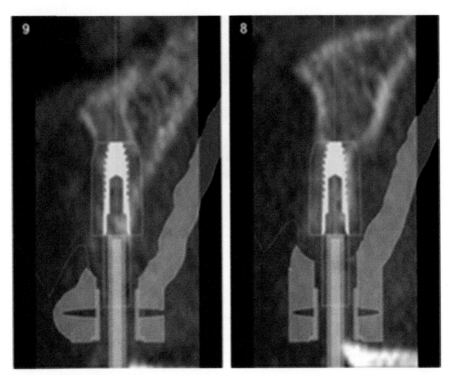

Fig. 6. Virtual Imaging of implant in bone.

be educated about periodontal disease, the "seeding" process of anaerobic bacteria invading the implants which could lead to peri-mucositis or peri-implantitis.[7,28] This does not mean that their teeth need to be extracted, instead the patient needs to be meticulous about their oral hygiene regimen. The goal of the GP should be to make the oral cavity as clean as possible to receive the initial implant(s), whereas the goal of the patient is to maintain the cleanliness of the oral cavity. Berglundh and colleagues[46] stated "there is strong evidence that there is an increased risk of developing peri-implantitis in patients who have a history of severe periodontitis, poor plaque control, and no regular maintenance care after implant therapy."

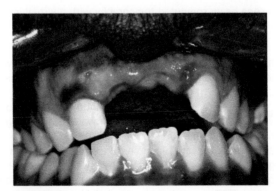

Fig. 7. Case #1 of the patients' occlusion.

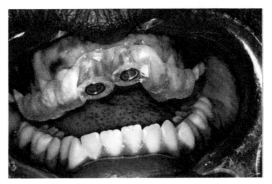

Fig. 8. Surgical guide fitted in the maxilla.

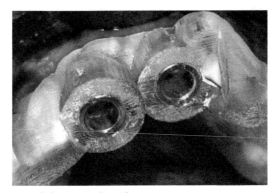

Fig. 9. Close up image of the surgical guide.

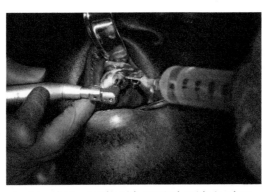

Fig. 10. Next, the osteotomy being made with surgical guide in place.

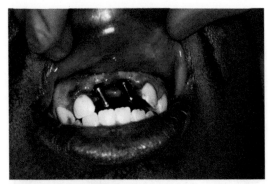

Fig. 11. Placement of the paralleling pins .

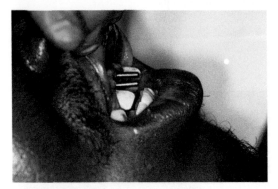

Fig. 12. Sagittal view with paralleling pins.

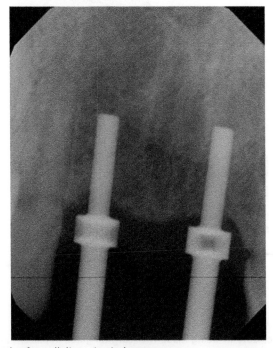

Fig. 13. Radiograph of paralleling pins in bone.

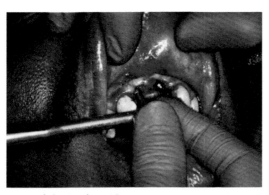

Fig. 14. Final placement of the implant #8.

In medicine, patient-reported outcomes are "any report of the status of a patient's health condition that comes directly from the patient, without interpretation of the patient's response by a clinician or anyone else."[47] In dentistry, patient-reported outcome measures are "subjective" reports of patients' perceptions of their oral health status and the impact on the patient's quality of life.[45,48,49] These are important criteria's in dental implantology, because patient expectations are increasing and the GP is left with making a decision that must satisfy the patient by the end of the treatment (which could result in additional costs if the patient is not satisfied). A deeper insight and discussion on patient-reported outcome measures is presented elsewhere in

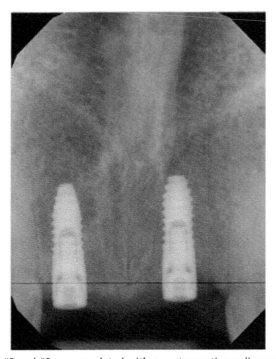

Fig. 15. Implants #8 and #9 are completed with a postoperative radiograph.

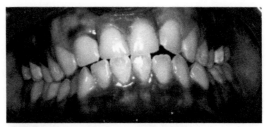

Fig. 16. Preexistng flipper before taken out of occlusion.

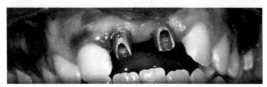

Fig. 17. Milled Gold custom (UCLA) abutments. (*Courtesy of* Milivoj Grego, CDT, MS.)

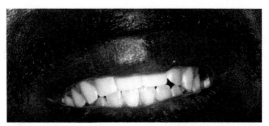

Fig. 18. The patient was satisfied with the aesthetic outcome. (*Courtesy of* Milivoj Grego, CDT, MS and Ricardo A. Boyce, DDS, FICD.)

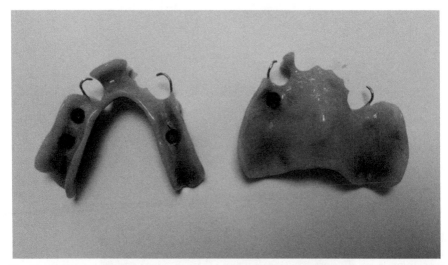

Fig. 19. Upper and lower acrylic removable partial dentures showing retentive elements on the intaglio surface of the RPD. This photo illustrates how the patient may choose to invest incrementally (in Implants) according to their financial budget.

this article. Misch[32] describes how often times the dental laboratory technician does not get the credit but are largely responsible for the final esthetic result. It is imperative for the restorative dentist or GP to choose a knowledgeable and experienced laboratory technician in the management of complex implant cases. Moreover, the GP should be skilled enough to envision the final outcome of a restoration or prostheses, know how to communicate this vision with the laboratory technician until the finished prosthesis is delivered and the patient is completely satisfied.

Edentulism is considered to be a disability according to the World Health Organizations.[50,51] The edentulous patient has a reduced quality of life, is at high risk for choking on foods, which could lead to digestive problems or even death. Prosthodontic rehabilitation/reconstruction of edentulism improves a patients' overall quality of life. In dentistry, the qualities of life include but are not limited to masticatory function, maintenance of weight, reduced gastrointestinal disturbances, psychological well-being, and enhanced esthetics.[52,53]

When there is an improvement in the retention and stability of the implant supported prostheses, it can lead to enhanced speaking, mastication, and swallowing, which can improve the patient's overall satisfaction.[54] The literature suggests for the dentist to consider the patient's past medical history, risk assessment, expectations, motoric skills, and financial costs before prosthodontic rehabilitation.[7,55] Even though mandibular implants are considered the standard of care for the edentulous patient, this is not always the case in the maxilla. Edentulous patients with good bony support in the maxilla may not need implant placement. In fact, de Albuquerque Júnior and colleagues,[56] stated that "maxillary implant prostheses *should not* be considered as a general treatment of choice in patients with good bony support," who are problem free with a maxillary conventional prostheses. This recommendation will be prudent advice for any patient that falls into the high risk category mentioned in **Box 1**. Removable implant overdentures, along with parts and systems (from the manufacturer or dental laboratory) serves to enhance retention, function, fixation, and stabilization.[57] In this particular Cochrane database systemic review, Payne and colleagues[52] described the 4 groups of attachment systems for removable implant overdentures as the (1) ball/stud attachment, (2) bar attachment, (3) magnet attachment, and (4) telescopic attachment. The decision of which attachment system to use solely depends on the clinician's expertise and personal preferences.[58] One systematic review brought to light some interesting pearls of wisdom for those who restore overdentures: (1) respect the manufacturers torqueing (screwing) guidelines, (2) share the likelihood of minor complications (ie, adjustments with patients) with the patient to facilitate communication of realistic expectations, (3) a strict follow-up with routine recall should be provided to maintain and improve denture adaptation, and (4) a denture that has to be fabricated after a decade, is not considered a failure; however, if it needs repair within 5 years success has not been achieved.[59] Some additional removable prosthodontic pearls for the different types of overdentures have been included in **Box 2**.

Patients should be informed that magnet, bar, and telescopic attachments will have higher fees owing to dental laboratory fees. Assaf and colleagues[59] stated that "there is no clear understanding of what the preferred retention system may be, nor which system should be designated as routine maintenance repairs vs complications, as the difference is quantitative and subjective."[60]

When the decision has been made by the GP to provide Oral Rehabilitation/Reconstruction for the completely edentulous patient, there should be a few questions to include in the treatment plan. The GP should determine (1) if there is a monetary budget, (2) whether the patient is comfortable with the thought of wearing dentures attached to the implants (some patients do not like the concept of a denture), (3)

> **Box 2**
> **Prosthodontic Pearls for various types of Overdentures**
>
> - The Ball/Stud (locator) attachment can be used with nonparalleled implants.
> - The Bar attachment (with clips or riders) have high retentive capacities and reduced loading forces over implants. Also, they can be used with nonparalleled implants.
> - The Bar attachments have an increased probability of plaque accumulation; therefore, good oral hygiene maintenance should be practiced. Also, gingival hyperplasia has been reported with bar attachments.
> - The magnet attachment is better suited for the elderly patient with limited dexterity. There are reduced loading forces over the implants and can be used with nonparalleled implants.
> - The magnet attachment can lose retention over time owing to intraoral corrosion.
> - The telescopic attachments allow for high retention and stability of the denture. Oral hygiene is more easily accessible.

whether the patient would prefer the ability to remove and clean your denture, and (4) whether the patient prefers the denture to stay in the mouth (without the ability to remove it)? Once these preferences are established, they will help with patient satisfaction at the time of delivery. It should be noted that once the patients' desires are confirmed, the ultimate plan will be determined by the patient's bone volume, soft tissue condition, anatomic structures, and interarch space.

The fundamental prosthodontic principles in dental implantology include (1) preliminary and definitive impressions, (2) jaw relation records, (3) wax try-in, (4) metal framework try-in (with and without artificial teeth), and (5) insertion of definitive prostheses.[61] The second half of this article discusses the fixed prostheses designed in 3 different ways. They will be displayed according to minimal complications for the clinician, allowing for a passive fit, and ease of hygiene for the patient to the most complex prostheses. Computer-aided designed/computer aided manufacturing are preferred by many clinicians based off of reported accuracy of fit.[61]

The maxillary posterior region is the most sensitive area of all 4 quadrants owing to its inadequate density and caution is warranted when placing implants in this region. Sinus lifts are commonly performed to facilitate implants in this region; however, many implants fail owing to type IV bone in the region. There are some patients who may be hesitant or afraid at the mere thought of dental implants at or near their sinuses. Should a patient decide not to obtain a sinus lift (when there is a need), or if the patient has pneumatization of the sinuses, then the consideration of intentionally tilted implants could be considered as an option. This option could be given to the patient who does not mind the concept of wearing a denture and prefer the prostheses to be fixed. The "fixed–hybrid" or "all-on-four" concept requires angulation, placement of 2 posterior implants, and placement of 2 anterior implants to allow the denture to attach, function, and the inability to be removed (unless done so by the operator or another trained clinician with the implant parts). Of course, other options can be suggested; nonetheless, the main reason behind offering this first is due to the 45° angulation of the posterior implant, which could limit the addition of other implants in the future **(Fig. 20)**. Morton and colleagues[28] stated "there is no statistically significant difference in primary outcomes (survival rates for implant prosthesis) or secondary outcomes (peri-implant marginal bone loss, soft and hard tissue complications, prosthetic complications and patient-centered outcomes) for implants placed in a tilted configuration when used to support full arch fixed partial dentures." The authors

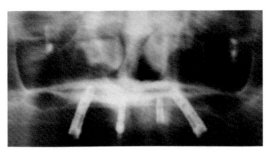

Fig. 20. 45° intentionally tilted posterior implants, just anterior to the maxillary sinuses.

went further to state that "the final prosthetic plan should be considered when developing a surgical plan for implant placement." Even though a 1-piece full-arch fixed prosthesis is acceptable, it may not be the best choice for those patients in the high-risk category for implant loss or complications (ie, smokers). The patient in high-risk categories can be offered a treatment plan with 6, 8, or more in an arch in case there are complications or failures (or simply decline the placement of implants).

The key prosthodontic points of all-on-four hybrid system are that (1) there are only 4 implants, (2) it is a prosthetically driven process, where the posterior abutments are torqued at 15 neutons and the anterior abutments are torqued at 30 neutons, (3) there is a collaboration between the restorative dentist and the oral surgeon, (4) the posterior regions are avoided owing to the intentionally (45°) tilted implant, (5) there is use of a cantilever, (6) the intaglio surface should be smooth and convex, (7) and maintenance will be with the use of Superfloss (see **Fig. 38**) or a floss threader or a Waterpik.

According to the Group 2 ITI Consensus Report, the prosthetic plan should include (a) the prosthetic material, (b) 1-piece (**Figs. 21–24**) and (**Figs. 30–37**) or segmented prostheses (**Figs. 25–29**), (c) aesthetic factors (ie, lip support, smile line), (d) the condition of the opposing dentition, (e) the available space for the prosthesis, (f) the anatomy of the edentulous ridge (maxilla, mandible, bone volume and quality, and anatomic limitations), (g) planned distribution and cantilever length, (h) space availability hygiene and maintenance (see **Figs. 38** and **39**).[28] Morton and colleagues[28] mentioned that "a minimum number of 4 appropriately distributed implants are recommended to support a one-piece full arch fixed prosthesis... the impact of future implant loss/complications on prosthesis support should be considered when choosing a number." The case with the classic implant roundhouse 1-piece, failed after stage 2 of the healing caps being placed on #3 (see **Fig. 31**). This patient refused to wear an implant overdenture and would only accept a treatment plan with a fixed bridge (see **Figs. 31–37**). The patient had a history of smoking 1 pack of cigarettes per day for 35 years. There are some patients who will not heed the warnings from

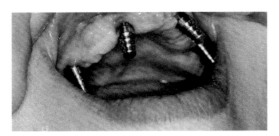

Fig. 21. Closed Tray impression copings. (*Courtesy of* Ricardo A. Boyce, DDS, FICD.)

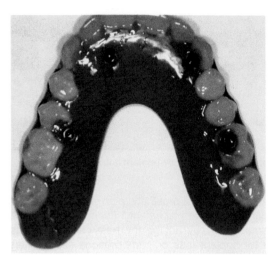

Fig. 22. Excess flanges of acrylic should be trimmed by the GP. These vents will be plugged with cotton pellets and sealed off. The choice of acrylic or composite can be used. (*Courtesy of* Ricardo A. Boyce, DDS, FICD.)

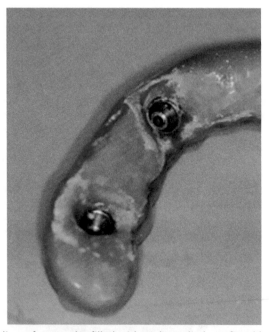

Fig. 23. The intaglio surface can be filled with pink acrylic (retrofitted by the GP) to make the prostheses cleansable for the patient. Special care should be made not to allow any acrylic to enter the metal coping on the intaglio surface, for the screws. The chair time will increase for the GP, but this particular "fixed hybrid" can be made affordable to the patient.

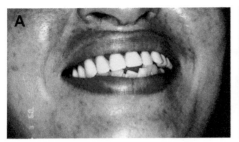
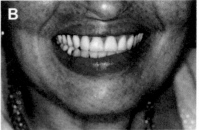

Fig. 24. The patient was extremely satisfied at the delivery date. The lower anterior teeth were extracted and treated with an immediate removable partial dentures on the day of delivery. (*A*) Before. (*B*) After.

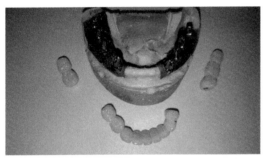

Fig. 25. This case displays the segmented cement retained fixed partial denture. (*Courtesy of* Milivoj Grego, CDT, MS.)

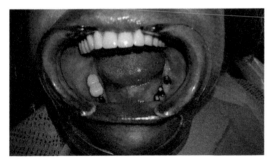

Fig. 26. The connected crowns were cemented first. (*Courtesy* of Ricardo A. Boyce, DDS, FICD.)

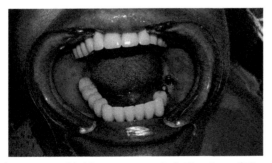

Fig. 27. Next, the long spanned bridge was cemented. (*Courtesy of* Ricardo A. Boyce, DDS, FICD.)

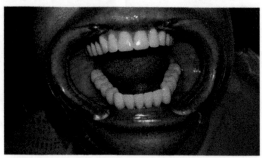

Fig. 28. Finally, the last bridge was cemented. (*Courtesy of* Ricardo A. Boyce, DDS, FICD.)

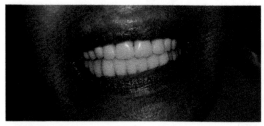

Fig. 29. The patient was satisfied on delivery. (*Courtesy of* Milivoj Grego, CDT, MS and Ricardo A. Boyce, DDS, FICD.)

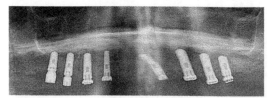

Fig. 30. Eight implants.

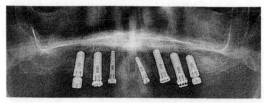

Fig. 31. Implant #3 failed, owing to the patients' history of cigarette smoking.

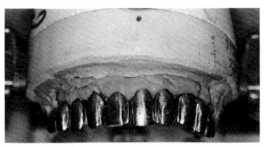

Fig. 32. The connected metal framework may fit perfect on the cast. (*Courtesy of* Milivoj Grego, CDT, MS.)

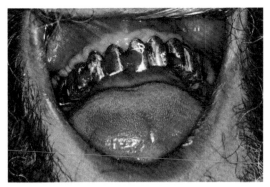

Fig. 33. One of the disadvantages of the "roundhouse" is misfit on delivery. Management of this problem could be to retake the impression or it could be sectioned, placed back in the mouth, splinted with inlay resin. Note: a pickup impression with PVS should be made, sent to the dental laboratory. (*Courtesy of* Ricardo A. Boyce, DDS, FICD.)

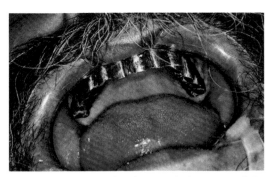

Fig. 34. The soldered "roundhouse" tried in the mouth. (*Courtesy of* Ricardo A. Boyce, DDS, FICD.)

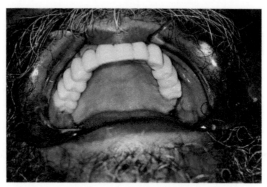

Fig. 35. The GP should request a Bisque–Bake appointment to adjust occlusion. An occlusal-protected appointment. (*Courtesy of* Ricardo A. Boyce, DDS, FICD.)

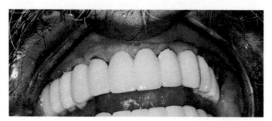

Fig. 36. Before cementation. (*Courtesy of* Ricardo A. Boyce, DDS, FICD.)

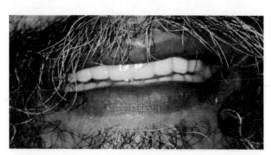

Fig. 37. Satisfied patient on delivery. (*Courtesy of* Milivoj Grego, CDT, MS and Ricardo A. Boyce, DDS, FICD.)

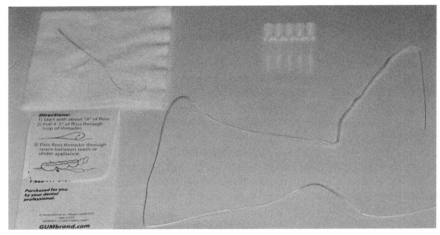

Fig. 38. Floss threader, soft picks, and super floss.

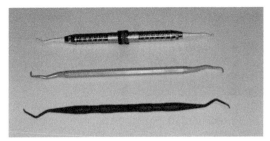

Fig. 39. Plastic, titanium, and graphite dental instruments.

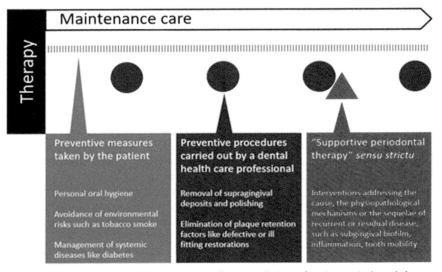

Fig. 40. The 3 components of maintenance after completion of active periodontal therapy and after dental implant therapy. (*From* Mombelli A. Maintenance therapy for teeth and implants. Periodontol 2000. 2019;79(1):191; with permission.)

the GP and choose various risks (ie, smoking), which could lead to complications or failure.

Mombelli[62] stated: "regarding dental implants, as the evolution from peri-implant mucositis to peri-implantitis may be gradual, maintenance therapy has the potential to intercept infection before the bone has been damaged extensively." He described 3 important components of maintenance care after completion of active periodontal therapy and after dental implant therapy (**Fig. 40**): (1) measures taken by the patient (ie, personal oral hygiene, avoidance of tobacco smoke, management of systemic diseases), (2) preventive procedures carried out by the dental health care professional (ie, removal of subgingival deposits, elimination of plaque retentive factors), and (3) supportive periodontal therapy sensu strictu (ie, interventions addressing the cause, the pathophysiologic mechanisms, or the sequelae of recurrent or residual disease.

Baseline radiographs and probing depths (with a plastic periodontal probe) should be taken on delivery of the implant-supported prostheses and at subsequent follow-up visits to establish the bone level and follow the remodeling process.[63–66]

Patient satisfaction (with overall treatment, aesthetics) is the primary goal of the dentist/GP providing any prosthodontic procedure and has been viewed equally important as implant survival.[45] The 4 most frequently used parameters for measuring the success of dental implants include (1) the implant level, (2) peri-implant soft tissue level, (3) prosthesis level, and (4) the patient's subject assessment.[67] Wittenben[45] used the visual analogue scale to determine the patient-reported outcome measures to evaluate how patients felt about their overall treatment and esthetics. Their systematic review concluded that (1) the aesthetics of implant-supported FDPs are highly rated by patients (visual analogue scale = 90.0; 87.9–92.2); (2) the appearance of the mucosa surrounding the implant-supported FDP's was highly rated (visual analogue scale = 84.7; minimum of 73.0 to maximum of 92.0) by patient-reported outcome measures; (3) patient-reported outcome measures ratings were higher with patients having soft tissue level implants compared with the ones with bone level type implants however without being statistically significant (P = .128); (4) individual restorative materials had no influence on ratings of PROMs focusing on the aesthetics of implant-supported FDPs; and (5) the use of a provisional restoration had no effect on aesthetic ratings of the definitive restorations on implant-supported FDPs evaluated by PROMs. An even more interesting point that was made when it comes to aesthetics, are that the studies that have proved the worse critics in the aesthetic outcome to be prosthodontists and general dentists, while patients shown to be less critical and often times highly satisfied with their overall treatment and aesthetics.[68–72]

SUMMARY

The current COVID-19 pandemic has been a challenge for dentists and their dental offices owing to the consequent economic recession. The modern day dentist may need to be more conservative (ie, down payments, offer payment plans) with their patients' treatment plans involving implants. All members of the dental health team should be wearing appropriate PPE and practicing hand hygiene throughout the day. Patients are requesting edentulous spaces to be restored with FDP. The 10-year survival rate of implant crowns and FDPs range between 89% and 94%. The GP is encouraged to implement an occlusal plan to provide an implant protective occlusion, to reduce biomechanical complications and improve clinical outcomes. There is no gold standard for implant placement after extraction(s). The GP can use their own techniques or choose between the immediate, early, or late protocols with the higher percentages of survival rates. The surgical plan will be determined by the patients' risk factors (past medical history, medications, social habits, etc), bone volume (need for bone grafting), soft tissue conditions, anatomic structures, and interarch space. The prosthetic plan should involve the prostheses (type, material), aesthetic factors, condition of the opposing dentition, space for the prostheses, anatomy of the edentulous ridge, planned distribution, hygiene, and maintenance. A nightguard is recommended as a part of the final delivery for crown(s) and long spanned prostheses. The modern-day dentist will need to provide patients who are interested in implants with evidenced-based knowledge, goals, and treatment to satisfy their needs and expectations.

CLINICS CARE POINTS

- All patients should be queried over the phone (before) and on the day of their arrival in the clinic (ie, recent travel histories and test results for coronavirus, fever, respiratory symptoms, etc.).
- The patient and family who accompany them should be instructed to wear masks to their appointments.
- The goal of the GP should be to protect all patients and staff from coronavirus.
- Attach dental floss to restorative tools to avoid an uneventful aspiration by the patient.
- Risk factors for failure or potential complications should be discussed with the patient before treatment.
- There is no gold standard for Implant placement after extraction(s); however, the implant placement and loading protocol should be planned before surgery.
- Respect the manufacturer's torqueing guidelines.
- The surgical plan will be determined by the patient' risk factors, bone volume, soft tissue conditions, anatomic structures, and interarch space.
- The prosthetic plan should involve the prostheses (type material), aesthetic factors, condition of the opposing dentition, space for the prostheses, anatomy of the edentulous ridge, planned distribution, hygiene, and maintenance.
- Nightguards should be recommended in long spanned and/or complex cases.

DISCLOSURE

The author has nothing to disclose.

REFERENCES

1. Zembic A, Tahmaseb A, Jung RE, et al. Patient reported outcomes of maxillary edentulous patients wearing overdentures retained by two implants from insertion to 4 years. Int J Oral Maxillofac Implants 2019;34:481–8.
2. Pjetursson BE, Zarauz C, Strasding M, et al. A systematic review of the influence of the implant abutment connection on the clinical outcomes of ceramic and metal implant abutments supporting fixed implant reconstructions. Clin Oral Implants Res 2018;29(Suppl.18):160–83.
3. Jung RE, Zembic A, Pjetursson BE, et al. Systemic review of the Survival rate and the incidence of biological, technical, and aesthetic complications of single crowns on implants reported in longitudinal studies with a mean follow-up of 5 years. Clin Oral Implants Res 2012;23(Suppl 6):2–21.
4. Givi B, Schiff BA, Chinn SB, et al. Safety Recommendations for Evaluation and Surgery of the Head and Neck during the COVID-19 Pandemic. JAMA Otolarygol Head Neck Surg 2020;146(6):579–84.

5. Izzetti R, Nisi M, Gabriele M, et al. COVID-19 transmission in the dental practice: brief review of prospective measures in Italy. J Dent Res 2020. https://doi.org/10.1177/0022034520920580.

6. Kern J-S, Kern T, Wolfart S, et al. A systemic review and meta-analysis of removable and fixed implant-supported prostheses in edentulous jaws: post- loading implant loss. Clin Oral Implants Res 2016;27:174–95.

7. Boyce RA, Klemons G. Treatment Planning for Restorative Implantology. Dent Clin North Am 2015;59:291–304.

8. Peng X, Xu X, Li Y, et al. Transmission routes of 2019-nCoV and controls in dental practice. Int J Oral Sci 2020;12(1):9.

9. Meng L, Hua F, Bian Z, et al. Response to the Letter to the Editor: how to deal with suspended oral treatment during the COVID-19 epidemic. J Dent Res 2020; 99(8):988.

10. Ekfelt A, Christiansson U, ErikssonT, et al. A Retrospective analysis of factors associated with multiple implant failures in the maxillae. Clin Oral Implants Res 2001;12:462–7.

11. Minsk L, Polson AM, Weisgold A, et al. Outcome failures of endosseous implants from a clinical training center. Compend Contin Educ Dent 1996;17:848–59.

12. Mombell A. Microbiology of the Dental Implant. Adv Dent Res 1993;7(2):202–6.

13. Balshi TJ. Analysis and management of fractured implants: a clinical report. Int J Oral Maxillofac Implants 1996;11:660–6.

14. Rose LF, Mealy B, Genco R, et al. Periodontics: medicine, surgery, and implants. St Louis (MO): Elsevier Mosby; 2004. p. 611–74.

15. Chappuis V, Avila-Ortiz G, Araújo MG, et al. Medication-related dental implant failure: systematic review and meta-analysis. Clin Oral Implants Res 2018; 29(Suppl. 16):55–68.

16. Heitz-Mayfield LJ, Aaboe M, Araujo M, et al. Group 4 ITI consensus report: risks and biologic complications associated with implant dentistry. Clin Oral Implants Res 2018;29(Suppl. 16):351–8.

17. Hämmerle CHF, Tarnow D. The etiology of hard- and soft-tissue deficiencies at dental implants. J Periodontol 2018;89(Suppl 1):S291–303.

18. Chiapasco M, Zaniboni M, Boisco M. Augmentation procedures for the rehabilitation of deficient edentulous ridges with oral implants. Clin Oral Implants Res 2006;17(Suppl. 2):136–59.

19. Sanz-Sanchez I, Carrilllo de Albornoz A, Figuero E, et al. Effects of lateral bone augmentation procedures on peri-implant health or disease: a systematic review and meta-analysis. Clin Oral Implants Res 2018;29(Suppl. 15):18–31.

20. Thoma DS, Bienz SP, Figuero E, et al. Efficacy of lateral bone augmentation performed simultaneously with dental implant placement: a systematic review and meta-analysis. J Clin Periodontol 2019;46(Suppl. 21):257–76.

21. Ogle OE. Implant Surface Material, Design, and Osseointegration. Dent Clin North Am 2015;59:505–20.

22. Pohl V, Thoma DS, Sporniak-Tutak K, et al. Short dental implants (6mm) versus long dental implants (11-15)mm) in combination with sinus floor elevation procedures: 3 year results from multicenter, randomized, controlled clinical trial. J Clin Periodontol 2017;44:438–45.

23. Bidez MW, Misch CE. Clinical biomechanics in implant dentistry. In: Misch CE, editor. Contemporary implant dentistry. 3rd edition. St. Louis (MO): Mosby; 2008. p. 543–55.

24. Ravidà A, Wang I-C, Barootchi S, et al. Meta-analysis of randomized clinical trials comparing clinical and patient-reported outcomes between extra –short ($\leq$ 6 mm) and longer ($\geq$10 mm) implants. J Clin Periodontol 2019;46:118–42.
25. Chen ST, Buser D. Clinical and esthetic outcomes of implants placed in posterior extraction sites. Int J Oral Maxillofac Implants 2009;24(Suppl):186–217.
26. Canellas JVDS, Medeiros PJD, Figueredo CMDS, et al. Which is the best choice after extraction, immediate implant placement or delayed placement with alveolar ridge preservation? A systematic review and meta-analysis. Craniomaxillofac Surg 2019;47(11):1793–802.
27. Gallucci GO, Hamilton A, Zhou W, et al. Implant placement and loading protocols in partially edentulous patients: a systemic review. Clin Oral Implants Res 2018 Oct;29(Suppl 16):106–34.
28. Morton D, Gallucci G, Lin W, et al. Group 2 ITI Consensus Report: prosthodontics and implant dentistry. Clin Oral Implants Res 2018;29(Suppl. 16):215–23.
29. Isidor R. Histological evaluation of peri-implant bone at implants subjected to occlusal overload or plaque accumulation. Clin Oral Implants Res 1997;8:1–9.
30. Rangert B, Krogh PH, Langer B, et al. Bending overload and implant fracture: a retrospective clinical analysis. Int J Oral Maxillofac Implants 1995;7:40–4.
31. Fuentealba R, Jofre J. Esthetic Failure in Implant Dentistry. Dent Clin North Am 2015;59:227–46.
32. Misch CE. Dental Implant Prosthetics. In: Misch C, editor. Rationale for dental implants. 2nd edition. St. Louis (MO): Elsevier (Mosby); 2015. p. 874–937.
33. Misch C, editor. Occlusal considerations for implant-supported prostheses. Contemporary implant dentistry. St. Louis (MO): Mosby; 1993.
34. Misch CE, Bidez MW. Implant protected occlusion: a biomechanical rationale. Compend Contin Dent Educ 1994;15:1330–43.
35. Papaspyridakos P, Chen C-J, Chuang SK, et al. A systematic review of biologic and technical complications with fixed implant rehabilitation for edentulous patients. Int J Oral Maxillofac Implants 2012;27(1):102–10.
36. Papspyridakos P, Bordin TB, Kim YJ, et al. Technical complications and prosthesis survival rates with implant-supported fixed complete dental prostheses: a retrospective study with 1 to 12 year follow-up. J Prosthodont 2020;29(1):3–11.
37. Varthis S, Tarnow D, Randi A. Interproximal open contacts between implant restorations and adjacent teeth. Prevalence – causes – possible solutions. J Prosthodont 2019;28:e806–10.
38. Sadid-Zadeh R, Kutkut A, Kim H. Prosthetic failure in Implant Dentistry. Dent Clin North Am 2015;59:195–214.
39. Goodacre CJ, Bernal G, Rungcharassaeng K, et al. Clinical complications with implants and implant prostheses. J Prosthet Dent 2003;90:121–32.
40. Romanos GE, Javed F, Delgado-Ruiz RA, et al. Peri-implant diseases: a review of treatment interventions. Dent Clin North Am 2015;59:157–78.
41. Scarfe W, Farman A, Sukovic P. Clinical applications of cone-beamed computed tomography in the dental practice. J Can Dent Assoc 2006;72(1):75–80.
42. Hutlin H, Svensson K, Trulsson M. Clinical advantages of computer-guided implant placement: a systemic review. Clin Oral Implants Res 2012;23(Suppl 6):124–38.
43. Block MS. Color Atlas of implant surgery. 3rd edition. Saunders (Elsevier); 2011. p. 58–114.
44. Aziz SR. Hard and soft tissue surgical complications in dental implantology. Oral Maxillofacial Surg Clin N Am 2015;27:313–8.

45. Wittneben J-G, Wismeijer D, Brägger U, et al. Patient-reported outcome measures focusing on aesthetics of implant- and tooth-supported fixed dental prostheses: a systematic review and meta-analysis. Clin Oral Implants Res 2018; 29(Suppl. 16):224–40.

46. Berglundh T, Armitage G, Araujo MG. Peri-implant diseases and conditions: consensus report of workgroup 4 of the 2017 World Workshop on the Classification of Periodontal and Peri-Implant Diseases and Conditions. J Periodontol 2018; 89(Suppl 1):S313–8.

47. Mittal H, John MT, Sekulić S, et al. Patient- Reported Outcome Measures for Adult Dental Patients: a systemic review. J Evid Based Dent Pract 2019;19(1):53–70.

48. Lang NP, Zitzmann NU. Working Group 3 of the VIII European Workshop on Periodontology. Clinical research in implant dentistry: evaluation of implant-supported restorations, aesthetic and patient-reported outcomes. J Clin Periodontol 2012;39(Suppl. 12):133–8.

49. Cosyn J, Thoma DS, Hämmerle CH, et al. Esthetic assessments in implant dentistry: objective and subjective criteria for clinicians and patients. Periodontol 2000 2017;73(1):193–202.

50. Petersen PE, Bourgeois D, Ogawa H, et al. The global burden of oral diseases and risks to oral health. Bull World Health Organ 2005;83(9):661–9.

51. Peterson PE, Yamamoto T. Improving the Oral health of older people: the approach of the WHO Global Oral Health Programme. Community Dent Oral Epidemiol 2005;33(2):81–92.

52. Payne AGT, Alsabeeha NHM, Atieh MA, et al. Interventions for replacing missing teeth : attachment systems for Implant over-dentures in edentulous jaws. Cochrane Database Syst Rev 2018;(10):CD008001.

53. Babush CA. Post-treatment quantification of patient experiences with full-arch implant treatment using a modification of the OHID – 14 questionnaire. J Oral Implant 2012;38(3):251–60.

54. Lopez CS, Saka CH, Rada G, et al. Impact of fixed implant supported prostheses in edentulous patients: protocol for a systemic review. BJM Open 2016;6: e009288.

55. Sykess D. Medico-legal aspects of dental implants. Ann R Australas Coll Dent Surg 2000;15:309–14.

56. de Albuquerque Júnior RF, Lund JP, Tang L, et al. Within-subject comparison of maxillary long-bar implant-retained prostheses with and without palatal coverage: patient-based outcome. Clin Oral Implants Res 2000;11:555–65.

57. Fero KJ, Morgano SM, Driscoll CF, et al. the Glossary of Prosthodontic Terms: Ninth Edition GPT-9. J Prosthet Dent 2017;117(5 Suppl):e1–105.

58. Naert I. The influence of attachment systems on implant-retained mandibular overdentures. In: Feine JS, Carsson GE, editors. Implant overdentures: the standard of care for the edentulous patients, vol. 13. Chicago, Illinois, USA: Quintessence Publishing Co Inc; 2003. p. 238–43.

59. Assaf A, Daas M, Boittin A, et al. Prosthetic maintenance of different mandibular implant overdentures: a systematic review. Prosthet Dent 2017;118(2):144–52.

60. Attard NJ, Zarb GA, Laporte A. Long-term treatment outcomes in edentulous patients with implant overdentures: the Toronto study. Int J Prosthodont 2004;17: 425–33.

61. Drago C, Howell K. Concepts for Designing and Fabricating Metal Implant Frameworks for Hybrid Implant Prostheses. J Prosthodont 2012;21:413–24.

62. Momelli A. Maintenance therapy for teeth and implants. Perodontol 2000 2019; 79:190–9.

63. Araujo MG, Lindhe J. Peri-implant health. J Periodontol 2018;89(Suppl 1): S249–56.
64. Heitz-Mayfiel LJA, Salvi GE. Peri-implant mucositis. J Periodontol 2018;(Suppl 1): S257–66.
65. Schwartz F, DerksJ Monje A, Wang H-L. Per-implamtitis. J Periodontol 2018; 89(Suppl1):S267–90.
66. Renevert S, Perrson GR, Pirih FQ, et al. Peri-implant health, peri-implant mucositis: case definitions and diagnostic considerations. J Periodontol 2018;89(Suppl 1):S304–12.
67. Papaspyridakos P, Chen CJ, Singh M, et al. Success criteria in implant dentistry: a systemic review. J Dent Res 2012;91(3):253–60.
68. Chang M, Odman P, Wennström JL, et al. Esthetic outcome of implant-supported single-tooth replacements assessed by the patient and by prosthodontists. Int J Prosthodont 1999;12(4):335–41.
69. Tettamanti S, Millen C, Gavric J, et al. Esthetic evaluation of implant crowns and peri-implant soft tissue in the anterior maxilla: comparison and reproducibility of three different indices. Clin Implant Dent Relat Res 2016;18(3):517–26.
70. Hartlev J, Kohberg P, Ahlmann S, et al. Patient satisfaction and esthetic outcome after immediate placement and provisionalization of single-tooth implants involving a definitive individual abutment. Clin Oral Implants Res 2014;25(11): 1245–50.
71. Cosyn J, Eghbali A, De Bruyn H, et al. Single implant treatment in healing versus healed sites of the anterior maxilla: an aesthetic evaluation. Clin Implant Dent Relat Res 2012;14(4):517–26.
72. Cosyn J, Eghbali A, Hanselaer L, et al. Four modalities of single implant treatment in the anterior maxilla: a clinical, radiographic, and esthetic evaluation. Clin Implant Dentistry Relat Res 2013;15(4):517–30.

Maxillofacial Bone Grafting Materials 2021 Update

Nabil Moussa, DDS*, Yijiao Fan, DDS, Harry Dym, DDS

KEYWORDS

- Bone • Tissue grafting • Bone regeneration • Osteoinductivity
- Regenerative materials • Tissue engineering • Bone morphogenetic protein

KEY POINTS

- This article provides a summary of the basic knowledge and fundamental principals of bone grafting in the setting of Oral and Maxillofacial Surgery.
- Autogenous bone graft is currently the gold standard in regards to grafting success.
- Available grafting materials include autograft, allograft, xenograft and alloplast.
- Bone morphogenic protein is predictable method for inducing bone formation.

INTRODUCTION

Successful outcomes in the use of bone grafting and reconstructive outcomes heavily depend on understanding the fundamentals and material properties. The purpose of grafting is to achieve regeneration of hard tissues. The regenerated bone must have the capacity to provide the same physiologic support as the original dentition. Such goals can be achieved through regenerating well-vascularized bone that will undergo normal remodeling and healing. Prosthetically, a variety of restorative options, including fixed, hybrid, and removable restorative options, have become available. These options restore functionality and quality of life to patients who may have both esthetic and functional disabilities. Regenerated bone must have histologically and physiologically identical characteristics to native bone. Implant integration and function depend on the composite characteristics and structural stability of native bone to function. This article provides an overview of the currently available bone regenerative materials, their advantages, and their uses in the current literature.

BIOLOGY OF BONE

Bone is a composite structure composed of a macrostructure of type I collagen with calcified components. Bone is a dynamic structure undergoing constant resorption

This article has been updated from a version previously published in Dental Clinics of North America, Volume 64, Issue 2, April 2020.
Department of Dentistry, Division of Oral and Maxillofacial Surgery, Brooklyn Hospital Center, 121 Dekalb Avenue, Brooklyn, NY 11201, USA
* Corresponding author.
E-mail address: moussanabil@gmail.com

and deposition by osteoclasts and osteoblasts. To maintain balance, the body orchestrates cell activity by secreting parathyroid hormone (PTH), vitamin D, and calcitonin. This dynamic system plays an important role in growth, adaptation to biomechanical stresses, and repair of macrofractures and microfractures.

Bone deposition, resorption, and maintenance are achieved through the actions of osteoblasts, osteoclasts, and osteocytes. Osteoblasts are derived from local differentiated osteoprogenitor cells in reaction to stimuli. Such osteoprogenitor cells are present in the periosteal and endosteal layers of the bone. These critical parenchymal tissues serve as a vital reservoir for undifferentiated stem cells in addition to serving as a blood supply to the native tissue. Minimizing the reflection of periosteum during dissection preserve vascularity to the local tissues, which leads to improved outcomes of bone regeneration. Osteoclasts are resorptive cells that, through the actions of alkaline phosphatase, resorb bone and release calcium. Through the coordinated actions of PTH, calcitonin, and vitamin D, bone turnover and calcium levels are maintained. Diseases that affect this balance can be detrimental to the body. Diseases such as Paget, rheumatoid arthritis, and osteopenia can compromise the integrity of the bony framework. Conditions such as release of parathyroid hormone–related proteins in squamous cell carcinoma and renal osteodystrophy can result in osteolytic lesions defects that make bone susceptible to fracture.

Bone is composed of 2 major components: cortical and trabecular bone. Cortical bone is a dense housing that forms the outer layers that encase the trabecular bone marrow. Harvesting and grafting each type affects the quality of the regenerated bone. Cortical bone is a dense structure made of haversian canal systems. Examination of cortical bone reveals bone resembling tubes with a central core containing osteocytes. Cortical bone is composed of multiple units of tubules, referred to as haversian canals. Trabecular bone is formed by an aggregate of bone loosely arranged in a meshlike fashion. Within this lattice, erythron and leukopoiesis takes place.

During bone formation, mesenchymal cells are stimulated by growth factors during development and differentiate into osteoblasts. Osteoblasts deposit bone in their immediate surrounding, encasing themselves within a mineralized matrix termed lacunae. As the bone grows, these osteoblasts mature into osteocytes. Groups of lacunae form into conical structures previously referred to as haversian canals. The individual osteocytes communicate with one another through the canals, which allow resorption and deposition in response to the needs of the body. Trabecular bone forms within the core of the developing cortical bone. A thin, fibrous tissue subsequently forms around the maturing bone. Periosteum is the layer that envelopes cortical bone. In comparison, endosteum envelopes trabecular bone. The tissue surrounding these bony structures provides vascular supply and nutrition (**Table 1**).

Bone is classified into several categories depending on the thickness and volume of cortical and cancellous bone. The composition changes depending on the load and demands on the bone. Branemark[1] described and classified bone based on the composition of cortical and trabecular bone. Type 1 bone is composed mainly of cortical bone with minimal amounts of trabecular bone. In contrast, type 4 bone is composed mainly of trabecular bone and little cortical bone. Types 2 and 3 bridge the gap between types 1 and 4, with more trabeculae present in type 3 bone. The mandible is typically characterized by a composition of type 1 and 2 bone. Type 3 bone primarily makes up the maxillary alveolus, with sections of type 4 bone posteriorly toward the tuberosity.

Implant placement and primary stability are affected by the type of bone in which it is placed. Implant placed in type 2 bone is likely to have good primary stability with good bone/implant interface, and such bone is typically found in the mandible. Type 3 bone may need an implant with a more aggressive thread design, and such bone

Table 1
Composition of bone

Type of Bone	Histologic Features
Organized matrix	40% of the dry weight of bone. Composed of 90% type 1 collagen, noncollagenous proteins, ground substance, water, proteoglycans, cytokines, and growth factors
Cells	Osteoprogenitor cells: osteoblasts osteocytes osteoclasts
Vascular and nutrient	Bone receives 5%–10% of cardiac output via arterial supply through the periosteum and endosteum.
Distribution	Microcirculation, lymphatics, and venous return
Neurologic	Bone is supplied by autonomic and neurosensory networks
Marrow	Serves hematopoietic and osteogenic functions
Periosteum	A source of osteoprogenitor cells, neurovascular distribution, and blood supply
Endosteum	A source of osteoprogenitor cells
Communication systems	A network including haversian and Volkmann canaliculi lacunae and extracellular fluid

From Moussa NT, Dym H. Maxillofacial bone grafting materials. Dental Clin North Am. 2020;64(2):474; with permission.

is typically found in the maxilla. Both types 1 and 4 bone have their own respective disadvantages and are not favorable for implant placement. Type 1 bone is dense with minimal trabecular bone present. Such bone has reduced vascularity and subsequently is more susceptible to necrosis and implant failure. Type 4 bone has minimal cortical bone present, and implants placed in such bone, although integrated, may not be able to support functional loads. The end result is implant failure and compromise in the foundation of the prosthesis.

BONE HEALING BIOLOGY

The mechanism of bone healing closely follows that of other tissues. Bone must proceed through the 3 phases of healing: inflammation, proliferation, and remodeling. Inflammation leads to blood coagulation and hematoma formation. Damage to endothelial cells leads to platelet aggregation and degranulation. Critical growth factors are released to promote angiogenesis and formation of a hematoma. Growth factors include fibroblastic growth factor and vascular endothelial growth factors. In the proliferative phase, fibroblasts are recruited and migrate into the surgical site. Fibrin deposition and angiogenesis result in organized tissue development, referred to as granulation tissues. The fibrin and collagen network paves the way for osteoblast migration and collagen deposition within 48 hours.

Initial collagen meshwork in bone is composed of type I and III collagen. The fibers are laid in a haphazard manner and the process of ossification begins. Calcification begins in what are referred to as ossification or maturation centers. Immature osteoid forms around these foci of calcified tissues, slowly growing in a concentric manner. Additional osteoblasts are recruited and surround the osteoid, further expanding the bone until ossification centers come into contact with one another and merge. Large blocks of osteoid are referred to as a soft callus, forming 4 to 7 days following the initial insult. As the soft callus matures and bone consolidates in the remodeling phase, osteoid begins to reorganize into organized matrices of cortical and trabecular bone. The remodeling phase starts at 8 weeks and forms what is known as a hard callus. The remodeling phase is orchestrated by the actions of osteoblasts and osteoclasts, which are responsible for bone deposition and resorption respectively. Type III collagen is replaced by the composite structure made of type I collagen. At the time of remodeling, the bone is most brittle and susceptible to fracture. Sixteen weeks following the insult is when bone maturation and remodeling is completed. The bone is considered to have the structural integrity for load-bearing forces.

EFFECTS OF BONE GRAFTING ON HEALING

The purpose of bone grafting and reconstruction is to regenerate tissues that are histologically identical to the native bone tissues. Aside from autogenous tissue, grafting materials are limited to those that are acellular. The remaining types of graft material are processed to maintain the macrostructure of bone or synthesized to mimic local scaffolding of bone to facilitate the movement and migration of local cells into the graft. This property of grafting materials is referred to as being osteoconductive. Techniques have been developed to preserve or add growth factors that add osteoinductive potential to the graft. The ability to facilitate and recruit cells into the graft material is referred to as being osteoinductive. Synthetic grafts such as calcium carbonate or even xenografts have been shown to have a slower rate of resorption and can act to resist compressive forces from wound contraction or masticator forces that may cause volume loss. Autografts have osteoinductive and osteoconductive properties. In addition, autografts transplant live osteoclasts, osteoblasts, and the pluripotent osteoprogenitor cells. Such tissues are considered to have osteogenic potential. The osteogenic potential of autografts has a significant positive impact on tissue healing and bone integration. Autografts are considered the gold standard of bone grafting materials.

IMPACTS ON BONE HEALING

Minimizing factors that can negatively affect bone healing leads to reduced risk of graft failure and increased volume of regenerated bone. Immobility and vascular perfusion are essential in bone healing. Micromotion in healing is considered an important contributing factor for nonunion. For example, fractured bone segments that are not immobilized result in micromotion and severance of the newly formed blood vessels. Compromises in the vascular supply lead to nonunion. In a similar fashion, grafted bone that receives pressure and is not immobilized has an increased incidence of failure, with greatly reduced bone volume regenerated. Pressure on grafted bone when placed under function can result in graft failure during the healing period due to compromised vascular supply.

Patients who have received radiation have drastically reduced angiogenic and cellular capacity for healing. Free radicals formed through radiation damage cell structure and cause sclerosis of vital vessels. The result is referred to as the 3 Hs: hypocellular, hypo-oxygenated, and hypovascular tissue. In such circumstances, patients must receive treatment to improve tissue oxygen perfusion in the form of hyperbaric oxygen. Hyperbaric oxygen treatment increases the oxygen tension of the tissues, subsequently stimulating angiogenesis with the goal of improving the chances of bone healing.

Systemic conditions that affect the vascular supply of tissues also have a negative effect on bone healing. Conditions such as diabetes and atherosclerosis reduce the flow of blood to the healing bone, subsequently reducing the nutritional supply to the healing tissues. In addition, modifiable risk factors such as smoking have devastating effects on the vascular supply to healing bone. The effects of nicotine on the vasculature last 5 hours (5 half-lives of 60 minutes) and compromise the blood flow to tissues. In addition, smokers have reduced oxygen carrying capacity through the formation of carboxyhemoglobin, which shifts the hemoglobin dissociation curve to the left. The result is a reduced proportion of hemoglobin molecules available for carrying oxygen. Patients that have stopped smoking have been found to have impaired macrophage and antimicrobial resistance for up to 6 months.

BASICS OF BONE GRAFTING

Clinical success in bone regeneration depends on good clinical practice and understanding the basics. Bone must have adequate blood supply and fixation. Several technical basics must be kept in mind when conducting patient care. Obtaining a good vascular supply is largely influenced by the clinician's ability to design and handle soft tissue gently. Mucosal and attached gingiva must be handled with care, and crush injuries must be avoided when using the tissue forceps. When designing a flap, the base of the flap must be wider than the free margin of the flap. Folding or kinking flaps must be avoided to optimize blood flow and perfusion pressure to the flap. The clinician must conduct appropriate release of the soft tissue and periosteum. Without primary closure, blood supply is compromised and the bone is exposed to the oral flora, giving rise to potential infections. However, it is important to maintain tension-free closure to avoid ischemic necrosis in the soft tissue. It is prudent to pay attention to detail in flap design and not create incisions that will result in closure over root prominences (eg, over the canine root). Such flaps conveniently place incisions over points of tension.

When grafting, primary stability of the grafted material is critical. Micromotion in bone grafting or any pressure applied to the graft can compromise the vascular supply to the grafted material. Often, fibrous nonunion and subsequent graft failure result. Grafts can be fixated with the use of fixation screws or pins. A minimum of 2 screws must be placed to prevent rotational forces. Titanium mesh is a reliable medium to secure and house particulate grafts. The material is able to maintain its shape, resist functional forces of deformation, and minimize motion. Materials such as polytetrafluoroethylene (PTFE) have been developed to provide protection in cases where primary closure is difficult or not possible. These membranes have the capacity to remain exposed in the oral cavity and can be stabilized with the use of titanium screws or pins. Both PTFE and titanium mesh are nonresorbable membranes and must be removed before additional fixture placement. The PTFE membrane is typically removed 4 weeks following placement once the soft tissue callus has formed.

BONE GRAFTING MATERIALS

Four basic types of bone grafting materials are available for use clinically to augment and reconstruct the maxillofacial skeleton (**Tables 2 and 3**).

AUTOLOGOUS BONE

Autologous bone refers to bone that is harvested form the individual's own tissue. Examples of harvest sites used in the oral surgery setting include the anterior and posterior hip, calvarium, tibia, and mandibular ramus and symphysis. Use of autologous bone and its popularity in the routine oral surgical setting has decreased because of the predictability and availability of allogenic bone. However, autogenous bone is still maintained as the gold standard for bone grafting.[2] This particular source of bone is the only graft material that boasts osteoconductive, osteoinductive, and osteogenic properties. In the contemporary setting, autogenous bone is typically reserved for large defects or situations where predictable results are hard to obtain; for example,

Table 2
Classes of bone graft materials

Bone Type	Description
Autograft (autogenous)	Transplant of viable cortical or cancellous bone from one location of the body to another within the same patient
Xenograft	Cross-species transplant of tissue: the use of organic bovine bone or porcine collagen
Alloplast	Implantation of synthetic material, such as apatite or tricalcium phosphate, bioactive glass, or polymers

From Moussa NT, Dym H. Maxillofacial bone grafting materials. Dental Clin North Am. 2020;64(2):475; with permission.

in continuity defects and alveolar clefts.[3] In patients with craniofacial dysplasia and oculoauriculovertebral spectrum disorders, rib grafts, with their respective cartilaginous components, have been used in the reconstruction of temporomandibular joints. Depending on the harvest site, different volumes and compositions of grafts can be harvested (**Table 4**).

As discussed previously, adequate vascular supply to the grafted bone is critical in the survival and integration of the graft. Defects ranging more than 6 to 8 cm are considered the limit for nonvascularized bone grafting. Reconstruction in defects large than 6 to 8 cm becomes challenging when using nonvascularized grafts because the nutritional and oxygen supply is inadequate. Nonvascularized grafts obtain their nutritional supply through a process known as imbibition. Subsequent inosculation of blood vessels to the graft provides new anastomosis and vascular network for the grafted tissues. The limitations of this process are reached when defects become bigger than 6 to 8 cm. When reconstructing large defects as a result of resections from ameloblastoma and squamous cell carcinoma or loss from traumatic injuries, vascularized grafts are indicated. A vascularized graft is needed to maintain nutrition and oxygen tension to the grafted tissue. Examples of vascularized bone grafts include free fibula, iliac crest, and scapular tip grafts.

Table 3
Bone grafting material overview

Bone Graft	Structural Strength	Osteoconduction	Osteoinduction	Osteogenesis
Autograft	—	—	—	—
Cancellous	No	+++	+++	+++
Cortical	+++	++	++	++
Allograft	—	—	—	—
Cancellous	—	—	—	—
Frozen	No	++	+	No
Freeze dried	No	++	+	No
Cortical	—	—	—	—
Frozen	+++	+	No	No
Freeze dried	+	+	No	No

From Giannoudis PV, Dinopoulos H, Tsiridis E. Bone substitutes: an update. Injury. 2005;36(Suppl3):S21; with permission.

Table 4 Typical noncompressed graft volumes available for harvest		
	Noncompressed Corticocancellous	**Cortical Block**
Tibia	25–40 cm^3	1×2 cm
Anterior Ilium	50 cm^3	3×5 cm
Posterior Ilium	100–125 cm^3	5×5 cm
Calvarium	Variable, minimal	Abundant

From Zouhary KJ. Bone graft harvesting from distant sites: concepts and technique. Oral Maxillofac Surg Clin North Am. 2010;22(3):303; with permission.

In planning for reconstruction, it is important to consider the volume and composition of the graft that can be harvested. It is generally accepted that a 1-cm defect require 10 cm^3 of bone for reconstruction. Depending on the harvest site, large volumes of cortical or trabecular bone may be harvested. For example, the symphysis of the mandible yields primarily cortical bone, which is useful in reconstructing alveolar defects in the area of lateral incisors or in gaining structural support (vertical and horizontal). In contrast, harvesting graft from the ilium (anterior or posterior) yields a large volume of trabecular bone, which is useful in guided tissue regeneration and reconstruction of alveolar clefts. Cortical blocks are often used for their structural integrity in reconstruction. Periosteum often constricts during the healing process. Cortical grafts resist compression forces placed on the graft material during the healing process. Such resistance is important to maintain the volume of regenerated tissue and achieve the appropriate dimensions for fixture placement. Trabecular bone is often favorable for filling defects. The handling characteristics make marrow bone ideal for filling walled defects and contouring the graft sites.

Autogenous graft is advantageous for the key reason that it is the host's own tissue. As mentioned previously, it has osteoinductive, osteoconductive, and osteogenic properties. Osteoconduction and osteoinduction refer to the graft's ability to facilitate movement of cells into the graft and induce differentiation of host monocytes into osteoblasts, respectively. When harvested, the graft maintains the original macrostructure and microstructure of the tissue, which includes the cytokines, growth factors, and cells of the tissue. The transplant of vital host cells is referred to as osteogenic grafting. Components of the graft give autograft distinct advantages of efficient signaling and differentiation of osteoprogenitor cells present within the periosteum and endosteum within the host site and the graft. These properties facilitate efficient new osteoid formation and graft integration.

Because the tissue is harvested from the host, there is no risk of immune rejection and disease transmission. Autogenous grafts eliminate risks in transmission of diseases, including human immunodeficiency virus and hepatitis B and C. There are still reported cases of disease transmission despite the manufacturers' efforts to appropriately screen, test, and process tissue in a disease-free condition.

The need for a secondary surgical site is the main disadvantage of autologous grafts. In addition, limited volume can be harvested and the process is associated with its own morbidity. For example, anterior and posterior iliac crest grafts have an associated risk of gait disturbance, which can result in difficulty ambulating. Complication rates have been reported to be 8.5% to 20%.[4–8] Other types of complications include hematoma formation, gastric ileus, blood loss, neurosensory disturbances, hernia formation, pelvic fracture, and chronic pain. Harvest sites such as the symphysis can result in cosmetic defects, droopy chin, and sensory disturbances in the distribution of the mental nerve. The invasive nature and risk of morbidity restrict its access to those clinicians that are appropriately trained in the harvest of autogenous graft. In addition, its use must be carefully planned so the risks of harvest are justified by the benefits of the graft. However, with the use of trephine burs and bone scrapers, local harvesting techniques have made obtaining grafts easier. In summary, autogenous bone is a superior graft material with numerous advantages, such as improved healing time and predictable results compared with other types of available grafting material. However, its use must be carefully considered and the risks must be weighed against the benefits.

Cleft lip and palate is a good example of an indication for the necessary use of autogenous bone grafting. Carlini and colleagues[9] report a case series of 16 patients with bilateral transincisive foraminal defects of the premaxilla. Following a period of orthodontic optimization and stabilization using a transpalatal appliance, the premaxillary segment was surgically repositioned and secured using an acrylic splint. The surgery involved invasive reflection and repositioning of soft and hard tissues (**Fig. 1**). Iliac crest bone (cortical and trabecular) was harvested and the cortical plates were used to fixate the premaxilla to the posterior alveolar segments with titanium screws to achieve primary stability. Medullary bone was subsequently used to fill the remaining void and contour the bone. In such cases where incisions and osteotomies compromise the vascular supply to the tissues, autogenous graft provides the appropriate stability, tissue volume, and growth potential to obtain a predictable result.[9] Precious

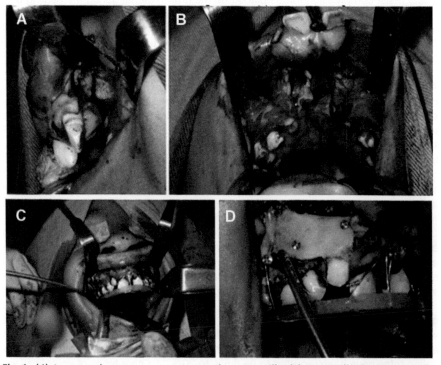

Fig. 1. (*A*) Access and osteotomy to separate the premaxilla; (*B*) premaxilla displacement for closure of the nasal mucosa; (*C*) suturing to remake the nasal fossa floor; and (*D*) cortical fixation with screws (1.5 mm) in the maxilla and premaxilla. (*From* Carlini JL, Biron C. Use of the iliac crest cortex for premaxilla fixation in patients with bilateral clefts. J Oral Maxillofac Surg. 2020;78(7):1192.e3; with permission.)

and colleagues[10] outlined repair of the cleft palate with the use of iliac crest bone graft. Repair and excellent results were achieved with the use of careful surgical planning, technique, and autogenous bone (**Fig. 2**).

Acocella and colleagues[11] evaluated the clinical, histomorphic, and histologic quality of bone in transplanted mandibular ramus grafts used for the regeneration of maxillary alveolar bone. The study population consisted of 15 patients with maxillary alveolar defects planned for implant placement and prosthesis fabrication. Reconstructive sites involved defects of both the anterior and posterior maxilla. The clinical procedures focused on horizontal augmentation. The mean width of augmentation was measured preoperatively and at time of reentry (**Fig. 3**).

The grafts were allowed to heal for a period of 3 to 9 months. Bone samples were harvested at the time of implant site preparation. The study reported a mean augmentation thickness of 4.6 mm, with a range from 3 to 6 mm. Following adequate healing, the mean thickness of bone remaining was 4.0 mm, which showed a loss of thickness to resorption of 0.6 mm. These findings were consistent with what is reported in the literature, with good volumetric stability of cortical grafting and minimal resorption. A total of 30 implants were placed with no reported failures. The histologic findings of the study are of particular interest because the investigators paid attention to the rate of neovascularization of bone. All of the samples collected in the study showed signs of remodeling and were free of inflammatory tissue. In addition, the investigators noted good neovascularized tissue present in the grafted bone, with good osseous integration of the host site with the grafted bone. However, the investigators did note a histologic change in the direction of lamella demarcating the margin of the grafted bone with the native bone. The histologic observations that vital bone contained osteocytes in a core of osteoid surrounded by neovascularized bone suggest that the host tissue recolonized the grafted bone (**Fig. 4**).

The study noted that neovascularized bone tissue represented an area of osteocytes that did not survive the transplant and required tissue reperfusion and remodeling for the graft to survive.[11] In comparison, Ellegaard and colleagues[12] found that, following disruption of blood vessels, many osteocytes do receive the nutrition necessary for osteocyte survival. In support of these findings, Ham and colleagues[13] noted that osteocytes require less than 0.1-mm proximity to haversian systems for survival. The literature provides evidence that, with adequate time, autogenous grafting

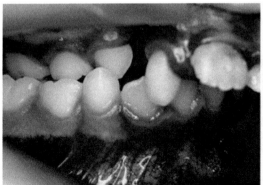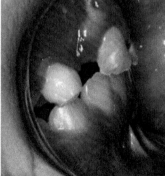

Fig. 2. Preoperative and postoperative results following bone grafting. Visible is the good soft tissue perfusion and integration of the graft with the host tissue. (*From* Carlini JL, Biron C. Use of the iliac crest cortex for premaxilla fixation in patients with bilateral clefts. J Oral Maxillofac Surg. 2020;78(7):1192.e4; with permission.)

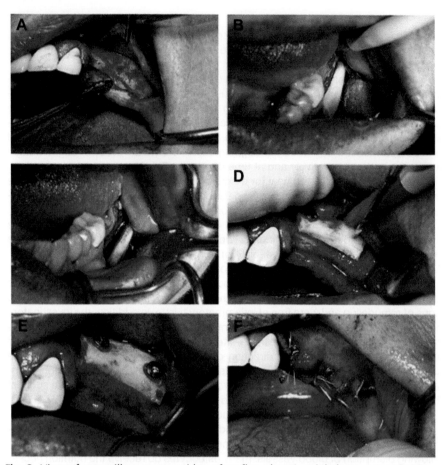

Fig. 3. View of a maxillary narrow ridge after flap elevation (*A*); bone osteotomies on mandibular buccal shelf (*B*); the monocortical is out-fractured (*C*); adaptation and fixation of the graft to the maxillary recipient site (*D*); gaps around the block grafts were filled with bone chips harvested from the donor site (*E*); primary flap closure without tension (*F*). (*From* Acocella A, Bertolai R, Colafrenceschi M, et al. Clinical, histological and histomorphometric evaluation of the healing of mandibular ramus bone block grafts for alveolar ridge augmentation before implant placement. J Craniomaxillofac Surg. 2010;38(3):225; with permission.)

supports neovascularization and survival of osteocytes in grafted autogenous bone. The regenerated bone provides a good foundation for implant placement and survival.

Harvesting bone from the hip provides large volumes of grafting material (see **Table 4**): between 50 and 100 cm³ based on harvest site. Fretwurst and colleagues[14] investigated the bone level changes around dental implants placed in autogenous bone grafted from iliac crest (**Figs. 5** and **6**). Both maxillary and mandibular regenerative tissues were evaluated. A total of 32 patients were recruited for the study, and 150 implants were placed into the regenerated tissues. Following a mean observation period of 69 months (12–165 months of healing), implant success rates were evaluated. The study reported a success rate of 96% in the maxilla and 92% in the mandible. The mean crestal bone loss was 1.8 mm, which is consistent with rates reported in the literature.[14]

In the reconstruction of large mandibular and maxillary defects, the fibula serves as a large source of available bone. The fibula is a non–weight-bearing bone and does not

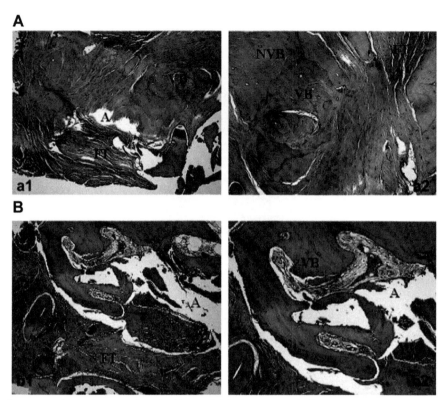

Fig. 4. Histologic changes of grafted bone. (*A*) (*a1*) Four months following surgery with substantial amount of fibrous tissue (FT) and minimal amounts of vital bone (VB), (*a2*) same specimen at a higher magnification. VB is surrounded by new vascularized bone (NVB) with empty lacunae representing creeping substitution. (*B*) (*b1*) Six months following surgery, active bone remodeling is appreciated with presence of larger amounts of VB, (*b2*) same specimen at higher power, with larger composition of VB containing osteocytes compared with 4 months. (*From* Acocella A, Bertolai R, Colafrenceschi M, et al. Clinical, histological and histomorphometric evaluation of the healing of mandibular ramus bone block grafts for alveolar ridge augmentation before implant placement. J Craniomaxillofac Surg. 2010;38(3):228; with permission.)

risk the patients' ability to ambulate when harvested. The graft can be harvested as a vascularized or nonvascularized graft. When reconstructing defects larger than 6 to 8 cm, vascularized grafts are necessary to maintain nutritional supply to the grafted bone. Duttenhoefer and colleagues[15] provided their results with grafting of atrophic mandibles. The investigators showed that atrophic mandibles (thickness <10 mm) could be predictably grafted with the use of avascular fibular grafts. In addition, the study showed long-term stability and osseointegration of implants placed in the regenerated bone. The patients were followed up to 15 years with stable results. The bone was sampled at the time of implant placement, which supported that autogenous bone successfully revascularized and retained cortical bone structure (**Fig. 7**).[15] The findings of Duttenhoefer and colleagues[15] were consistent with other reports in the literature. Nelson and colleagues[16] reported their results on 10 patients augmented with avascular fibular graft in a vertical fashion. Vertical grafting is very technique sensitive and has a significant risk of volumetric loss. However, the study

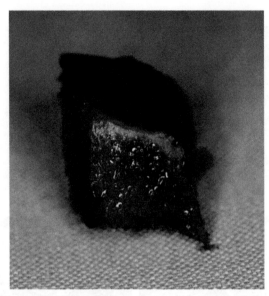

Fig. 5. Harvested iliac crest bone graft. (*From* Fretwurst T, Nack C, Al-Ghrairi M, et al. Long-term retrospective evaluation of the peri-implant bone level in onlay grafted patients with iliac bone from the anterior superior iliac crest. J Craniomaxillofac Surg. 2015;43(6):957; with permission.)

reported a loss of 7.2% of the gained vertical height with a mean follow-up period of 6.25 years. The bone height was then observed to stabilize with minimal vertical loss subsequently (**Fig. 8**).[16]

ALLOGENEIC BONE

Because of increasing popularity in dental implants and the ease of placement, an increasing number of general practitioners have incorporated implant dentistry into their practices. In a similar fashion, the availability of allogenic graft material has increased. The graft has shown a 15-fold increase in use. In the year 2000, it

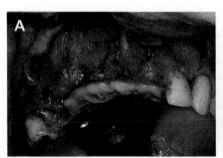
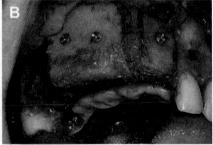

Fig. 6. Maxillary iliac crest bone grafting. Maxillary defect shown with horizontal and vertical deficiencies (*A*). Reconstruction of the maxillary defect with iliac bone graft (*B*). (*From* Misch CM. Maxillary autogenous bone grafting. Oral Maxillofac Surg Clin North Am. 2011;23(2):230; with permission.)

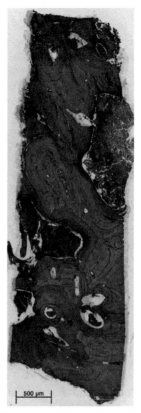

Fig. 7. Histologic specimen of fibular bone 10 years following grafting to the mandible and implant loading. (*From* Duttenhoefer F, Nack C, Doll C, et al. Long-term peri-implant bone level changes of non-vascularized fibula bone grafted edentulous patients. J Craniomaxillofac Surg. 2015;43(5):614; with permission.)

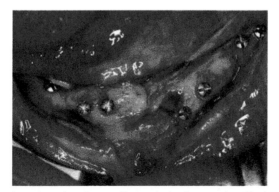

Fig. 8. Intraoperative view showing well-vascularized avascular fibular graft 3 months following surgery and before implant placement. (*From* Nelson K, Glatzer C, Hildebrand D, et al. Clinical evaluation of endosseous implants in nonvascularized fibula bone grafts for reconstruction of the severely atrophied mandibular bone. J Oral Maxillofac Surg. 2006;64(9):1429; with permission.)

represented one-third of all grafting material in the medical community.[17] Allogenic bone graft refers to bone that is harvested from the same species (ie, human cadavers). The donated bone is screened for any transmissible diseases and processed and prepared using several different techniques. Depending on the processing technique and degree of processing, various types of bone grafting material can be prepared. The properties of the bone change based on the remaining components.

Types of available bone include fresh, fresh-frozen, freeze-dried, and demineralized types of bone. Demineralized graft material no longer contains the calcium phosphate mineral component of bone, leaving the collagen network of the composite material. Following the processing, a minimal risk remains of disease transmission, and this risk increases and is inversely related to the degree of processing the material undergoes. If any cellular components are remaining within the graft, there is an additional risk of the host mounting an immunologic reaction to the graft material. Fresh bone samples have the least amount of processing and must undergo a rigorous screening process to ensure little to no transmission disease. Freeze-dried bone, which is heavily processed, has very little risk of disease transmission but has little to no osteoconductive or osteoinductive potential. Fresh bone may be prepared to contain the maximum amount of growth factors and, in some cases, viable cells. Vivigen, sold by DePuy Synthes, is fresh bone that is advertised to contain lineage-committed bone cells for differentiation. Freeze-dried demineralized bone grafting materials receive the most processing and may provide only osteoconductive benefits to grafting. Growth factors normally found in bone, such as bone morphogenetic protein (BMP), are removed as a consequence of the processing. The growth factor BMP induces differentiation of neighboring bone mesenchymal cells to differentiate into osteoblasts. However, the remaining macrostructure continues to promote migration and angiogenesis of bone at the graft site.

Particle size has a strong influence on the osteoconductive properties of allogenic bone. Goldberg and colleagues[18] published their work to show that a particle size of 100 to 300 μm has the greatest osteoconductive potential. This size allows osteoclasts and osteoblasts to migrate into the macrostructure of the grafted bone. In comparison, a particle size of 1000 to 2000 μm does not promote predictable osteoconduction. Moreover, particles of less than 100 μm have been associated with eliciting a macrophage response that results in resorption of the graft. Using a graft that is not optimal for osteoconduction results in resorption of the grafted material with decreased volume of gained regenerative bone.

The major advantage of allogenic bone compared with autogenous bone is that no harvest site is required to obtain the graft. Patient experience and acceptance of treatment improved without the need for a harvest site. In addition, supply of allogenic bone is limited by the quantity available for purchase. With regard to success and achievable bone volume, allogenic bone yields comparable results with autogenous bone when used for alveolar bone regeneration. Limitations may be encountered with larger defects (eg, segmental reconstructions) when using allogenic bone alone. Chaushu and colleagues[19] conducted a split-mouth study to compare volumetric changes after sinus augmentation of completely edentulous maxilla with autogenous and allogenic fresh-frozen bone particles. Harvested bone from the mandibular ramus was placed concurrently with allogenic bone to compare volumes of regenerated bone at 1 week, 6 months, and 12 months following the graft. Allogenic bone showed no statistically significant difference in grafted bone volume compared with autogenous bone. The investigators noted that autogenous bone had a distinct disadvantage of added donor site morbidity. The study concluded that allogenic bone was clinically effective in providing comparative results in regenerated bone volume in the maxillary sinus.[20]

Monje and colleagues[21] investigated the stability and predictability of allogenic block grafts in the edentulous maxilla. The investigators conducted a systematic review of the literature and studied the results of 361 cases of allogenic block grafting to the maxilla followed by a mean follow-up of 4 to 9 months after surgery. The study reported that, of the 361 cases, 9 grafts failed within 1 to 2 months, representing a 2% failure rate. The study additionally reported a mean horizontal width gain of 4.79 mm from 119 graft sites. The study concluded that block grafting with allogenic blocks to gain horizontal width is predictable And, furthermore, that it provides enough augmentation to facilitate implant placement.[21] As previously noted, the goal of grafting is to regenerate histologically identical tissue to the native host site. Acocella and colleagues[11] provided histologic evidence that regenerated tissue structure was consistent with that of the host tissues. The investigators sampled clinical specimens of bone regenerated through the use of allogenic bone grafted for the regeneration of atrophic maxillary ridges. Samples were taken at 4, 6, and 9 months postoperatively. At 4 months, creeping substitution from vital host bone into the allograft was observed with scant osteoclasts and poor neovascularization. At 6 months, cellular activity was still poor; however, graft resorption and regeneration with native bone was observed. After 9 months of healing, the histology showed significant progression, showing invasion of new vital bone surrounding nonvital bone. The process seemed to show continued regeneration and resorption at this time.[2] Bone is considered clinically stable for implant placement at 3 months and 6 months following grafting to the mandible and maxilla respectively. Although clinical success is achieved and the study shows invagination and regeneration of new bone, it suggests that bone is still actively being regenerated after 9 months of healing. It is imperative to use good clinical judgment when examining the grafted bone at the time of placement and to examine the radiodensity of bone before conducted surgery because the site may not be stable for implant placement even though the expected healing time has passed.

Failure rates reported with allogenic bone grafting are similar to those reported in autogenous grafting. Chaushu and colleagues[19] reported a failure rate of 7% in a sample pool of 137 graft sites. The study reported an infection rate of 13%; however, not all infected grafts failed. This finding included both partial and full removal of the grafted material in both the maxilla and mandible. Additional complications rates were also reported in the study. Soft tissue complications, specifically soft tissue dehiscence and membrane exposure, were reported at 30%. In their conclusions, the investigators noted that soft tissue coverage is often difficult to achieve. Failure to achieve primary closure is suspected to have contributed to their complication rates. The investigators noted that maintaining good technique, careful handling of soft tissues, and maintenance of blood supply are critical in preventing graft and membrane exposure and reducing complication rates.[19] Similar studies in the literature reported similar complications and rates.[22,23]

As mentioned earlier, processing of bone material has important impacts on their compositions. Vivogen, a fresh-frozen bone graft, requires strict screening to prevent possible disease transmission. However, the bone is able to maintain vital mesenchymal precursor cells within the grafts. Barone and colleagues[24] conducted a study to investigate the success and stability of implants in augmented ridges using fresh-frozen bone. Twenty-four alveolar ridges were grafted with corticocancellous blocks that were secured with screws (**Figs. 9** and **10**). Soft tissue compromise in the form of dehiscence was observed in 2 of the grafted sites. The grafts necessitated removal because of infection. The remaining grafts showed good integration with the recipient

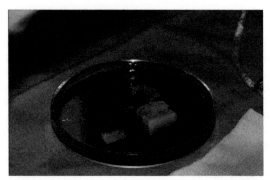

Fig. 9. Corticocancellous block; allogenic block allograft restored in rifamycin. (*From* Barone A, Varanini P, Orlando B, et al. Deep-frozen allogeneic onlay bone grafts for reconstruction of atrophic maxillary alveolar ridges: a preliminary study. J Oral Maxillofac Surg. 2009;67(6):1302; with permission.)

sites, and implants showed good success following prosthetic restoration. The study followed implant stability and 2 implants were deemed failures and had to be removed. The study concluded that fresh-frozen bone grafts provided predictable and long-term stable regeneration of bone to augment the maxilla.

XENOGENEIC BONE

Xenograft refers to tissues transplanted between animals of different species. Typically grafts are often obtained from bovine or equine sources. The tissues are completely devitalized and any cellular or immunogenic materials are removed. This process is important to prevent disease transfer and rejection. Reducing risk of immunologic reactions to xenografts is important because these grafts are harvested from a different species. Similar to allografts, xenograft availability is dictated by the supply. However, costs are often notably less than that of cadaveric bone.

Use of xenogenic bone has been extensively reported in the literature and its success has been documented. Xenografts possess poor osteoinductive properties because of the rigorous processing of the tissues. All of the organic constituents of

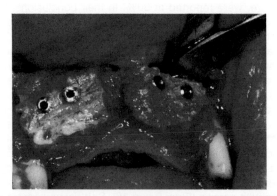

Fig. 10. Horizontal onlay augmentation. (*From* Barone A, Varanini P, Orlando B, et al. Deep-frozen allogeneic onlay bone grafts for reconstruction of atrophic maxillary alveolar ridges: a preliminary study. J Oral Maxillofac Surg. 2009;67(6):1302; with permission.)

the material must be removed to prevent immune reactions from the host. For example, temperature deorganification is used to process and burn away organic components of the donor tissue. Simple osteoconductive properties are maintained because of preservation of the macrostructure of the graft. Often xenograft is mixed with autogenous graft to augment the volume of autograft. The osteoinductive and osteogenic properties of autogenous bone combined with the osteoconductive properties of xenograft makes for a successful regeneration of substantial volume of bone.[22] Factors such as BMP or platelet-rich plasma (PRP) must be used to supplement xenografts. In addition, xenografts may have poor handling properties, requiring placement of a membrane to ensure stability of the graft.

Split-mouth studies were used to investigate the success, predictability, and stability of xenografts used in augmentation for the purposes of implant placement. Lima and colleagues[25] compared the volumetric stability of autologous grafts and xenografts with subsequent implant placement. The study compared augmented anterior maxilla with autologous and xenogenic block grafts. The graft sites were split in the midline where 1 side was grafted with each respective graft. Particulate grafts were used to contour the irregular margins, and autogenous bone was processed through a bone mill to harvest particular autogenous graft. Measurements were conducted clinically and radiographically with the use of three-dimensional imaging. The grafts were allowed to heal for a period of 6 months and the radiographic thicknesses of the grafts were recorded. The grafts did not show a statistically significant difference in the achieved thickness of the grafts. Higher insertion torques were achieved when implants were placed in autogenous graft, suggesting a higher density of bone in autogenous grafts. The study concluded that graft stability and predictability in achieving horizontal augmentation were comparable.[25]

Histologic examination of grafted xenogenic bone was completed by Li and colleagues.[26] The investigators examined the histology of horizontally augmented atrophic ramus using block grafts following 9 months of healing. The histology revealed consistent vital bone invasion of the block xenograft following augmentation.[26] Vertical augmentations were investigated by Simion and colleagues.[27] The investigators vertically grafted atrophic mandible with a mixture of 1:1 xenograft with allograft. The autograft was harvested with the use of bone trephine burs. Implants were placed simultaneously with the graft with a PTFE membrane using a tenting technique. Histologic examination of the graft sites showed formation of cortical and lamellar bone consistent with that of the host tissues. However, the core section of the regenerated tissue revealed speculum of residual xenogenic bone. The contact point of the graft showed histologic continuity with the host lamellar bone. The histology additionally revealed good vascular penetration of the graft to the core. The study concluded that autogenous bone grafted with xenograft provides better outcomes in bone regeneration than xenograft alone.[27]

ALLOPLASTIC BONE

When grafting in the oral cavity, challenges such as handling properties, lack of structural support, and pressure from contraction of tissues during healing can make obtaining predictable results difficult. Alloplastic grafting materials have been engineered for improved handling properties and specialized use. Alloplastic bone grafts are defined as grafting materials or bone substitutes made synthetically or derived from coral of algae hydroxyapatite. Examples of alloplastic materials include coralline calcium carbonate, bioceramic alloplasts (β-tricalcium phosphate), and bioactive glass. Alloplastic materials are often combined with allogeneic grafts when grafting the maxillary sinus. The grafts have properties of being radiopaque and not resorbing, which provide support to the graft against the contractile forces of the sinus membrane when healing.

The grafting success of hydroxyapatite materials depends on the total surface area that is available for the body to interact with. Porous materials allow osteoblasts and osteoclasts to invade and allow space for vascular invasion to incorporate the material into the host's tissue. The biological basis of why coral-based hydroxyapatite works lies in the material's macromolecular structure. The structure of the material is very similar to that of the bone's macromolecular structure. Coral, which is composed of calcium carbonate, is processed by manufacturers to produce calcium carbonate, which has a similar structure to hydroxyapatite. Engineers have even developed a subtype of calcium phosphate that allows it to be more resorbable. Resorbable hydroxyapatite has been synthesized at a particle size that allows the macrophages of the body to remove the particles, essentially making the material resorbable. Biphasic calcium phosphate is such a type of alloplast. The material is engineered from a combination of hydroxyapatite and tricalcium phosphate or from pure tricalcium phosphate. Depending on the ratio of hydroxyl apatite to tricalcium phosphate, the degree of resorption of the material changes.

Alloplasts can have the unique ability of allowing bone to bond to its surface. Silica-based materials, also known as bioactive glass. have this property. BioGran and PerioGlas are two such examples. The bone creates a chemical bond between the bone and glass interface. Maintaining the particle size within a very narrow range allowed the materials to degrade enough to allow cells to access the particulate and lay down new bone in the material. The glass gets lost through degradation processes over time.

Calcium sulfates were developed as bone void filler. Their excellent handling properties made them useful as a binder with other materials or as a barrier laid on top of bone graft. First, the material is synthesized in its hemihydrate form ($CaSO_4$ ½ H_2O). Mixing with water yields a partially hydrated solid form of plaster of Paris. In addition, polymeric bone graft is composed of polymethyl methacrylate (PMMA) and has an inner core of PMMA. This material is less than ideal in a bone graft because it is nonresorbable (**Table 5**).

To compare the clinical effects of alloplast, Bechara and colleagues[28] conducted a study comparing the predictability of nonceramic hydroxyapatite when used as a graft with autogenous bone graft. The investigators conducted a split-mouth study to evaluate the stability of the grafted sites. The study used a sandwich osteotomy technique to reconstruct the vertical height of bone by placing graft material between the osteotomized segments. Autogenous bone graft was harvested from the ramus of the host and hydroxyapatite was placed in the contralateral mandible. The segments were stabilized with titanium plates and screws (**Fig. 11**). The bone was sampled at 6 months and histologic examination revealed residual graft material in the experimental group (**Fig. 12**). In addition, bone marrow density and marrow spaces were similar between the test and control. The study concluded that alloplastic hydroxyapatite graft material is a suitable substitute for grafting the mandible using a sandwich technique. Orsini and colleagues[29] also conducted a split-mouth study to regenerate periodontal defects with calcium sulfate and autogenous bone graft. Twelve patients were treated in this study using guided bone regeneration. Autogenous bone graft was harvested from the mandible and coated with a collagen membrane or calcium sulfate. The graft was exposed in 6 of 12 patients and covered with membrane, and in 4 of 12 patients it was covered with calcium sulfate. The

Table 5
Bone selection and properties

Type	Graft	Osteoconduction	Osteoinduction	Osteogenesis	Advantages
Bone	Autograft	3	2	2	Gold standard
	Allograft	3	1	0	Availability in many forms
Biomaterials	DBM	1	2	0	Supplies osteoinductive BMPs, bone graft extender
	Collagen	2	0	0	Good as delivery vehicle system
Ceramics	TCP, hydroxyapatite	1	0	0	Biocompatible
	Calcium phosphate cement	1	0	0	Some initial structural support
Composite grafts	p-TCP/BMA composite	3	2	2	Ample supply
	BMP/synthetic composite	—	3	—	Potentially limitless supply

DMB, demineralized bone; TCP, tricalcium phosphate.
From Giannoudis PV, Dinopoulos H, Tsiridis E. Bone substitutes: an update. Injury. 2005;36(Suppl3):S22; with permission.

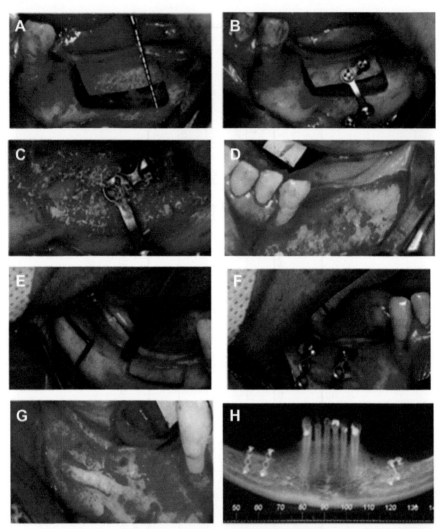

Fig. 11. (*A*) Osteotomized mandible bone segments. (*B*) Elevated bone segment fixated with a titanium plate for immobility. (*C*) Alloplast graft packed into defect. (*D*) Six months following healing of the grafted segment. (*E*) Harvested ramus graft before delivery. (*F*) Fixated elevated bone segment with titanium plate for immobility. (*G*) Healed segment following ramus autogenous graft. (*H*) Radiograph showing comparable regenerative height achieved with autograft (*right*) and alloplast (*left*). (*Adapted from* Bechara K, Dottore AM, Kawakami PY, et al. A histological study of non-ceramic hydroxyapatite as a bone graft substitute material in the vertical bone augmentation of the posterior mandible using an interpositional inlay technique: A split mouth evaluation. Ann Anat. 2015;202:2–3; with permission.)

grafted sites healed following the exposure by secondary intention with good tissue coverage and quality of soft tissue. There was no statistical difference in the regeneration of periodontal defects. This study suggested that alloplastic materials can act as a barrier surface to prevent soft tissue invasion.[29]

The current consensus for grafting with alloplastic materials is for its use as an adjunct used in conjunction with autograft or allograft. The mechanical properties of

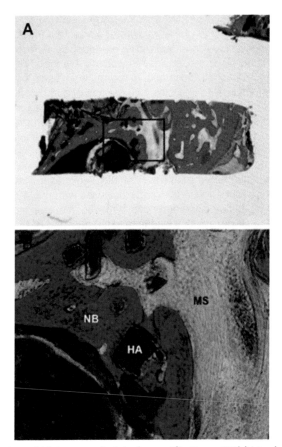

Fig. 12. Low-power and high-power (original magnification ×100) histophotographs of hydroxyapatite (HA)-incorporated bone graft material. The hydroxyapatite particles are surrounded by newly formed bone. (*A*) lower power microscopic view. (*B*) high power microscopic view. MS, marrow space, NB, new bone. (*From* Bechara K, Dottore AM, Kawakami PY, et al. A histological study of non-ceramic hydroxyapatite as a bone graft substitute material in the vertical bone augmentation of the posterior mandible using an interpositional inlay technique: A split mouth evaluation. Ann Anat. 2015;202:5; with permission.)

the alloplastic material make it ideal for handling. The predictability of the graft when used alone is suspect.

BONE MORPHOGENETIC PROTEIN

The bulk of osseous regeneration is focused on a strategy of providing the host osteoblasts and osteoclasts with a scaffold for new bone construction. Biologically active agents have been developed to bridge the gap and provide predictable and dependable stimulation for bone formation. BMPs, specifically BMP2 and 7, have been developed to promote osteoinduction in grafted materials. BMPs have been extensively studied and have received US Food and Drug Administration approval for sinus augmentation.[30] The literature reports that BMP contains the capacity to stimulate endochondral and intramembranous bone formation from mesenchymal cells in situ.[31]

The osteoinductive potential of BMP was investigated by Boyne and colleagues,[30] who grafted recombinant human bone morphogenic protein (rhBMP2) into sinus lift sites without conjunctive bone grafting. Collagen sponges were soaked in rhBMP2 and placed under lifted sinus membranes in patients planned for maxillary implant placement (**Fig. 13**).[26] Concentrations of 0.75 mg/mL were used to soak membranes. The study evaluated volumetric changes with the use of computed tomography pre-operatively and at 4 and 6 months postoperatively. Results were compared with volumetric changes achieved in a control group receiving conventional allografting. After a period of 4 months, 11.3 mm of bone height was noted in the test group. In comparison, the control group showed a mean height gain of 10.2 mm. There were no statistically significant differences between the heights gained with rhBMP2-soaked sponges alone and allografted sinuses. The histologic examination of the study revealed mature bone formation in the grafted sinuses with rhBMP2. Comparison of the bone showed no histologic differences between the test and control groups (**Figs. 14** and **15**). The study provides evidence to suggest that BMP carries the potential to induce bone formation without the need for a grafted scaffolding. Furthermore, the study advocates that the induced bone can be predictably used for implant placement and loading for oral rehabilitation.[26]

Evidence of the predictability of bone inductions has been well documented in the literature. Triplett and colleagues[31] conducted a similar study in which the maxillary sinus was augmented with BMP2-soaked collagen sponges. The investigators conducted a split-mouth study using BMP and autograft harvested from the hip. The investigators used computed tomography scans not only to measure augmented height but to investigate the bone density (**Fig. 16**).[31] After a healing period of 6 months, a mean of 7.8 mm of height was regenerated with BMP alone compared with 9.4 mm with allograft material. Histologic examination revealed no significant differences in the regenerated bone, which closely resembled native bone. The study did not report any complications that were unique to BMP-grafted sites. In comparison, the autograft was associated with expected complications and morbidity associated with its harvest (pain, gait disturbance, and paresthesia). The study restored the

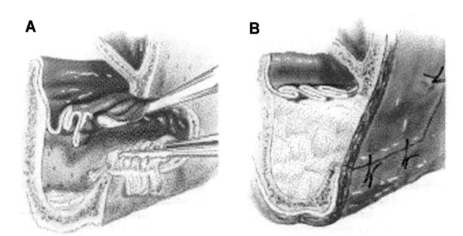

A   **B**

Fig. 13. (*A*) Completed Schneiderian membrane elevation. (*B*) Augmented Schneiderian membrane with BMP-infused sponge. (*From* Boyne PJ, Lilly LC, Marx RE, et al. De novo bone induction by recombinant human bone morphogenetic protein-2 (rhBMP-2) in maxillary sinus floor augmentation. J Oral Maxillofac Surg. 2005;63(12):1695; with permission.)

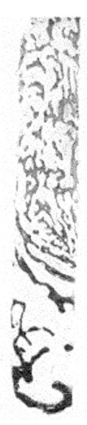
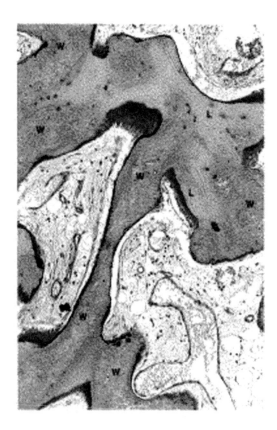

Fig. 14. Histology from patient treated with 0.75 mg/mL rhBMP2. Twenty-eight weeks post-operative (Goldner stain, original magnification ×10). (*From* Boyne PJ, Lilly LC, Marx RE, et al. De novo bone induction by recombinant human bone morphogenetic protein-2 (rhBMP-2) in maxillary sinus floor augmentation. J Oral Maxillofac Surg. 2005;63(12):1701; with permission.)

arches of 160 patients, and a total of 251 and 241 implants were placed in BMP and autografted sites, respectively. The postoperative failure rate was reported to be 42 of 241 in the BMP-regenerated bone and 50 of 251 implants in autogenous bone. No statistical differences in implant success and survivability were noted. The investigators concluded that BMP alone achieved similar results to what can be achieved with autogenous bone.

COLLAGEN-INFUSED BONE GRAFT MATERIALS

A newer development in bone grafting is the addition of collagen to the graft material proper. Unlike most other developments in bone grafting material, the addition of collagen is not designed to increase bone growth or osteointegration. Instead, embedding bone material in a collagen matrix gives cohesion to the bone graft material, providing markedly improved workability intraoperatively. This advantage is especially applicable for xenografts, where the preparation of bone graft material and collagen can be easily and abundantly assembled and packaged for use for immediate availability. Traditionally, organic components are removed from a variety of xenografts to

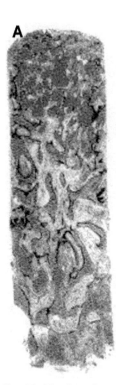
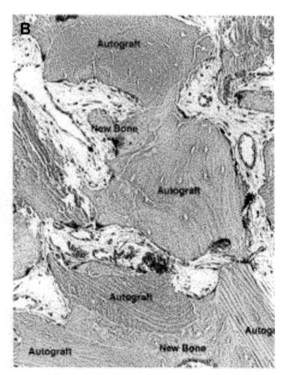

Fig. 15. Histology from patient treated with combination of demineralized, freeze-dried allograft, and autograft 34 weeks postoperative (Goldner stain, original magnification ×10). High-power (*A*) and low-power (*B*) pictomicrograph of sampled bone from BMP-augmented sinus alone. (*From* Boyne PJ, Lilly LC, Marx RE, et al. De novo bone induction by recombinant human bone morphogenetic protein-2 (rhBMP-2) in maxillary sinus floor augmentation. J Oral Maxillofac Surg. 2005;63(12):1701; with permission.)

reduce risk of triggering an immune reaction against the graft and to reduce risk of transfer of potential infectious agents.[32,33] The remaining graft material is brittle and granular owing to its lack of structural framework, and is demanding to use during surgeries. Renewed interest in reintroducing treated fibrillar collagen in small amounts allows increased graft material workability by holding the graft together in a way that better contours to the surgical defect. Fibrillar collagen has been shown to carry and deliver BMP2 in a workable form; for example, in alveolar cleft reconstruction.[34] Bio-Oss (Geistlisch Pharmaceutical) is an example of adaptation of this technology. Traditional Bio-Oss is a product of deproteinized bovine cancellous bone used in many standard bone grafting applications. Bio-Oss Collagen is cancellous bone granules in a matrix of 10% collagen fibers in block form. The collagen in this case is treated with gamma radiation to mitigate adverse immunologic effects of organic material in the graft.[32] Intuitively, anecdotally, and through personal experience, the consistency of Bio-Oss Collagen is vastly superior to Bio-Oss because of its ability to be adapted to osseous defects and ease of handling. The company claims the material is indicated for a variety of therapeutic areas, including ridge preservation, bone augmentation, and periodontal surgeries, and it claims that the collagen is absorbed after a few weeks, allowing predictable osteointegration.[35] Wong and colleagues[32] evaluated Bio-Oss Collagen for osteointegration in rabbits and found it to be a viable bone grafting material producing

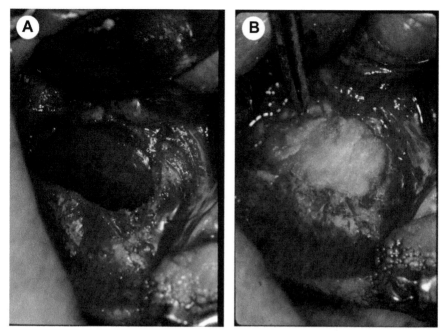

Fig. 16. (A) Osteotomy site ready to receive BMP sponge. (B) Osteotomy site with delivered BMP-soaked sponge. (*From* Triplett RG, Nevins M, Marx RE, et al. Pivotal, randomized, parallel evaluation of recombinant human bone morphogenetic protein-2/absorbable collagen sponge and autogenous bone graft for maxillary sinus floor augmentation. J Oral Maxillofac Surg. 2009;67(9):1951; with permission.)

339% more new bone versus collagen graft alone. Clinically, socket preservation studies in the form of randomized controlled clinical trials in human subjects consistently found collagen-infused bone graft to be viable. Jung and colleagues[36] found that collagen-infused demineralized bovine bone with or without a soft tissue graft outperformed control and a traditional mineral phosphate graft in terms of residual bony dimensions at the extraction site. Nart and colleagues[37] showed that deproteinized bovine bone mineral and deproteinized bovine bone material with 10% collagen performed statistically indistinguishably following a socket preservation procedure. Ergo, collagen-infused bone graft material seems promising in that it is both successful as a bone graft material and provides the advantage of improved intraoperative handling. Contraindications to grafting with Bio-Oss and similar materials include an infected wound and patients with known allergy to collagen.

PLATELET RICH CONCENTRATES

Platelet-rich concentrates are autologous filtrates that are rich in growth factors such as platelet-derived growth factor (PDGF) and transforming growth factor (TGF) beta and are made from centrifuging a patient's own blood, which can be added to a bone graft material to potentially enhance its success. They contain a patient's own growth factors (largely from blood-borne platelets) and white blood cells. Their proposed mechanism of action is supersaturating a wound with these growth factors, thereby promoting tissue regeneration, including osteointegration. They are easily produced chairside at the time of surgery, and there is a growing mass of literature substantiating their use in bone grafting in dentistry. There are 2 varieties of platelet-rich concentrates now used. PRP is whole blood centrifuged to remove red blood cells, leaving behind a suspension rich in white blood cells and plasma rich in growth factors. PRP is used as a liquid that is applied over a bone grafting site and bone graft material. There is anticoagulant in the centrifuge tubes to keep the blood products in suspension form so that they can be separated. In contrast, platelet-rich fibrin (PRF) omits the anticoagulation and, through controlled slow centrifugation, produces a moldable solid composed of a fibrin matrix containing abundant growth factors. Per unit quantity, PRP has a greater initial concentration of growth factors, and PRF has more delayed sustained release of growth factors.[38]

PRF can be further subdivided into 2 forms: a solid and a liquid. Both are routinely used and allow sustained delayed release of growth factors.[38] Solid PRF is the most common and allows upfront consolidation of the fibrin matrix. In this form, PRF can be used as a mass to fill large defects, flattened to a wafer to produce a membrane analogue, or divided and mixed with bone as a particulate bone substitute. Liquid PRF, also known as injectable PRF, is produced as a liquid by using very low centrifuge force for a shorter period of time. The resultant liquid is used as an injection by itself or used to wet a bone graft.[38]

To produce PRP/PRF, start with venipuncture.[38] Collect blood in 10-mL cylinders. Glass cylinders activate clotting more than plastic cylinders. Either can be used, depending on the type of platelet concentrate needed. Transfer the blood to the centrifuge immediately. A PRF/PRP centrifuge is used to spin the blood product, typically at preprogrammed settings.

In the setting of bone grafting in dentistry, Marx and colleagues[39] showed that PRP can be an osteoinductive force by retaining a high concentration of PDGF and TGF-beta, which act to promote mitogenesis of stem cells nearby and to promote chemotaxis of inflammatory cells. This process resulted in a 2-fold increase in bone density. Fennis and colleagues[40] used PRF in reconstruction of mandibular continuity defects in animal models. Garg and colleagues[41] and Kim and colleagues[42] showed that PRF can successfully be used to bone graft around implants with good success. In ridge-preservation procedures, a PRF graft shaped as a plug to fit into an extraction socket showed minimal ridge width loss of 7.38% and ridge height loss of 7.13% versus 11.59% and 17.79%, respectively, in groups in which only a bone graft with a collagen membrane was used.[43] In some cases, PRF was used alone without a bone graft with successful osseous healing of the bone graft. Dhote and colleagues[44] showed that PRF alone could be used to graft a defect after removal of a radicular cyst in a 10-year-old patient. On 2-year follow-up, the defect was healed and there was also eruption of a nearby displaced premolar.[44] Essentially, platelet-rich concentrates are associated with promotion of wound healing and show promise as an adjunct in all bone grafting applications.

SUMMARY

Autogenous bone has been the staple and gold standard for grafting purposes. Recent trends in bone grafting practice have seen increased use of allograft combined with growth factors such as PRF and BMPs. However, although clinically effective, these methods come with risks and complications, such as harvest site morbidity with autogenous grafts and risks of disease transmission with allografts. Recent advances in engineering have shown promise in resorbable synthetic grafting materials. Newer materials show the promise of clinically significant volumes of bone augmentation with resorbable membranes, which would eliminate important complications and increase patient comfort and safety. Autogenous bone grafts will most likely remain the gold standard of grafting materials and will continue to be essential in reconstruction of the maxillofacial skeleton. New materials will most likely shift the bone grafting philosophies of clinicians toward synthetic resorbable materials in the future.

CLINICS CARE POINTS

- Bone is a composite and dynamic structure undergoing constant resorption and deposition by osteoclasts and osteoblasts.
- Bone deposition, resorption, and maintenance are achieved through the actions of osteoblasts, osteoclasts, and osteocytes.
- Branemark described and classified bone based on composition of cortical and trabecular bone.
- Autologous bone refers to bone that is harvested form the individual's own tissue.
- Allogenic bone graft refers to bone that is harvested from the same species (ie, human cadavers).
- Alloplastic bone grafts are defined as grafting materials or bone substitutes made synthetically or derived from coral of algae hydroxyapatite.
- Xenograft refers to tissues transplanted between animals of different species.
- BMP, specifically BMP2 and BMP7, have been developed to promote osteoinduction in grafted materials through stimulation of endochondral and intramembranous bone formation from mesenchymal cells.
- Platelet-rich concentrates are autologous filtrates that are rich in growth factors such as PDGF and TGF-beta and that can be added to a bone graft material.

DISCLOSURE

The authors have nothing to disclose.

REFERENCES

1. Brånemark P-I, Zarb GA, Albrektsson T. Tissue-Integrated Prostheses. In: Brånemark P-I, Zarb GA, Albrektsson T, editors. Osseointegration in Clinical Dentistry. 1985.
2. Acocella A, Bertolai R, Ellis E 3rd, et al. Maxillary alveolar ridge reconstruction with monocortical fresh-frozen bone blocks: a clinical, histological and histomorphometric study. J Craniomaxillofac Surg 2012;40(6):525–33.
3. Chiapasco M, Zaniboni M, Boisco M. Augmentation procedures for the rehabilitation of deficient edentulous ridges with oral implants. Clin Oral Implants Res 2006;17(Suppl 2):136–59.
4. Arrington ED, Smith WJ, Chambers HG, et al. Complications of iliac crest bone graft harvesting. Clin orthop Relat Res 1996;(329):300–9.
5. Banwart JC, Asher MA, Hassanein RS. Iliac crest bone graft harvest donor site morbidity. A statistical evaluation. Spine 1995;20(9):1055–60.
6. Ross N, Tacconi L, Miles JB. Heterotopic bone formation causing recurrent donor site pain following iliac crest bone harvesting. Br J Neurosurg 2000;14(5):476–9.
7. Seiler JG 3rd, Johnson J. Iliac crest autogenous bone grafting: donor site complications. J South Orthop Assoc 2000;9(2):91–7.
8. Skaggs DL, Samuelson MA, Hale JM, et al. Complications of posterior iliac crest bone grafting in spine surgery in children. Spine 2000;25(18):2400–2.
9. Carlini JL, Biron C. Use of the iliac crest cortex for premaxilla fixation in patients with bilateral clefts. J Oral Maxillofac Surg 2020;78(7):1192.e1–13.

10. Precious DS. A new reliable method for alveolar bone grafting at about 6 years of age. J Oral Maxillofac Surg 2009;67(10):2045–53.
11. Acocella A, Bertolai R, Colafranceschi M, et al. Clinical, histological and histomorphometric evaluation of the healing of mandibular ramus bone block grafts for alveolar ridge augmentation before implant placement. J Craniomaxillofac Surg 2010;38(3):222–30.
12. Ellegaard B, Karring T, Löe H. The fate of vital and devitalized bone grafts in the healing of interradicular lesions. J Periodont Res 1975;10(2):88–97.
13. Ham AW. Some histophysiological problems peculiar to calcified tissues. J Bone Joint Surg Am 1952;24(3):701–28.
14. Fretwurst T, Nack C, Al-Ghrairi M, et al. Long-term retrospective evaluation of the peri-implant bone level in onlay grafted patients with iliac bone from the anterior superior iliac crest. J Craniomaxillofac Surg 2015;43(6):956–60.
15. Duttenhoefer F, Nack C, Doll C, et al. Long-term peri-implant bone level changes of non-vascularized fibula bone grafted edentulous patients. J Craniomaxillofac Surg 2015;43(5):611–5.
16. Nelson K, Glatzer C, Hildebrand D, et al. Clinical evaluation of endosseous implants in nonvascularized fibula bone grafts for reconstruction of the severely atrophied mandibular bone. J Oral Maxillofac Surg 2006;64(9):1427–32.
17. Boyce T, Edwards J, Scarborough N. Allograft bone. The influence of processing on safety and performance. Orthop Clin North Am 1999;30(4):571–81.
18. Goldberg VM, Stevenson S. The biology of bone grafts. Seminars in arthroplasty 1993;4(2):58–63.
19. Chaushu G, Mardinger O, Peleg M, et al. Analysis of complications following augmentation with cancellous block allografts. J Periodontol 2010;81(12):1759–64.
20. Xavier SP, Silva ER, Kahn A, et al. Maxillary sinus grafting with autograft versus fresh-frozen allograft: a split-mouth evaluation of bone volume dynamics. Int J Oral Maxillofac Implants 2015;30(5):1137–42.
21. Monje A, Pikos MA, Chan HL, et al. On the feasibility of utilizing allogeneic bone blocks for atrophic maxillary augmentation. Biomed Research International 2014; 2014:814578.
22. Bahat O, Fontanesi FV. Complications of grafting in the atrophic edentulous or partially edentulous jaw. Int J Periodontics Restorative Dent 2001;21(5):487–95.
23. Keith JD Jr, Petrungaro P, Leonetti JA, et al. Clinical and histologic evaluation of a mineralized block allograft: results from the developmental period (2001-2004). Int J Periodontics Restorative Dent 2006;26(4):321–7.
24. Barone A, Varanini P, Orlando B, et al. Deep-frozen allogeneic onlay bone grafts for reconstruction of atrophic maxillary alveolar ridges: a preliminary study. J Oral Maxillofac Surg 2009;67(6):1300–6.
25. Lima RG, Lima TG, Francischone CE, et al. Bone volume dynamics and implant placement torque in horizontal bone defects reconstructed with autologous or xenogeneic block bone: a randomized, controlled, split-mouth, prospective clinical trial. Int J Oral Maxillofac Implants 2018;33(4):888–94.
26. Li J, Xuan F, Choi BH, et al. Minimally invasive ridge augmentation using xenogenous bone blocks in an atrophied posterior mandible: a clinical and histological study. Implant Dent 2013;22(2):112–6.
27. Simion M, Fontana F, Rasperini G, et al. Vertical ridge augmentation by expanded-polytetrafluoroethylene membrane and a combination of intraoral autogenous bone graft and deproteinized anorganic bovine bone (Bio Oss). Clin Oral Implants Res 2007;18(5):620–9.

28. Bechara K, Dottore AM, Kawakami PY, et al. A histological study of non-ceramic hydroxyapatite as a bone graft substitute material in the vertical bone augmentation of the posterior mandible using an interpositional inlay technique: A split mouth evaluation. Ann Anat 2015;202:1–7.
29. Orsini M, Orsini G, Benlloch D, et al. Comparison of calcium sulfate and autogenous bone graft to bioabsorbable membranes plus autogenous bone graft in the treatment of intrabony periodontal defects: a split-mouth study. J Periodontol 2001;72(3):296–302.
30. Boyne PJ, Lilly LC, Marx RE, et al. De novo bone induction by recombinant human bone morphogenetic protein-2 (rhBMP-2) in maxillary sinus floor augmentation. J Oral Maxillofac Surg 2005;63(12):1693–707.
31. Triplett RG, Nevins M, Marx RE, et al. Pivotal, randomized, parallel evaluation of recombinant human bone morphogenetic protein-2/absorbable collagen sponge and autogenous bone graft for maxillary sinus floor augmentation. J Oral Maxillofac Surg 2009;67(9):1947–60.
32. Wong RW, Rabie AB. Effect of bio-oss collagen and collagen matrix on bone formation. Open Biomed Eng J 2010;4:71–6.
33. Jung RE, Philipp A, Annen BM, et al. Radiographic evaluation of different techniques for ridge preservation after tooth extraction: a randomized controlled clinical trial. J Clin Periodontol 2013;40(1):90–8.
34. Chin M, Ng T, Tom WK, et al. Repair of alveolar clefts with recombinant human bone morphogenetic protein (rhBMP-2) in patients with clefts. J Craniofac Surg 2005;16(5):778–89.
35. Fan Y, Perez K, Dym H. Clinical Uses of Platelet-Rich Fibrin in Oral and Maxillofacial Surgery. Dent Clin North Am 2020;64(2):291–303.
36. Jung RE, Philipp A, Annen BM, et al. Radiographic evaluation of different techniques for ridge preservation after tooth extraction: a randomized controlled clinical trial. J Clin Periodontol 2013;40(1):90–8.
37. Nart J, Barallat L, Jimenez D, et al. Radiographic and histological evaluation of deproteinized bovine bone mineral vs. deproteinized bovine bone mineral with 10% collagen in ridge preservation. A randomized controlled clinical trial. Clin Oral Implants Res 2017;28(7):840–8.
38. Fan Y, Perez K, Dym H. Clinical uses of platelet-rich fibrin in oral and maxillofacial surgery. Dent Clin North Am 2020;64(2):291–303.
39. Marx RE, Carlson ER, Eichstaedt RM, et al. Platelet-rich plasma: growth factor enhancement for bone grafts. Oral Surg Oral Med Oral Pathol Oral Radiol Endod 1998;85(6):638–46.
40. Fennis JP, Stoelinga PJ, Jansen JA. Mandibular reconstruction: a clinical and radiographic animal study on the use of autogenous scaffolds and platelet-rich plasma. Int J Oral Maxillofac Surg 2002;31(3):281–6.
41. Garg AK. The use of platelet-rich plasma to enhance the success of bone grafts around dental implants. Dent Implantol Update 2000;11(3):17–21.
42. Kim SG, Chung CH, Kim YK, et al. Use of particulate dentin-plaster of Paris combination with/without platelet-rich plasma in the treatment of bone defects around implants. Int J Oral Maxillofac Implants 2002;17(1):86–94.
43. Tanasković N. Use of platelet-rich fibrin in maxillofacial surgery. Contemp Mater 2016;VII-1:45–50.
44. Dhote VS, Thosar NR, Baliga SM, et al. Surgical management of large radicular cyst associated with mandibular deciduous molar using platelet-rich fibrin augmentation: a rare case report. Contemp Clin Dent 2017;8(4):647–9.

Update on Maxillary Sinus Augmentation

Natasha Bhalla, DDS*, Harry Dym, DDS

KEYWORDS

- Transcrestal sinus lift • Lateral window sinus lift • Osseodensification
- Schneiderian membrane

KEY POINTS

- Over time, the maxillary sinus undergoes a process called pneumatization.
- Over time, the alveolar bone of the posterior maxilla will undergo resorption.
- Augmentation of the maxillary sinus can be performed by using a transcrestal sinus lift or a lateral approach.

INTRODUCTION

A common clinical finding facing the implant surgeon when planning for implant placement in the posterior maxilla is lack of adequate bone height either due to low lying maxillary sinus or due to atrophy of the alveolous following extraction. Augmentation of the site can be performed by using a transcrestal sinus lift or a lateral approach. Both techniques are discussed in this chapter.

ANATOMY OF THE MAXILLARY SINUS

The maxillary sinus is an air space that occupies the maxilla bilaterally[1] and is surrounded by the nasal cavity mesially, the maxillary tuberosity laterally, the orbit superiorly, and the alveolar bone inferiorly.[1] The volume of the maxillary sinus is approximately 20 mL[1] and is usually present at birth completing its development at 18 years of age.[1]

The maxillary sinus is also lined with ciliated pseudostratified epithelium, and there are cilia lining the membrane of the maxillary sinus as well,[1] the purpose of which is to clear the paranasal sinus cavity of pathogens and debris that are continually inspired in normal respiration.[1]

Department of Dentistry/Oral and Maxillofacial Surgery, The Brooklyn Hospital Center, 121 DeKalb Avenue, Brooklyn, NY 11201, USA
* Corresponding author.
E-mail address: natashaa95@gmail.com

Dent Clin N Am 65 (2021) 197–210
https://doi.org/10.1016/j.cden.2020.09.013
0011-8532/21/© 2020 Elsevier Inc. All rights reserved.
dental.theclinics.com

The maxillary sinus is robustly supplied by multiple arteries,[1] which include the infraorbital artery, greater palatine artery, lesser palatine artery, sphenopalatine artery, and the posterior superior alveolar artery.[1]

INDICATIONS

Over time, the maxillary sinus undergoes a process called pneumatization. This process occurs when an individual loses their posterior maxillary teeth and in response to this loss of teeth the maxillary sinus will enlarge and encompass a larger portion of the posterior maxillary alveolous. Pictured in **Fig. 1** is a pneumatized maxillary sinus. Over time, the alveolar bone of the posterior maxilla will undergo resorption. The pneumatization of the maxillary sinus and resorption of the maxillary alveolar bone results in difficulty placing dental implants in the maxillary sinus. A maxillary sinus lift is conducted in order to facilitate the placement of dental implants in an environment with diminished vertical bone height. In order to have a successfully integrated dental implant, the recommendation is to place at least a 10-mm long implant with a width of 3 mm.[1]

WORKUP

The diagnostic and surgical workup for those patients who may require a sinus lift begins as most other surgical workups do, beginning with obtaining the following needed information: chief complaint, medical history, medications, allergies past surgical

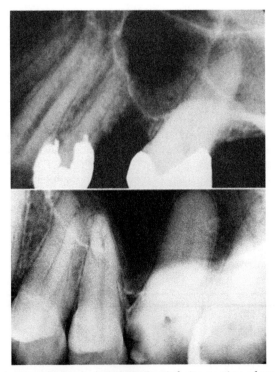

Fig. 1. Posteroanterior radiograph demonstrating inferior portion of pneumatized maxillary sinus.

history, and dental history. A patient who may require a maxillary sinus lift may indicate that they lost their maxillary posterior teeth many years ago and have trouble eating. Other patients with big smiles may indicate that they do not smile as much as the missing posterior teeth are noticeable.

An important part of the medical history is for the practitioner to ascertain that the patient does not have a history of bleeding problems.[2] This is especially important as one of the complications of a maxillary sinus lift is perforation of the maxillary sinus intraoperatively, which can lead to bleeding, which would be worse in a patient with a history of bleeding problems.[2] A patient with a history of bleeding problems may report a history of frequent nose bleeds, heavy menstrual bleeding (in females), easy bruising, and a history of prolonged bleeding after a wisdom tooth extraction.[2] A patient on blood thinners such as Warfarin or PO Heparin is also prone to excessive bleeding intraoperatively.[2]

Another important factor relevant to the medical questionnaire is learning about a possible history of rhinosinusitis. Rhinosinusitis is associated with nasal congestion, postnasal drip, headaches, and sore throat,[3] and evidence of rhinosinusitis may be seen on dental imaging. Later in this text, the author will discuss the implication of radiographic findings associated with the maxillary sinus.

Following the medical history, a physical examination must be conducted. The author recommends starting the examination with a complete head and neck examination to rule out any gross abnormalities followed by the intraoral examination. Specifically, it is important to note the buccal/palatal width of the maxillary alveolar bone, presence of keratinized tissue, and intraocclusal distance for the final prostheses. In order to place an implant of 3 mm diameter the buccal palatal length of the maxillary bone must be 4 mm.[1]

Following completion of the physical examination a radiographic examination is performed. Generally, a panoramic imaging study is adequate; however many practitioners may include a cone beam computed tomography (CBCT) study as well in order to accurately assess a patient. The 3-dimensional CBCT allows one to obtain information necessary information about the buccal/lingual width of the maxillary alveolar bone, and one can also determine the exact distance from the crest of the alveolar bone to the maxillary sinus. In addition, the CBCT study can also reveal whether there are septa within the planned sinus surgical site. Normally, septa with low height (less than 2 mm) do not require further attention because the membrane can usually be elevated without difficulty.[2] However, high septa with partial or complete separation of the sinus cavity may involve the preparation of 2 windows during sinus lift surgery.[2] Finally, the clinician can observe possible sinus mucosal thickening, sinus polyps, and air fluid levels.[3] This chapter, in a later section, discusses the implications of these findings on the success of a maxillary sinus lift and ultimately, the placement of a dental implant.

A maxillary sinus augmentation is recommended when there is less than 10 mm of space available from the alveolar crest to the maxillary sinus,[1] and the clinician and patient wish not to use small implants to reconstruct the area. As part of the discussion with the patient, the length of treatment time should be discussed with the understanding that the patient may or may not have a single stage or possible 2-stage implant procedure.

In a 1-stage implant placement, the implant can be placed at the same appointment as the sinus augmentation, whereas in a 2-stage implant placement, the sinus augmentation is performed first and the dental implant is placed 4 to 6 months later. Later in this chapter, the recommendations based on evidence-based medicine for one procedure versus the other are discussed.

During this appointment, the risks, benefits, and alternatives to the procedure must also be discussed with the patient, and it is recommended that a formal consent be obtained and signed by the patient as well.

ABNORMAL RADIOGRAPHIC FINDINGS

Upon review of the imaging studies, the practitioner may notice abnormal maxillary sinus findings including, but not limited to, mucosal thickening, sinus polyps, mucosal perforation, opacification of the maxillary sinus, and obstruction of the osteomeatal complex.[3] The reported rate of incidental radiologic sinus abnormalities in asymptomatic patients is as high as 60%.[3]

An air fluid level would be the most typical imaging finding of mucosal thickening (**Fig. 2**).[3] A sinus polyp would be viewed as a hypodensity in the maxillary sinus (**Fig. 3**).[3] Opacification as the name suggests would be seen as an opacified maxillary sinus (**Fig. 4**).[3] Lastly, the obstruction of an osteomeatal complex would be seen as opacification of the maxillary sinus.[3]

If any of these pathologies are viewed on the patient's radiograph, additional discussion with the patient is warranted. This discussion should rule out any history of rhinosinusitis. Rhinosinusitis can be divided into acute and chronic states,[3] with acute being defined as symptoms lasting less than 4 weeks.[3] These symptoms include nasal mucopurulent drainage, facial pressure and/or feeling of fullness, nasal congestion, and possible loss of sense of smell,[3] whereas chronic rhinosinusitis is defined as symptoms lasting greater than 4 weeks.[3]

If a patient denies any symptoms of rhinosinusitis, the radiographic findings can be considered to be incidental findings and is not a contraindication to performing maxillary sinus augmentation.[3] The most common augmentation complication is maxillary sinusitis and has been reported in 27% of cases.[3] Incidental radiographic findings with no clinical symptoms do not increase the risk of developing maxillary sinusitis.[3] It is important to note that patients who do have symptoms of acute or chronic sinusitis should be referred to an ear, nose, and throat doctor for possible treatment,[3] as these patients are at possible increased risk for postaugmentation maxillary sinusitis.[3]

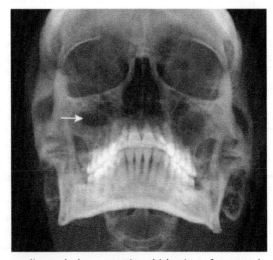

Fig. 2. Waters view radiograph demonstrating thickening of mucosa (*arrow*).

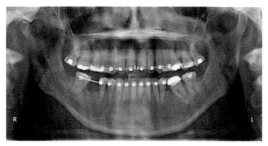

Fig. 3. Panoramic radiograph showing a sinus polyp on the floor of right maxillary sinus (*arrow*).

BONE GRAFTING MATERIALS

During the maxillary sinus augmentation technique, bone grafting material is placed inferior to the sinus membrane. Before this, the sinus membrane is elevated on the medial and lateral walls. The options of bone graft materials available include the following:

1 .Autograft—bone graft from the patient
2 .Allograft—bone graft from the same species (but not from the patient)

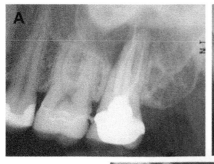
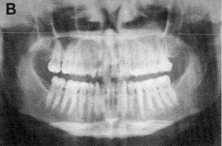
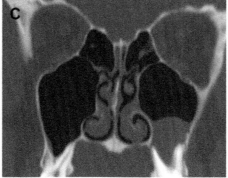

Fig. 4. (*A*) Periapical film showing opacification of the inferior portion of the left maxillary sinus. (*B*) Panoramic radiograph showing opacification of the inferior portion of the left maxillary sinus. (*C*) CT Maxillofacial (axial cut) showing opacification of the inferior portion of the left maxillary sinus.

3 .Alloplast—a graft material that is engineered, it is derived from a nonanimal source
4 .Xenograft—bone graft from a different species

The graft material that is the gold standard and has the highest success rate is the autogenous bone graft.[1] In situations where large amounts of bone graft is required, the anterior iliac crest is an option.[1] From this site, one can obtain approximately 50 cc of corticocancellous bone[1]; however, if even more bone graft is required the options are either anterior iliac crest or the posterior iliac crest. If a small amount of bone is needed, there are several options. These include the maxillary tuberosity, mandibular ramus, or mandibular symphysis.

As an alternative to autogenous bone grafting, nonautogenous bone grafts are also a viable option[1] and are advantageous because there is no associated donor site morbidity, they are associated with good success rates, are easily obtained, and are easy to use.[1]

SURGICAL PROCEDURE

A lateral maxillary window sinus lift is generally performed on patients who require more than 3 mm of augmentation.[2] Generally, when a large amount of bone is required to place an implant, the lateral window sinus lift is recommended[2] rather than a transcrestal sinus lift.

An incision is made over the alveolar crest from the maxillary midline to where the implant osteotomy site is planned. The incision should extend past the osteotomy site so that the incision can be closed on sound bone. While making the osteotomy, one should keep principles of surgical access and good visualization in mind. A dental bur or a piezoelectric device is used to create an oval or rectangular osteotomy over the lateral maxillary sinus wall[2] (**Fig. 5**). It is important to not perforate the sinus membrane during this step. Once the lateral window has been made, the sinus membrane is teased off the floor of the sinus and from the surrounding walls (**Fig. 6**). The bone graft is then placed under the sinus membrane. The practitioner should aim for having 12 mm of bone after the sinus lift is completed,[2] keeping in mind that the length of the implant will be at least 10 mm. The few extra millimeters of bone are in order to account for bone resorption during the healing process.

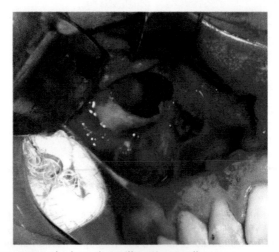

Fig. 5. An osteotomy over the lateral maxillary sinus wall.

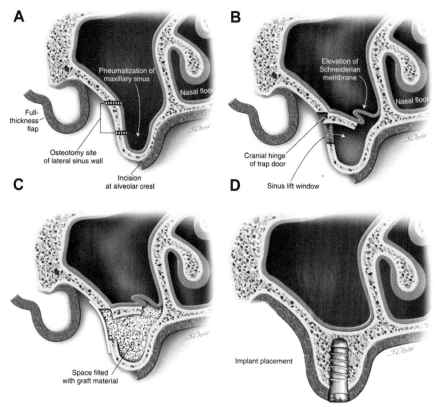

Fig. 6. The lateral approach involves elevation of a full-thickness buccal flap and osteotomy through the lateral wall. (*A*) Full thickness mucoperiosteal flap raised in order to gain access to osteotomy site. (*B*) Osteotomy. (*C*) Augmentation. (*D*) Placement of implant. (*From* Louis PJ. The maxillary sinus lift. In: Kademani D, Tiwana PS, editors. Atlas of oral & maxillofacial surgery. St. Louis: Elsevier Saunders; 2016. p. 199–209; with permission.)

Once the bone graft has been placed, the incision is primarily closed with resorbable sutures.

The healing process for a maxillary sinus augmentation procedure is approximately 6 months. The authors usually take radiographic imaging after the sinus lift procedure and then again 5 months later in order the evaluate the height of the alveolar crest.[2]

PLATELET-RICH FIBRIN

Platelet concentrates have been used in dentistry since the 1980s as a way to achieve better clinical outcomes. In order to generate platelet-rich fibrin (PRF), the patient's blood is put through a centrifuge without any anticoagulant.[4,5] The advantage to the patient is better potential bone and wound healing.[4,5] The disadvantage may include discomfort to the patient during the drawing of blood, additional financial costs, and longer length of surgery.[4,5]

In a systematic review conducted by Ortega-Mejia and colleagues, it was found that the use of PRF in sinus augmentation procedures did not demonstrate any significant increase in bone formation.[4] The review proposed that perhaps the use of PRF may improve the healing period and bone formation after a sinus augmentation procedure.[4]

ONE-STAGE VERSUS TWO-STAGE IMPLANT PLACEMENT

For many decades, the recommendation has been to conduct a 2-stage implant placement if the height of the maxillary alveolar bone is less than 4 to 5 mm. In a 2-stage implant placement, the sinus augmentation is carried out initially and the surgical site is allowed to heal for 4 to 6 months and then the implant is placed in a second surgical appointment. The disadvantage of a 2-stage procedure is the length of time it takes for completion of the procedure. It can take longer than a year for a patient to receive their implant and final prosthesis.

In the recent past, there have been a number of studies that have examined the success rate of an implant placement when placed in alveolar bone less than 5 mm. One study followed-up patients for up to 2 to 6 years after implant placement and found a 98% implant survival and 100% prosthesis survival in implants placed in less than 6 mm maxillary alveolar bone.[6,7] In another study, patients were followed up to 9 years after implant placement.[6] Implants were placed in residual bone less than 5 mm, and the success rate of the implants was 97.9%.[6]

Kim and colleagues conducted a study that compared implant survival in 1-stage versus 2-stage implant placement in residual bone less than 4 mm,[6] and they found no statistical difference in the survival of implants in each stage,[6] with the patients followed-up for 10 years. However, if time is a consideration for a patient, the practitioner may choose to conduct a 1-stage implant placement for their patients[6] if clinically acceptable.

COMPLICATIONS AND MANAGEMENT

It is important to review the patient's past medical history, as it can relate directly to postsurgical possible complications. Specific things that the practitioner is looking to glean is whether the patient has uncontrolled diabetes mellitus and other possible immunodeficient diseases,[2] as these medical conditions can interfere with wound healing and may decrease the chance of the dental implant ultimate osseointegration.[2] If a patient has been on bisphosphonate or denosumab therapy, a medical consult from their medical doctor is also recommended.[2] Other conditions that would require a medical consult are chronic liver disease and radiation therapy to the head and neck region.[2]

Other important medical considerations include a patient's alcohol intake and use of cocaine.[2] A patient who is a chronic alcohol drinker has a greater chance of bleeding postoperatively,[2] and a patient who uses cocaine will likely have damage to their nasal passageways and sinuses.[2] Finally, if a patient is a smoker it is recommended for the patient to quit smoking 1 week before the procedure and for 8 weeks following the procedure. If the patient is undergoing a 1-stage procedure with placement of dental implant, this will possibly help increase the chance of success of osseointegration.[2]

Membrane Perforation

The Schneiderian membrane is the membrane that lines the maxillary sinus.[2] During the maxillary sinus lift, it is not unusual for a small perforation of the membrane to occur,[2] with the resulting defect being covered with a resorbable membrane.[2] Alternatively, the practitioner can choose to use bone morphogenic protein (BMP)-infused collagen to cover the perforated membrane[2] before filling the sinus with bone graft material. Larger perforations will require using larger absorbable membranes fixated to the superior bony wall of the maxillary opening with bone tacks or screws before bone augmentation. However, it is important to keep in mind that if not done correctly, the BMP graft can extravasate into the maxillary sinus.[2] This can lead to an increased risk of infection of the maxillary sinus and possible loss of the bone graft.[2] If the tear is exceedingly large and one is unable to stabilize a long-lasting resorbable membrane, there may be a need to possibly abort the procedure at this time.[2]

Antral Septae

The presence of antral septae can sometimes complicate lateral sinus augmentation procedures,[2] the reason being that it is challenging to lift the sinus membrane from a septa without tearing it.[2] The presence of antral septae can be detected on the preoperative imaging,[2] and the practitioner can modify the planned procedure based upon the precise location of the septa.[2] The initial lateral bony window can be made larger to lessen the probability of perforating the membrane in this clinical situation.[2] Another alternative is to create 2 lateral window osteotomies so that the practitioner does not have to operate over the maxillary septa.[2]

Bleeding

As mentioned earlier, the maxillary sinus is robustly supplied by multiple arteries,[2] and it is for this reason that an artery can be encountered and damaged during the planned sinus surgical procedure, which can lead to profuse bleeding within the maxillary.[2] This is an issue that can complicate the procedure, as it will certainly decrease the visualization of the surgical field and may prove challenging if not impossible to control the bleeding.[2] In the author's experience when profuse bleeding has occurred during lateral approach to the maxillary sinus, packing the sinus with ½ inch iodoform gauze and applying digital pressure for 5 minutes has led to cessation of bleeding in all cases when this situation was in fact encountered.

TRANSCRESTAL OR INTRAORAL SINUS LIFT APPROACH

The previous section in this chapter dealt with the more often performed lateral window surgical approach to the maxillary sinus for the augmentation of the deficient posterior maxilla before the placement of endosseous implants.

The disadvantages of this technique, however, is that it is a relatively large surgical operation; a need for specialized instrumentation and the procedure takes time to do well, so clinician patience is required to avoid possible Schneiderian membrane perforation. The technique is also often accompanied by postoperative symptoms and high costs.

A less invasive procedure, often referred to as the transcrestal osteotome sinus floor elevation technique, was first presented by Dr Summers[8] in 1994 and is a viable alternative in certain clinical settings to the lateral window sinus lift procedure.

Alveolar bone loss that occurs in the posterior maxilla can be demarcated into 3 main categories:

1 .An alveolar ridge containing 5 to 10 mm of bone before encroaching upon the sinus
2 .An alveolar ridge equal to or less than 5 mm of bone
3 .A complete absence of alveolar bone between the sinus floor and alveolar crest

In the opinion of one of the authors (HD), the lateral maxillary sinus window approach for categories 2 and 3 is absolutely indicated, with category 1 being more amenable to the Summers technique for sinus lift elevation and augmentation, which is discussed in the following section.

SUMMERS/CRESTAL SINUS LIFE TECHNIQUE

As in the traditional lateral sinus window approach, a prior imaging study of the planned surgical posterior maxillary area with a clear view of the sinus should be available before the initiation of the procedure. The imaging study can be a panoramic view or cone beam study or a CT scan or even a quality periapical film. The patient must be made aware of the risks of the procedure, which can include the standard surgical complications one sees with almost all oral surgical procedures including pain, postoperative swelling and edema, possible infection in the sinus (maxillary sinusitis), and possible infection of the grafted material placed. Local anesthesia is often all that is necessary for this procedure although of course sedation, either oral, intravenous, or via inhalation, can also be used.

One necessary piece of equipment required for this procedure is a set of surgical osteotomes of varying incremental increasing diameter size. A set of 4 or 5 osteotomes is all that is necessary and can be obtained from multiple specialized dental and oral surgical supply houses. The osteotomes (Ace Surgical or Salvin Dental) contain graduated markings on the side to allow you to be aware of the depth of the insertion at all times. They are available as either straight or off-set osteotomes.

If the bone is soft in the area in which the transcrestal sinus augmentation is planned then the entire procedure can be done with a series of osteotomes. The osteotomes have a concave tip and are introduced into the maxillary soft bone. By controlled upward pressure they cause the soft bone to be retained and displaced and compacted laterally and also moved apically toward the antral floor. The antral floor can be flexed upward and elevated with repeated pressure from the osteotome tip as the trapped bone particles and fluids are pushed upward. Summers writes[9] that adding hydrated bone into the osteotomy site, the combined bone plus trapped fluids will act as a hydraulic plug to push up the sinus membrane with less likelihood of membrane tear. However, if the bone is a bit more dense, the first osteotomy will require using a standard pilot drill. In the technique described by Dr Summers,[8] after having determined the height of the residual crest the first length of the 2 mm initial drill bit is drilled to a depth that is 1 mm beneath the sinus floor. Then, sequentially a 2.8 mm and a 3.3 mm diameter osteotomes are introduced and malleted into place. Before inserting the final osteotome, the grafting material that is planned to be used to augment the sinus floor is inserted in a slurry form into the osteotomy site. The last osteotome should always be 0.7 to 1.0 mm less in diameter than the planned implant diameter for better implant stability.

A novel technique using osteotomes, as described by Summers, followed by hydraulic pressure from saline syringe to elevate the sinus membrane has also been described in the literature.[10]

OSSEODENSIFICATION-ASSISTED TRANSCRESTAL SINUS LIFT

Osseodensification is a technique that involves plastic deformation of bone that is created by rolling and sliding contact using a densifying bur that is fluted in such a manner that it densifies and compacts the bone with minimal heat elevation.

A rather new implant site/osteotomy preparation technique was developed in 2013, which densifies the bone as it prepares the implant site by means of a nonsubstractive drilling technique referred to as by its innovator Dr Huwais[11] as osseodensification. This is a surgical technique that uses specialized designed fluted burs (DENSAH burs) that help densify the bone as they prepare the osteotomy site. Standard drills excavate bone during site preparation, whereas the DENSAH burs allow for bone preservation and condensation through compaction that occur during the preparation, thus increasing the bone density in the periimplant area and improving mechanical stability.[12,13] The drills are used at high speed (1200 RPM) in a counter clockwise direction with a steady external irrigation referred to as the densifying mode.

Increasing bone density is a critical factor in ensuring primary implant stability. Trisi and colleagues[13] found a statistically significant correlation between periimplant bone density, insertion torque, and micromotion. Increasing bone density was directly related to significant increase in implant insertion torque and a concomitant reduction in micromotion. This technique was introduced for horizontal augmentation in narrow alveolar ridges but can also be used to gain vertical height with an internal sinus lift via a transcrestal approach described in **Boxes 1** and **2**.

According to the inventor's DENSAH protocol,[11] if additional lift beyond the 3 mm is needed, an allograft material can be added and gently pushed into the sinus to achieve additional 2 mm increase in height. Well-hydrated cancellous bone is used to fill the osteotomy of the final diameter drilled site and then the last diameter DENSAH drill used is run at 150 to 200 REM with no irrigation in a counter clockwise direction to propel the allograft into the sinus. The final drill diameter should be 7 mm to 1 mm less than the planned implant diameter.

Following the lift, the implant is placed into the site with the appropriate torque wrench.

The osseodensification procedure can, according to the published literature, not only expand osteotomy sites both horizontally and vertically but also help to improve maxillary bone density leading to an increase in bone-to-implant contact, thereby improving implant stability.[12]

ALTERNATIVE METHOD FOR TRANSCRESTAL APPROACH
Dentium-Advanced Sinus Kit System

The senior author (HD) has written[14] about this system in the past, and it is a viable alternative with a click learning curve for augmenting the maxillary sinus via a transcrestal approach. Similar to the other techniques, a series of varying size of drill bits are used to achieve the desired osteotomy diameter, leaving a 1 mm ceiling of bone between final drill and sinus floor. Then the specialized (DASK System) DASK drill is introduced into the osteotomy, which due to its unique dome shape and diamond finish will thin out the antral floor bone without causing a perforation in the Schneiderian

---

Box 1
Technique for vertical augmentation of 3 mm or more

Step 1: measure the bone height to the sinus floor

Step 2: flap the soft tissue using instruments and techniques as usual

Step 3: begin with DENSAH bur 2.0 diameter in osseodensification (OD) mode (counterclockwise drill speed 800 to 1500 RPM with copious irrigation). Continue running bur until you are at the sinus floor but not further and confirm position with a radiograph.

Step 4: use the next drill diameter 3.0 at the same drill speed with a pumping motion and advance past the sinus floor 1 mm in increments up to 3 mm. Bone will be pushed toward the apical end and will begin to gently lift the membrane. Confirm the drill position with a radiograph.

Step 5: depending on the diameter of the implant you wish to place, continue with the next size diameter drill bit.

> **Box 2**
> **Osseodensification technique for transcrestal sinus lift**
>
> Step 1: measure height of maxillary sinus
>
> Step 2: rotate pilot drill in standard clockwise direction to 1 mm short of sinus floor
>
> Step 3: next DENSAH drill bits at 800 to 1220 RPM in counterclockwise direction
>
> Step 4: final drill is advanced past sinus floor at maximum of 3 mm
>
> Step 5: if posterior bone height is 4 to 5 mm add slurry of bone to osteotomy site and advance drill (maximum of 3 mm) running at 150 to 200 RPM
>
> NOTE: always undersize the osteotomy site by 0.7 mm to 1.0 mm drill bits to planned implant diameter.

membrane. The membrane is then elevated and bone graft is then introduced (**Fig. 7**).

Transcrestal Sinus Lift Complications

The most common complications related to the transcrestal sinus flaps elevation procedure are similar to the lateral window surgical approach: sinus membrane perforation and maxillary sinusitis. However, unlike the lateral maxillary approach, the sinus

Crestal Approach (Sinus Lifting)

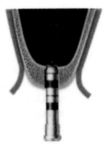
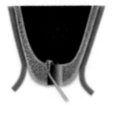
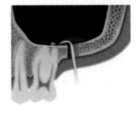

After Ø3.8 Final drilling, eliminate the residual bone (1mm) using a DASK Drill #1 or #2 (in hard bone) until you feel a slight drop

Detach sinus membran using the dome-shape sinus curette

Detaching the sinus membrane to create adequate space for graft material

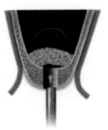
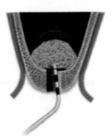
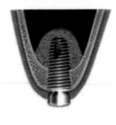

Fig. 7. DASK system transcrestal sinus augmentation technique with simultaneous implant placement. (*Courtesy of* Dentium.)

membrane perforations in the transcrestal approach can sometimes go unnoticed due to the lack adequate visibility. The most reliable method for identifying sinus membrane perforation during transcortical sinus lift procedures would be flexible endoscope examination. This technique is unlikely to ever become the standard of care due to the expensive nature of the equipment and its infrequent use. Most clinicians rely on using the Valsalva maneuver (which involved moderate forceful exhalation against a closed airway) as a reliable clinical method for detecting sinus membrane perforation. The patient's nostrils are gently squeeze shut while advising patient to breathe out. A positive result will be recognized by bubbling seen at the perforated sinus membranes at the prepared implant site or viewing the membrane flutter through the prepared implant site. Perforations via the transcortical approach can occur while infracturing the floor or while inserting the implant or while placing the graft material.

If a small sinus membrane perforation occurs the clinician is faced with a few clinical options. Number one would be to proceed with the planned procedure: placing a collagen sponge into the socket followed by the bone graft material and the implant. However, the patient will require frequent follow-up to monitor for possible development of sinusitis. If the perforation is rather large, equal to more than half the size of the osteotomy, the other option would be to perform a lateral window in the usual manner and lift the sinus membrane into position and then seal the perforation with a large collagen membrane. The other option would be to place the implant 2 mm into the sinus with no grafting, thus engaging the cortical floor of the sinus. The literature[15] has shown that in canine studies, implants protruding 2 mm or less in the maxillary sinus will lead to complete healing of the sinus membrane and bone formation with no sinusitis developing. The literature has also shown in human studies that implants protruding an average of 4 mm (some were 6 mm) did not lead to a clinical maxillary sinusitis and bone and implant failure or loss of osseous integration, but the likelihood of being covered by the maxillary Schneiderman membrane would be lessened.

SUMMARY

Augmenting the posterior alveolous before implant placement is often required to obtain solid implant stability. Two time-tested techniques—lateral and transcrestal sinus lifts—are presented in this chapter above with the most common complications. Sinus augmentation of the atrophic posterior maxilla via either the transalveolar or lateral window approach is a highly predictable procedure associated with a success rate of 90% or better.[16,17]

DISCLOSURE

The authors have nothing to disclose.

REFERENCES

1. Carrao V, DeMatteis I. Maxillary sinus bone augmentation techniques. Oral Maxillofacial Surg Clin N Am 2015;27(2):245–53.
2. Kao DW. Clinical maxillary sinus elevation surgery. Ames (IA): John Wiley & Sons; 2014. Accessed May 23, 2020.
3. Ritter A, Rozendorn N, Avishai G, et al. Preoperative maxillary sinus imaging and the outcome of sinus floor augmentation and dental implants in asymptomatic patients. Ann Otol Rhinol Laryngol 2020;129(3):209–15.

4. Ortega-Mejia H, Estrugo-Devesa A, Saka-Herrán C, et al. Platelet-rich plasma in maxillary sinus augmentation: systematic review. Materials 2020;13(3):622.
5. Attia S, Narberhaus C, Schaaf H, et al. Long-term influence of platelet-rich plasma (prp) on dental implants after maxillary augmentation: implant survival and success rates. J Clin Med 2020;9(2):391.
6. Kim HJ, Yea S, Kim KH, et al. A retrospective study of implants placed following 1-stage or 2-stage maxillary sinus floor augmentation by the lateral window technique performed on residual bone of <4 mm: results up to 10 years of follow-up. J Periodontol 2020;91(2):183–93.
7. Pai UY, Rodrigues SJ, Talreja KS, et al. Ossseodensification: a novel approach in implant dentistry,. J Indian Prosthodont Soc 2018;18(3):196–200.
8. Summers R. A new concenpt in maxillary implant surgery: the osteotome technique. Compend Contin Educ Dent 1994;15:152.
9. Summers R. Sinus lift elevation with osteotomes. J Esthet Dent 2007;10(3): 164–71.
10. Sotirakis EG, Gonshor A. Elevation of the maxillary sinus floor with hydraulic pressure. J Oral Implantol 2005;31(4):197–204.
11. Huwais S. Enhancing implant stability with osseodensification – a case report with 2 year follow-up. Implant Pract 2018;8(1):34.
12. Lipton D, Neiva R, Trahan W, et al. Osseodensification as a novel implant preparation technique that facilitates ridge expansion by compaction autografting, American Academy of Periodontology. Scientific Annual Meeting, Orland, FL, 2015
13. Trisi P, Berardini M, Falco A, et al. New osseodensification implant site preparation method to increase bone density in low density bone: in vivo evaluation in sheep. Implant Dent 2016;25(1):24–31.
14. Mohan N, Wolf J, Dym H. Maxillary sinus augmentation. Dent Clin North Am 2015; 59:275–388.
15. EL Zahwy M, Awad S, Kamel HM, et al. Clinical and radiographic evaluation of dental implants penetrating the maxillary sinus. J Int Dental Med Res 2017; 10(2):207–13.
16. Tan WC, Lang NP, Zwahlen M. A systemic review of the success of sinus floor elevation and survival of implants inserted in combination with sinus floor elevation part II: transalveolar technique: J Clin Periodontol 2008;35(suppl 8):241–54.
17. PJetursson BE, Tan WC, Zwahlen M. A systemic review of the success of sinus floor elevation and survival of implants inserted in combination with sinus floor elevation. J Clin Periodontol 2008;35(suppl 8):216–40.

All-on-4 Concept Update

Michael H. Chan, DDS[a,b,*], Yoav A. Nudell, DDS, MS[b]

KEYWORDS

- All-on-4 • All-on-4 concept • Atrophic maxilla • Atrophic mandible • Tilted implants
- Immediate function prosthesis • Full fixed arch restoration

KEY POINTS

- Using the All-on-4 concept is biomechanically sound with implant survival rates for the maxilla ranging from 93.9% to 100% with up to 13 years of follow-up. The cumulative survival rate for the mandible is 91.7% to 100% with up to 18 years of follow-up.
- Immediate loading provisional prosthesis survive well when implants are torqued between 30 to 50 Ncm ideally with no cantilever and with a one tooth cantilever maximum if necessary. If possible, use metal reinforced acrylic prosthesis to decrease incident of fracture.
- Final cantilever length to Anterior-Posterior spread (CL/AP ratio <1) should not exceed ratio <0.9 to minimize prosthetic fracture.
- Final restoration can have 10 to 12 teeth for proper esthetics and function. Final prosthesis survival rates using the "All-on-4" concept range from 97.06% to 100.0% in the maxilla with up to 13 years of follow-up and between 98.8% and 100% with up to 18 years in the mandible.
- Patient satisfaction was 95.6% surveyed by questionnaire.

INTRODUCTION

For the past 17 years, the All-on-4 concept has been used to rehabilitate the edentulous jaws with a full fixed arch prosthesis and immediate function. The intent of this article is to highlight some of the current data, contraindications/exclusion criteria, complications and remedies, occlusion and cantilever trends, implant size, and controversial topics. Conforming to the amount of material allowable to be written for this publication, please refer to the "Contemporary All-on-4 Concept" article for more descriptive surgical indications, and detailed stepwise procedures for surgery and prosthesis (**Fig. 1**).[1]

[a] Oral & Maxillofacial Surgery, Department of Veterans Affairs, New York Harbor Healthcare System (Brooklyn Campus), 800 Poly Place (Bk-160), Brooklyn, NY 11209, USA; [b] Oral & Maxillofacial Surgery, Department of Oral and Maxillofacial Surgery, The Brooklyn Hospital Center, 121 DeKalb Avenue (Box-187), Brooklyn, NY 11201, USA
* Corresponding author. 800 Poly Place (Bk-160), Brooklyn, NY 11209.
E-mail address: chanoms@yahoo.com
Twitter: @YoavNudell (Y.A.N.)

Dent Clin N Am 65 (2021) 211–227
https://doi.org/10.1016/j.cden.2020.09.014
0011-8532/21/Published by Elsevier Inc.

dental.theclinics.com

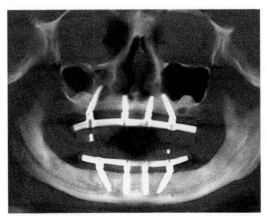

Fig. 1. Panoramic image of maxillary and mandibular all-on-4 prosthesis. (*From* Graves S, Mahler BA, Javid B, et al. Maxillary all-on-four therapy using angled implants: a 16-month clinical study of 1110 implants in 276 jaws. Oral Maxillofac Surg Clin North Am. 2011;23(2):282; with permission.)

IMPLANT SURVIVAL RATE

Data revealing implant survival within the All-on-4 concept are demonstrable by multiple investigators with continuous positive outcomes. Studies reported on maxillary implant survival ranges from 93.9% to 100% (up to 40 months to 13 years),[2–14] whereas the mandible registered between 91.7% and 100% (up 3 years to 18 years)[2,4,6–8,10–12,15–20] of follow-up. It is noteworthy, the lowest survival rate has been associated with the longest follow-up period for both arches.[14,20]

The lack of standardization used for implant success and survival criteria by numerous investigators makes interpreting data heterogeneous. Furthermore, most investigators choose to use survival rate's metrics over success primarily for the ability of these implants to ultimately support the prosthesis as the end goal resulting in better overall percentages commonly known as cumulative survival rate. In addition, the definition for survival is broader and generally refers to an implant remaining in the jaw; whereas, success has a defined set of subjective and objective parameters.[6] Nevertheless, some investigators reference Albrektsson's criteria as the gold standard (**Box 1**).[5,14,21,22] In the future, Papaspyridakos and colleagues[21] suggest a more uniform set of success criteria evaluating implant-prosthetic complex as a unit rather as a separate entity.[21]

Box 1		
Albrektsson and colleague (1986) criteria for implant success		
1	Absence of pain, paresthesia or Infection	Success
2	Absence of peri-implant radiolucency	Success
3	Absence of mobility	Success
4	Vertical bone loss must be less than 0.2 mm annually after first year of function	Success
5	Implant success rate of 85% at end of 5 years and 80% at end of 10 year period	Success

CONTRAINDICATIONS AND/OR EXCLUSION FOR ALL-ON-4 CONCEPT

- Insufficient bone volume[7,12]
- Poor oral hygiene[2,4,5,9,15]
- Patients noncompliant to follow-up[2,4,5,9,15]
- Parafunctional habits
  - That is, bruxers, clinchers, or oromandibular dystonia[2,4,5,9,13,15,19]
- Acute infection at prospective implant site[2,4,5,13,15,19]
- Smoking
  - Risk factor[2,14,20]
  - >10 cigarettes/d = [9]
  - >20 cigarettes/d = [19]
- Drug abuse[9,13]

Systemic conditions may not be amenable to implant placement

- Recent cardiovascular incident
  - Myocardial infarction <6 months is contraindicated[13]
  - Peri-implantitis risk[20,23,24]
- Diabetes
  - Peri-implantitis risk[16,20,23,25]
  - Uncontrolled diabetes as exclusion criteria for All-on-4 implant placement[2,5,10,13,15]
- Autoimmune disease
  - that is, rheumatoid arthritis, and other low-grade inflammatory disease[26]
- Metabolic bone disease
  - Antiresorptive (AR) Therapy
    - General exclusion criteria from longitudinal studies[9,19]
    - Oral bisphosphonate (BP) is a risk factor for implant loss[13,16]
    - High dose/intravenous contraindicated[10,13]
- Disease of immune system[4,5,13]
- Chemotherapy or head and neck radiation
  - Previous chemotherapy and radiation therapy[9,13]
  - Active chemotherapy and radiation therapy[12]
  - Radiation within 1 year[20]
  - Radiation within 5 years[9,19]
  - Chemotherapy or radiation therapy within 1 years[2,5,15]
  - Chemotherapy or radiation therapy within 5 years[5]
- Coagulopathy[4,5,13,15]
- Hematological disease[4,5,15]
- Pregnancy or lactation[5,8–10,15]
- Psychiatric illness[9,13]
- American Society of Anesthesiologist (ASA III and IV)[9]
- Steroid Therapy[9,19]

WHAT ARE SOME RISK FACTORS REPORTED FOR AILING OR IMPLANT FAILURES?

In general, implant failures can be categorized into 2 groups: early and late. Early failures are attributed to lack of osseointegration. Although some failures are universally accepted within the range of surgical failure, it is only natural to speculate what these factors are. Some postulate post-extractive sites (extraction with immediate implant placement) with presence of periapical infection as a contributing factor.[17] Another suggested inexperienced clinicians with fewer than 50 cases have more failures than experienced ones.[18] A recent prospective randomized control trial investigated high insertion torque (>50 Ncm) implants had approximately 50% more peri-implant bone remodeling and approximately 2 times the buccal soft tissue recession than implants inserted with regular torque (<50 Ncm) at 12 months.[27]

Numerous investigators have documented peri-implantitis as a late complication for implant failures. Many have attributed poor oral hygiene as the primary etiologic factor for development of mucositis (gingival redness and swelling without bone loss) to eventual peri-implantitis (peri-implant soft tissue inflammation with evidence of persistent bone loss).[5,7–9] Derks and colleagues[28]showed early peri-implantitis (66%) can be seen on radiographs at 3 years with greater than 0.5 mm bone loss in 81% of patients and will cause continuous bone loss over time. They reported the progression to moderate/severe peri-implantitis with an average marginal bone loss to be 3.5 ± 1.5 mm with mean follow-up of 8.6 ± 0.7 years.[28] Clinicians should have a regular maintenance recall schedule to intercept the disease at the earliest signs to prevent disease progression.

Parafunctional Habits

Excessive and constant jaw motion have many investigators report an overall negative impact to this full-arch prosthesis design. Multiple investigators recommend avoidance of patients with severe parafunctional habits (ie, bruxing, clenching, and/or oromandibular dystonia) to prevent future prosthetic and implant-related complications.[2,4,5,9,12,13,15,19] Additionally, Lopes and colleagues[12] have found 7.2% of patients with bruxism leading to peri-implantitis resulting in failures.

Smokers

Smoking is controversial with some investigators reporting a direct correlation to marginal bone loss, peri-implantitis, and/or implant failure for All-on-4 cases,[6,12,14,16,18] while others did not find any difference with implant survival rates above 98.6%.[4,5,13] Although there is an intuitive cause-and-effect relationship of the negative effects of smoking, more control studies are need to quantify the number of cigarettes (ie, fewer than or more than 10 cigarettes/d), length of smoking history, and a larger sample size with long follow-up period to get a better assessment for this All-on-4 design. Peri-implantitis requires lifelong maintenance to salvage some ailing cases.

Cardiovascular

In 2019, Maló and colleagues[14] revealed 80% of cardiovascular patients are at risk to develop peri-implantitis but warned not to draw these conclusions given the small sample size and lack of experimental control. However, a comprehensive systematic review performed by Ting and colleagues[23] concluded cardiovascular and uncontrolled diabetics were at high risk of developing peri-implantitis. Dhadse and colleagues[24] also reported cardiovascular patients were at a higher risk of developing peri-implantitis and 3 times more likely to be associated with Epstein-Barr virus.

Diabetes

Generally, people with diabetes are at higher risk for peri-implantitis. It has been shown poorly controlled group has greater probing depths and peri-implant bone loss than control group.[23,25] In addition, the longitudinal All-on-4 study of Malo and colleagues[16] found diabetic individuals with more biological complications (ie, abscess, infection, and peri-implantitis) leading to implant failure.[14] Numerous investigators listed uncontrolled diabetes as an exclusion criteria for All-on-4 implant placement.[2,5,10,13,15]

ANTIRESORPTIVE THERAPY

Antiresorptives (AR) are widely used to treat osteoporosis and cancer with 2 common classes encountered by clinicians: Bisphosphonate (BP) and Denosumab (Receptor Activator of Nuclear factor-KB ligand [RANKL] inhibitor). Although both medications prevent bone resorption, they work on different pathways. BP binds to the lattice structure of the hydroxyapatite found on bony surfaces. When osteoclast ingests bone saturated with BP, the ability for osteoclast to bind to bone has been nullified resulting its ability to resorb bone. On the other hand, RANKL inhibitor is a humanized monoclonal antibody that exerts its antiresorptive effects by blocking RANKL to RANK essential to initiate osteoclast differentiation. Unlike BP that binds to bone directly, RANKL inhibitors work on osteoclast "precursors" ultimately disabling production of mature osteoclasts.[29] The disruption of osteoclast's function with these medications could in theory cause more implant failures, increased marginal bone loss, and medication-related osteonecrosis of the jaw (MRONJ). It is also theoretically possible to discontinue denosumab (6 months) before implant placement because the mechanism of action does not affect bone directly but needs to await for new production of osteoclasts after the drug's biological inactivity. Cumulative dosages and relative drug potency are more important than the mode of administration with low dose typically prescribed for osteoporosis and high for malignancies (**Table 1**).[26,29,30]

A recent review by Stavropoulos and colleagues[26] investigated the outcome and complication rate of implant therapy with and without antiresorptive drug treatment. They concluded low-dose oral BP for osteoporosis treatment does not increase the rate of implant failures, marginal bone loss, peri-implantitis, and MRONJ when compared with the non-medication group. However, minimal clinical data are available to effectively assess patients on high-dose BP or denosumab but only to categorize this high-risk group for those who are on oral BP for a prolonged period with concurrent comorbidities or high-dose AR used for malignancies.[26]

Controversially, in another recent systematic review, Chappuis and colleagues[31] also found no increased risk of implant failure with oral BP but emphasize the absolute contraindication with intravenous BP. Interestingly, the investigators did find an association between proton pump inhibitors (PPIs) and serotonin reuptake inhibitors (SSRIs) with an increased risk for implant failures. PPIs impair calcium absorption from the intestine and therefore disrupt bone formation. SSRIs disrupt osteoclasts activation and differentiation thus having a negative influence on osseointegration.[31]

A more nuanced view taken by De-Freitas and colleagues[32] mirrors the American Association of Oral and Maxillofacial Surgeons recommendations by highlighting the importance of taking patient's concomitant risks into consideration. Ingesting oral BP for less than 4 years with no other risk factors can proceed with implant placement with specific informed consent explaining possible long-term implant failure and a low risk of osteonecrosis of the jaws. However, if patients have taken oral BP for less than 4 years, but have also been taking corticosteroids or antiangiogenic medications or if patients who have taken oral BP for more than 4 years, a drug holiday for at least 2 months before implant placement is suggested. This recommendation is based on the drug's half-life and urinary excretion to render the medication biologically as inactive suggested by Damm and Jones.[33] If possible, BP should be held until osseointegration is achieved.[33]

Table 1 Comparative examples of antiresorptive therapy				
Name	Class	Relative Potency to Etidronate = 1	Route of Administration and Dosage	Indication
Alendronate (Fosamax)	BP	500	70 mg po weekly (low dose)	Osteoporosis
Denosumab (Prolia)	Denosumab	?	60 mg sc 6 mo (low dose)	Osteoporosis
Denosumab (Xgeva)	Denosumab	?	120 mg sc 4 wk (high dose)	Cancer
Ibandronate (Boniva)	BP	1000	150 mg po monthly (low dose)	Osteoporosis
Ibandronate (Boniva)	BP	1000	50 mg po qd or 1500 mg monthly total (high dose)	Cancer

Abbreviations: BP, bisphosphonate; IV, intravenous; po, oral; sc, subcutaneous.
Data from Refs.[26,29,30]

Furthermore, a prospective cohort study by Tallarico and colleagues[34] on patients taking alendronate (Fosamax) 35 to 70 mg weekly for at least 3 years with a 6-month drug holiday reported implant success rate of 98% with a marginal bone loss of 1.35 ± 0.21 mm. Conversely, 2 All-on-4 longitudinal studies have correlated implant failure with oral BP as a risk factor without a drug holiday.[13,16]

Many investigators listed BP therapy as an exclusion criteria.[5,9,19] Although oral BP still lacks general consensus, the IV version is widely regarded as an absolute contraindication for dental implant placement.[10,13,33]

CHEMOTHERAPY AND RADIATION THERAPY

In a longitudinal study, Niedermaier and colleagues[13] revealed a patient with a history of chemotherapy as a risk factor for the All-on-4 design without achieving osseointegration. The investigators mentioned interpreting these results with caution because 2 other studies reported successful outcomes and further investigation is needed in particular with immediate load.[13] Currently, there is no clear consensus on the exclusion criteria for patients with past treatments with various investigators listed within 1 to 5 years.[2,4,5,9,10,12,13,15,19,20]

STEROID THERAPY

The use of corticosteroids have been documented to cause impaired cellular healing, hyperglycemia, increased rate of infection with overall negative effects on osseointegration.[35,36] Osteoporosis is a known consequence of chronic glucocorticoids therapy. Bone formation is thought to be disrupted by altering the Wingless-related integration site (Wnt) signaling through upregulating the Wnt antagonists, specifically sclerostin (SOST), and dickkopfrelated protein 1 (Dkk1). These Wnt antagonists decrease the production of osteoblasts resulting in less bone formation and increased osteoclastic activity with bone resorption creating an osteoporotic milieu.[37]

Generally, chronic steroids are listed as an exclusion criteria.[9,19] This, however, does not preclude use of short course of steroids (ie, medrol-dose pack) for nonsteroid users to help decrease postsurgical edema.[11]

PROSTHETIC SURVIVAL RATE

Similar to the implant survival criteria, prosthetic survival does not have a universally accepted standard, but most clinicians adopt the ability to fabricate a final prosthesis on existing osseointegrated implants. According to Malo and colleagues,[20] prosthetic survival is based on function, with the necessity of replacing the prosthesis classified as failure.

Nevertheless, final prosthesis survival rate also yields a successful outcome with the maxilla ranging from 97.06% to 100.0% (up to 36 months to 13 years),[2–13] whereas the mandible registers between 98.8% and 100% with (up to 3 years to 18 years)[2,4,6–8,10–12,15–20] of follow-up by multiple investigators.

MARGINAL BONE LOSS

Marginal bone loss data are based on radiographic bone measurements on the mesial and distal site for each implant. Specifically, the difference is calculated between the implant/abutment interface and existing bone level for pre and post loading.[9,13]

Adell and colleagues[38] first reported an average crestal bone loss for loaded implants to be 1.2 mm during the first year and 0.1 mm annually with these parameters during the implant's life expectancy. This finding was consistent with Niedermayer and colleagues,[13] who reported 1-mm bone loss with 0.2 mm annually.

Recent studies with short-term (up to 3 years), medium-term (between 3 and 7 years), and long-term (beyond 7 years) marginal bone loss range from 0.14 mm $\pm$ 0.59 to 1.19 mm $\pm$ 0.33 (mean $\pm$ SD/mm), 0.39 mm $\pm$ 0.18 to 1.9 mm $\pm$ 1.1, and 1.30 mm $\pm$ 0.63 SD to 2.30 mm for short-term, medium-term, and long-term, respectively, with 15-year follow-up.[4,9–13,18–20]

While comparing among different size diameter implants, Babbush and colleagues[11] demonstrated narrow (3.5 mm) diameter implants had statistically more bone loss but emphasized that the results were not clinically relevant up to 3 years of follow-up.

Maló and colleagues[20] reported 3 risk factors associated with advanced bone loss (>3 mm) at 10 years particularly with biological complication, previous implant failure, and smokers. In addition, through the binary logistic regression model, Malo and colleagues[20] found male gender, smoking, biological complication, and age to play a role for greater than 2.8 mm bone loss at 5 years.[14] Simply put, the likelihood of the amount of bone loss observed in a given period will occur with the preceding variables when compared with the absence of exposure.

Another often overlooked reason for marginal bone loss has been documented by Durkan and colleagues.[39] They described improper occlusion, implant, or prosthetic design will often burden the rest of the healthy implants with undue stress resulting in crestal bone loss.[39]

WHAT ARE THE TECHNICAL COMPLICATIONS ASSOCIATED WITH ALL-ON-4?

Technical complications are defined as the complications related to prosthetic components (**Table 2**). Acrylic prosthesis fracture is the most common complication followed by provisional screw loosening (abutment and/or prosthetic) for the provisional period. Bruxers are responsible for a good majority of the cases while opposing implant-supported bridge are attributed by the non-bruxer group.[12,40] Prosthetic repair, occlusal adjustment, and nightguard fabrication along with decrease in occlusal load (ie, softer diet) remedied the fracture situation while retightening the

Table 2
Technical complications and their remedies

Complications	Remedy	Notes
Provisional prosthesis		
Fracture of provisional prosthesis (66/111 pt) (59.4%) (Lopes et al,[12] 2017)	1. Repair prosthesis 2. Occlusal adjustment 3. Occlusal Nightguard	1. Bruxer(47/111 pt) (42.3%) 2. Non-Bruxer(25/111 pt) (22.5%) = Opposing implant-supported dentition
Abutment screw loosening (67/111 pt) (60.3%) (Lopes et al,[12] 2017)	1. Tighten screw 2. Occlusal adjustment 3. Occlusal Nightguard	1. Bruxer(47/111 pt) (42.3%) 2. Non-Bruxer(25/111 pt) (22.5%) = Opposing implant-supported dentition
Prosthetic screw loosening (7/111 pt) (6.3%) (Lopes et al,[12] 2017)	1. Tighten screw 2. Occlusal adjustment 3. Occlusal Nightguard	1. Bruxer(47/111 pt) (42.3%) 2. Non-Bruxer(25/111 pt) (22.5%) = Opposing implant-supported dentition
Fracture of provisional prosthesis (acrylic) (4/40 pt) (10%) (Tallarico et al,[9] 2016 Retro)	1. Repair prosthesis 2. Occlusal adjustment	Suggested metal reinforced provisional
Fracture of provisional prosthesis (acrylic) (2/40 pt) (5%) (Tallarico et al,[10] 2016 RTC)	1. Repair prosthesis 2. Occlusal adjustment	
Prosthetic screw loosening (3/40 pt) (7.5%) (Tallarico et al,[9] 2016 Retro)	1. Retighten screw 2. Occlusal adjustment	Parafunctional habit
Prosthetic Screw loosening (2/40 pt) (5%) (Tallarico et al,[10] 2016 RTC)	1. Retighten screw 2. Occlusal adjustment	
Detachment of veneering material (10.5% pt) (Francetti et al,[8] 2015)	1. Repair fractured veneer 2. Occlusal adjustment	1. Short facial height 2. Drastic changes from soft to hard diet 3. Parafunctional habit
Fracture of provisional prosthesis (8.1% pt) (Francetti et al,[8] 2015)	1. Repair prosthesis 2. Occlusal adjustment	1. Short facial height 2. Drastic changes from soft to hard diet 3. Parafunctional habit
Detachment of veneering material (20.6% pt) (Cavalli et al,[5] 2012)	1. Repair fractured veneer 2. Occlusal adjustment	Most common complication
Fracture of provisional prosthesis (14.7% pt) (Cavalli et al,[5] 2012)	1. Repair prosthesis 2. Occlusal adjustment	none

(continued on next page)

Table 2
(continued)

Complications	Remedy	Notes
Final prosthesis		
Fractured of final prosthesis (acrylic resin) (23/111 pt) (20.7%) (Lopes et al,[12] 2017)	1. Repair prosthesis 2. Occlusal adjustment 3. Occlusal Nightguard	1. Bruxers(18/111pt) (16.2%) 2. Non-Bruxers(15/111pt) (13.5%) = Implant-supported prosthesis as opposing arch
Abutment screw loosening (8/111 pt) (7.2%) (Lopes et al,[12] 2017)	1. Retighten screw 2. Occlusal adjustment 3. Occlusal Nightguard	1. Bruxers(18/111 pt) (16.2%) 2. Non-Bruxers(15/111pt) (13.5%) = Implant-supported prosthesis as opposing arch
Combination of prosthetic screw fracture and loosening (1/111 pt) (0.9%) (Lopes et al,[12] 2017)	1. Replace and Retighten screw/abutment 2. Occlusal adjustment 3. Occlusal Nightguard	1. Bruxers(18/111 pt) (16.2%) 2. Non-Bruxers(15/111pt) (13.5%) = Implant-supported prosthesis as opposing arch
Abutment fracture (1/111 pt) (0.9%) (Lopes et al,[12] 2017)	1. Replace and Retighten screw/abutment 2. Occlusal adjustment 3. Occlusal Nightguard	1. Bruxers(18/111 pt) (16.2%) 2. Non-Bruxers(15/111pt) (13.5%) = Implant-supported prosthesis as opposing arch
Fracture of veneering material (acrylic or ceramic) (3/40 pt) (7.5%) (Tallarico et al,[9] 2016 Retro)	1. Repair fractured veneer 2. Occlusal adjustment	Possible parafunctional habits
Fracture of veneering material (4/40 pt) (10%) (Tallarico et al,[10] 2016 RTC)	1. Repair fractured veneer 2. Occlusal adjustment	
Detachment of veneering material (23.2% pt) (Francetti et al,[8] 2015)	1. Repair fractured veneer 2. Occlusal adjustment	Most common complication 1. Short facial height 2. Drastic changes from soft to hard diet 3. Parafunctional habit
Screw loosening or fracture (19.8% pt) (Francetti et al,[8] 2015)	1. Retighten screw 2. Occlusal adjustment	None
Fracture of final prosthesis (7.0% pt) (Francetti et al,[8] 2015)	1. Repair fractured veneer 2. Occlusal adjustment	1. Short facial height 2. Drastic changes from soft to hard diet 3. Parafunctional habit
Detachment of veneering material (30.4% pt) (Lopes et al,[12] 2015)	1. Repair prosthesis 2. Occlusal adjustment 3. Occlusal Nightguard	Heavy Bruxer
Abutment screw loosening (7.2% pt) (Lopes et al,[12] 2015)	1. Retighten screw	Opposing implant-supported dentition

(continued on next page)

Table 2 (continued)		
Complications	Remedy	Notes
Detachment of veneering material (17.7% pt) (Cavalli et al,[5] 2012)	1. Repair fractured veneer 2. Occlusal adjustment	Most common complication
Fracture of provisional prosthesis (Acrylic) (2.9% pt) (Cavalli et al,[5] 2012)	1. Repair prosthesis 2. Occlusal adjustment	None

Abbreviation: pt, patient.

screw corrected the latter.[9,10,12,40] To counter acrylic resin fractures, Tallarico and colleagues[9] suggested metal reinforced provisional prosthesis.

As for final prosthesis, detachment of the veneering material is the most common complication. This was remedied with repair and occlusal adjustment.[5,7–10] Increased occlusal force and loss of proprioception are thought to be the contributing factors and patients need to retrain their bite strength.[40]

WHAT ARE THE BIOLOGICAL COMPLICATIONS ASSOCIATED WITH ALL-ON-4?

Biological complications refer to problems arising from dental implants (**Table 3**). This often provides a conundrum for the clinician.[5,7–10,12,17] Lopes and colleagues[12] reported smokers and bruxers have a higher implant failure rate both initial and long term with peri-implantitis as the cause for late development. Nevertheless, we should treat each patient with an end goal in mind to maintain full-arch prosthesis. Following are 3 different scenarios presented by Lopes and colleagues[12] and their outcome for each case.

Scenario 1

55 year-old man with failed maxillary implant #4.[12]
Remedy = Provisional prosthesis was kept in function with 3 implants and the denture shortened on the side of the failure for 6 months. A new implant was inserted.
Final outcome = Successful "All-on-4" restoration with 4 implants.

Scenario 2

63-year-old man (bruxer) with 3 mandibular implants, #20, #24, #29, failed to integrate.[12]
Remedy = Prosthesis was removed from function and 3 new implants were inserted 6 months later. Two of the new implants failed and another implant was reinserted.
Final outcome = Final prosthesis was supported by 3 implants "All-on-3."

Scenario 3

70-year-old woman (smoker and cardiovascular condition) with 3 maxillary implants, #4, #7, #12 failed to integrate with the fourth implant noted to have failed during the second surgical attempt and was replaced concurrently.[12]
Remedy = Four new implants were reinserted, which also failed to integrate.
Final outcome = Patient reverted back to removable denture.

The most common complication directly related to the mucositis, peri-implantitis, and late implants loss (Implant failure) is poor oral hygiene. Good home care with a

Table 3
Biological complications and their remedies

Complications	Remedy	Notes
Provisional prosthesis		
Failed implant integration (1/224 implants) (1.8%) (Tallarico et al,[9] 2016 Retro)	1. Remove implant 2. Shorten provisional prosthesis to right maxillary canine 3. Replace new implant in 3 months	Smoker = (1 pt)
Poor oral hygiene (53.5% pt) (Francetti et al,[8] 2015)	1. Improve oral hygiene 2. Plaque removal 3. Antimicrobial rinse	Most common complication Closer hygiene recall for prevention
Failed implant integration (3/ 876 implants) (0.3%) (Butura et al,[17] 2011)	1. Remove and immediately replace new implant in adjacent site with immediate loaded prosthesis	1. Implants were placed in post-extractive sites with periapical pathology = (2 pt) 2. Smoker = (1 pt) 3. Successful final prosthesis
Final prosthesis		
Peri-implantitis (25 pt) (22.5%) (Lopes et al,[12] 2017)	1. Treated either through nonsurgical (see mucositis section) and surgical intervention (see below) 2. Flap reflection (surgical only) 3. Mechanical debridement 4. Peridex to implant surface 5. Removal of granulation tissue	1. Smoking = (11 pt) (9.9%) 2. Bruxers = (19 pt) (17.1%) It failed to resolved for 11 pt (19 implants)
Mucositis (5/111 pt) (4.5%) (9/532 implants) (1.7%) (Lopes et al,[12] 2017)	1. Nonsurgical Intervention 2. Scaling 3. Antimicrobial rinse 4. Oral hygiene reinforcement	1. Closer hygiene recall 2. Treatments were successful except 1 patient lost 2 implants
Implant infection (7/111 pt) (6.3%) (10/532 implants) (1.8%) (Lopes et al,[12] 2017)	1. Nonsurgical intervention 2. Scaling 3. Antimicrobial rinse 4. Oral hygiene reinforcement	1. Closer hygiene recall 2. Treatments were successful except 1 patient lost 2 implants
Peri-implantitis (3/56 pt) (5.4%) (Tallarico et al,[9] 2016 Retro)	1. Mechanical debridement 2. Glycine-based air power abrasive device 3. Local application of antimicrobial agent 4. Reinforce oral hygiene	Treatment stopped progression of bone loss
Peri-implantitis (3/40 pt) (7.5%) (Tallarico et al,[10] 2016 RTC)	1. Mechanical debridement 2. Glycine-based air power abrasive device 3. Local application of antimicrobial agent 4. Reinforce oral hygiene	Treatment stopped progression of bone loss

(*continued on next page*)

Table 3 *(continued)*		
Complications	**Remedy**	**Notes**
Mucositis (30.2% pt) (Francetti et al,[8] 2015)	1. Improve oral hygiene 2. Plaque removal 3. More frequent recall 4. Antimicrobial rinse	Closer hygiene recall for prevention
Peri-implantitis (10.4% pt) (Francetti et al,[8] 2015)	1. Improve oral hygiene 2. Plaque removal 3. More frequent recall 4. Antimicrobial rinse	Closer hygiene recall for prevention
Implant loss (Late implant failure) (2.3% pt) (Francetti et al,[8] 2015)	1. Remove implant 2. Improve oral hygiene 3. Replace implant	Untreated or poorly treated mucositis or peri-implantitis
Peri-implantitis (2/23 pt) (8.7%) (2/92 implants) (2.2%) (Lopes et al,[8] 2015)	1. Intense oral hygiene 2. Surgical debridement	1. Closer hygiene recall for prevention 2. Resolved with treatment
Poor oral hygiene (38.2% pt) (Cavalli et al,[5] 2012)	1. Improve oral hygiene 2. Antimicrobial rinse	Most common complication Early interception is crucial
Peri-implant mucositis (11.8% pt) (Cavalli et al,[5] 2012)	1. Improve oral hygiene 2. Plaque removal 3. More frequent recall 4. Antimicrobial rinse	Early interception is crucial
Peri-implantitis (5.9% pt) (Cavalli et al,[5] 2012)	1. Improve oral hygiene 2. Plaque removal 3. More frequent recall 4. Antimicrobial rinse	Early interception is crucial

Abbreviation: pt, patient.

regular maintenance schedule can limit these issues.[5,7–10,12] Smokers and bruxers have also been implicated in contributing to peri-implantitis. Despite surgical intervention in one case series, approximately 44% (11/25 pt) of the patients failed to resolve their disease progression.[12]

WHAT IS THE CURRENT CANTILEVER TREND?

In 2005, Rangert's earlier calculations for the All-on-4 concept showed a cantilever length for the mandibular to be 2 times the A-P spread.[1] Others such as English reduced it to 1.5 times A-P-spread for the lower arch and limited it to 6 to 8 mm for the maxilla.[41] Complications associated with lengthy cantilevers can lead to either prosthetic fracture and/or screw loosening.[42] Recently, for provisional prosthesis, a 4-year clinical retrospective analysis by Drago[43] indicated cantilever length should not exceed one tooth size (author did not specify exact measurements) while the final prosthesis must have cantilever length/anterior posterior spread ratio less than 1 (CL/AP ratio <1). When keeping ratio at 0.9, he reported less than 1% complication rate with only one denture base fracture.[43] For example, if the maxillary implant A-P spread is 15.0 mm, then the cantilever cannot exceed 12.5 mm.

WHAT IS THE RECOMMENDATION FOR OCCLUSION?

Proper occlusion is essential for prosthetic longevity. Improper design can increase implant stress with eventual peri-implant bone loss, including various technical complications as stated previously.[41] Full-arch prosthesis should include a minimum of 10 to 12 teeth for proper esthetics and function.

We found a variety of occlusal designs for provisional and definitive prosthesis (**Fig. 2**). Most investigators choose mutually protected occlusion whereby the posterior teeth during centric occlusion disallow the anterior teeth to have any contact and the reverse is applied during lateral excursive movements for the posterior teeth (**Fig. 3**).[44]

Important points to remember about occlusion include the following:

1. Mutually protected occlusion
2. Minimal or no cantilever on provisional prosthesis
3. Lateral excursion = Canine or anterior guidance
4. Final prosthesis should have minimum 10 to 12 teeth per arch

DOES SIZE REALLY MATTER?

Various implant diameters and lengths are offered by manufacturing companies with narrow and wide implants are defined as less than 3.5 mm, and greater than 4.5 mm, respectively, whereas 8 mm or less is considered short.[13]

A 7-year retrospective analysis of immediately loaded implant-supported full-arch provisional prostheses by Niedermaier and colleagues[13] 2017 found no statistically significant differences in implant-related survival rates between the different implant diameters (3.5, 4.3, and 5 mm) and lengths (<8, 10, 11, 13, 15, 16, 18, and >20 mm). In addition, marginal bone loss for axial and tilted implants was identical with both recorded at 1.30 mm (± 0.35 SD/mm) in 5 years.

Another retrospective study by Babbush and colleagues[11] in 2016 reported using Nobel Active (platform switched) narrow, regular, and wide implants; all had cumulative implant survival of 99.8% at 3 years.

DOES ALL-ON-4 VERSUS ALL-ON-6 MATTER CLINICALLY?

In a recent 5-year randomized controlled trial by Tallarico and colleagues,[10] the All-on-4 group (98.75%) fare slightly better than the All-on-6 group (95.0%) in implant survival rate. However, the All-on-4 group has more technical and biological complications. Overall, there are no clinical or statistical differences in marginal bone loss between the All-on-4 (1.71 ± 0.42 mm) and All-on-6 (1.51 ± 0.36 mm) group, complications rates or worsening peri-implant conditions.[23]

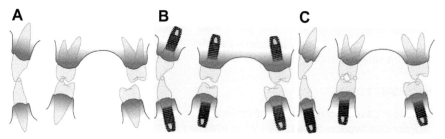

Fig. 2. Occlusion schemes. (*A*) Group function. (*B*) Mutually protected occlusion. (*C*) Bilateral balanced occlusion. (*From* Resnik RR, Misch CE. Occlusion complications. In: Resnik RR, Misch CE, editors. Misch's avoiding complications in oral implantology. St. Louis: Elsevier; 2018. p. 721–2; with permission.)

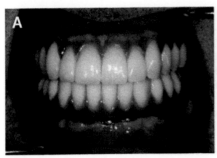 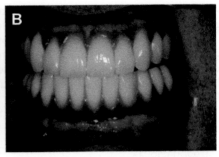

Fig. 3. Simultaneous bilateral point contacts on canine and posterior teeth and grazing contacts on incisor. Implant-supported full arch prosthesis with mutually protected occlusion. (*From* Misch CE. Occlusal considerations for implant-supported prostheses: implant-protective occlusion. In: Misch CE, editor. Dental implant prosthetics, 2nd edition. St. Louis: Mosby; 2015. p. 891; with permission.)

Failure of one of the inserted implants to meet the minimum 35 Ncm torque requirement is the main reason why these clinicians would place an additional 5th or 6th implant to qualify for immediate load protocol.[10]

CAN PATIENTS RECEIVE ALL-ON-4 TREATMENT EVEN WITH A HISTORY OF ADULT GENERALIZED PERIODONTITIS?

Patients with previously generalized aggressive adult periodontal disease appear to have success up to 5 years of follow-up with survival rate in an All-on-4 design reported at 98.75%. In addition, 100% of the final prostheses survived and marginal bone loss was recorded at 1.2 mm up to 7 years, respectively.[45]

ARE PATIENTS SATISFIED WITH THE OUTCOME?

In general, patients are very satisfied with the full-arch prosthesis when surveyed either by questionnaire forms or visual analog scale (VAS) scoring scale on the following categories: (1) esthetics, (2) phonetics, (3) function, (4) psychology (omitted in the VAS). Scores of 95.6% were recorded based on those surveyed.[40]

SUMMARY

The All-on-4 concept is still an excellent treatment option for the edentulous population despite a small percentage of unsuccessful cases needing to revert back to removable dentures. Understanding risk factors for potential failures and solutions for complications that arise will limit the number of problems. Long-term predictable outcomes always start with good case selection and realistic patient expectations through transparent doctor-patient discussion.

CLINICS CARE POINTS

- Proper case selection is critical for long term success.
- Poor oral hygiene remains the most common complication for peri-implantitis.
- Parafunctional habits contributes to prosthetic complication.
- Decreasing cantilever length can decrease prosthetic complications.
- Proper occlusion is essential for full arch restoration functional longevity.
- Implant size does not influence implant survival rate up to 5 years.

DISCLOSURE

The authors have nothing to disclose.

REFERENCES

1. Chan MH, Holmes C. Contemporary "All-on-4" concept. Dent Clin North Am 2015; 59(2):421–70.
2. Capelli M, Zuffetti F, Del Fabbro M, et al. Immediate rehabilitation of the completely edentulous jaw with fixed prostheses supported by either upright or tilted implants: a multicenter clinical study. Int J Oral Maxillofac Implants 2007; 22(4):639–44.
3. Maló P, de Araújo Nobre M, Lopes A, et al. "All-on-4" immediate-function concept for completely edentulous maxillae: a clinical report on the medium (3 years) and long-term (5 years) outcomes. Clin Implant Dent Relat Res 2012;14(Suppl 1): e139–50.
4. Francetti L, Romeo D, Corbella S, et al. Bone level changes around axial and tilted implants in full-arch fixed immediate restorations. Interim results of a prospective study. Clin Implant Dent Relat Res 2012;14(5):646–54.
5. Cavalli N, Barbaro B, Spasari D, et al. Tilted implants for full-arch rehabilitations in completely edentulous maxilla: a retrospective study. Int J Dent 2012;2012: 180379.
6. Balshi TJ, Wolfinger GJ, Slauch RW, et al. A retrospective analysis of 800 Brånemark System implants following the All-on-Four™ protocol. J Prosthodont 2014; 23(2):83–8.
7. Lopes A, Maló P, de Araújo Nobre M, et al. The NobelGuide® All-on-4® treatment concept for rehabilitation of edentulous jaws: a prospective report on medium- and long-term outcomes. Clin Implant Dent Relat Res 2015;17(Suppl 2):e406–16.
8. Francetti L, Corbella S, Taschieri S, et al. Medium- and long-term complications in full-arch rehabilitations supported by upright and tilted implants. Clin Implant Dent Relat Res 2015;17(4):758–64.
9. Tallarico M, Canullo L, Pisano M, et al. An up to 7-year retrospective analysis of biologic and technical complication with the All-on-4 concept. J Oral Implantol 2016;42(3):265–71.
10. Tallarico M, Meloni SM, Canullo L, et al. Five-year results of a randomized controlled trial comparing patients rehabilitated with immediately loaded maxillary cross-arch fixed dental prosthesis supported by four or six implants placed using guided surgery. Clin Implant Dent Relat Res 2016;18(5):965–72.
11. Babbush CA, Kanawati A, Kotsakis GA. Marginal bone stability around tapered, platform-shifted implants placed with an immediately loaded four-implant-supported fixed prosthetic concept: a cohort study. Int J Oral Maxillofac Implants 2016;31(3):643–50.
12. Lopes A, Maló P, de Araújo Nobre M, et al. The NobelGuide(®) All-on-4(®) treatment concept for rehabilitation of edentulous jaws: a retrospective report on the 7-years clinical and 5-years radiographic outcomes. Clin Implant Dent Relat Res 2017;19(2):233–44.
13. Niedermaier R, Stelzle F, Riemann M, et al. Implant-supported immediately loaded fixed full-arch dentures: evaluation of implant survival rates in a case cohort of up to 7 years. Clin Implant Dent Relat Res 2017;19(1):4–19.
14. Maló P, de Araújo Nobre M, Lopes A, et al. The All-on-4 concept for full-arch rehabilitation of the edentulous maxillae: a longitudinal study with 5-13 years of follow-up. Clin Implant Dent Relat Res 2019;21(4):538–49.

15. Agliardi E, Panigatti S, Clericò M, et al. Immediate rehabilitation of the edentulous jaws with full fixed prostheses supported by four implants: interim results of a single cohort prospective study. Clin Oral Implants Res 2010;21(5):459–65.
16. Malo P, de Araújo Nobre M, Lopes A, et al. A longitudinal study of the survival of All-on-4 implants in the mandible with up to 10 years of follow-up. J Am Dent Assoc 2011;142(3):310–20.
17. Butura CC, Galindo DF, Jensen OT. Mandibular all-on-four therapy using angled implants: a three-year clinical study of 857 implants in 219 jaws. Dent Clin North Am 2011;55(4):795–811.
18. Maló P, de Araújo Nobre M, Lopes A, et al. All-on-4® treatment concept for the rehabilitation of the completely edentulous mandible: a 7-year clinical and 5-year radiographic retrospective case series with risk assessment for implant failure and marginal bone level. Clin Implant Dent Relat Res 2015;17(Suppl 2): e531–41.
19. Sannino G, Barlattani A. Straight versus angulated abutments on tilted implants in immediate fixed rehabilitation of the edentulous mandible: a 3-year retrospective comparative study. Int J Prosthodont 2016;29(3):219–26.
20. Maló P, de Araújo Nobre M, Lopes A, et al. The All-on-4 treatment concept for the rehabilitation of the completely edentulous mandible: A longitudinal study with 10 to 18 years of follow-up. Clin Implant Dent Relat Res 2019;21(4):565–77.
21. Papaspyridakos P, Chen CJ, Singh M, et al. Success criteria in implant dentistry: a systematic review. J Dent Res 2012;91(3):242–8.
22. Albrektsson T, Zara G, Worthington P, et al. The long-term efficacy of current used dental implants: A review and proposed criteria of success. Int J Oral Maxillofacial Implants 1986;1:11–25.
23. Ting M, Craig J, Balkin BE, et al. Peri-implantitis: a comprehensive overview of systematic reviews. J Oral Implantol 2018;44(3):225–47.
24. Dhadse P, Gattani D, Mishra R. The link between periodontal disease and cardiovascular disease: How far we have come in last two decades ? J Indian Soc Periodontol 2010;14(3):148–54.
25. Dreyer H, Grischke J, Tiede C, et al. Epidemiology and risk factors of peri-implantitis: a systematic review. J Periodontal Res 2018;53(5):657–81.
26. Stavropoulos A, Bertl K, Pietschmann P, et al. The effect of antiresorptive drugs on implant therapy: systematic review and meta-analysis. Clin Oral Implants Res 2018;29(Suppl 18):54–92.
27. Barone A, Alfonsi F, Derchi G, et al. The effect of insertion torque on the clinical outcome of single implants: a randomized clinical trial. Clin Implant Dent Relat Res 2016;18(3):588–600.
28. Derks J, Schaller D, Håkansson J, et al. Peri-implantitis - onset and pattern of progression. J Clin Periodontol 2016;43(4):383–8.
29. Drake MT, Clarke BL, Khosla S. Bisphosphonates: mechanism of action and role in clinical practice. Mayo Clin Proc 2008;83(9):1032–45.
30. Lin T, Wang C, Cai XZ, et al. Comparison of clinical efficacy and safety between denosumab and alendronate in postmenopausal women with osteoporosis: a meta-analysis. Int J Clin Pract 2012;66(4):399–408.
31. Chappuis V, Avila-Ortiz G, Araújo MG, et al. Medication-related dental implant failure: systematic review and meta-analysis. Clin Oral Implants Res 2018; 29(Suppl 16):55–68.
32. De-Freitas NR, Lima LB, de-Moura MB, et al. Bisphosphonate treatment and dental implants: a systematic review. Med Oral Patol Oral Cir Bucal 2016;21(5): e644–51.

33. Ruggiero SL, Dodson TB, Fantasia J, et al. American Association of Oral and Maxillofacial Surgeons. American Association of Oral and Maxillofacial Surgeons position paper on medication-related osteonecrosis of the jaw–2014 update. J Oral Maxillofac Surg 2014;72(10):1938–56 [Erratum appears in J Oral Maxillofac Surg. 2015;73(7):1440; J Oral Maxillofac Surg. 2015;73(9):1879].
34. Tallarico M, Canullo L, Xhanari E, et al. Dental implants treatment outcomes in patient under active therapy with alendronate: 3-year follow-up results of a multicenter prospective observational study. Clin Oral Implants Res 2016;27(8):943–9.
35. Fu JH, Bashutski JD, Al-Hezaimi K, et al. Statins, glucocorticoids, and nonsteroidal anti-inflammatory drugs: their influence on implant healing. Implant Dent 2012;21(5):362–7.
36. Ouanounou A, Hassanpour S, Glogauer M. The influence of systemic medications on osseointegration of dental implants. J Can Dent Assoc 2016;82:g7.
37. Adami G, Saag KG. Glucocorticoid-induced osteoporosis: 2019 concise clinical review. Osteoporos Int 2019;30(6):1145–56.
38. Adell R, Lekholm U, Rockler B, et al. A 15-year study of osseointegrated implants in the treatment of the edentulous jaw. Int J Oral Surg 1981;10(6):387–416.
39. Durkan R, Oyar P, Deste G. Maxillary and mandibular all-on-four implant designs: A review. Niger J Clin Pract 2019;22(8):1033–40.
40. Soto-Penaloza D, Zaragozí-Alonso R, Penarrocha-Diago M, et al. The all-on-four treatment concept: Systematic review. J Clin Exp Dent 2017;9(3):e474–88.
41. Taruna M, Chittaranjan B, Sudheer N, et al. Prosthodontic perspective to all-on-4® concept for dental implants. J Clin Diagn Res 2014;8(10):ZE16–9.
42. Ben Hadj Hassine M, Bucci P, Gasparro R, et al. Safe approach in "All-on-four" technique: a case report. Ann Stomatol (Roma) 2015;5(4):142–5.
43. Drago C. Ratios of cantilever lengths and anterior-posterior spreads of definitive hybrid full-arch, screw-retained prostheses: results of a clinical study. J Prosthodont 2018;27(5):402–8.
44. Tiwari B, Ladha K, Lalit A, et al. Occlusal concepts in full mouth rehabilitation: an overview. J Indian Prosthodont Soc 2014;14(4):344–51.
45. Li S, Di P, Zhang Y, et al. Immediate implant and rehabilitation based on All-on-4 concept in patients with generalized aggressive periodontitis: a medium-term prospective study. Clin Implant Dent Relat Res 2017;19(3):559–71.

Zygomatic Implants

A Solution for the Atrophic Maxilla: 2021 Update

Jonathan Rosenstein, DDS[a], Harry Dym, DDS[b],*

KEYWORDS

• Alveolar • zygomatic • Endosseous • Implant • Maxillary bone • Maxillary sinus

KEY POINTS

• Atrophic maxilla following extraction of teeth is a commonly seen dilemma faced by implant surgeons. Inadequate bone foundation requires bone augmentation which can be a lengthy and complex process. Zygomatic implants offer the implant surgeon a viable alternative.

• Zygomatic implants can by themselves (if 2 implants are placed on either side of the maxilla, referred to as quad implants) offer a viable alternative for retention of dentures in an otherwise atrophic jaw.

• Zygomatic implants can easily be prosthetically managed as any other endosseous implant for the capable restorative dentist.

INTRODUCTION

Endosseous dental implants have quickly become the mainstay for restoration of edentulous spaces and an adjunct to the restoration of completely edentulous patients. The major limitation in the use of endosseous implants is the availability of sufficient alveolar bone. In patients with severely limited bone due to resorption, resection, or degenerative disease, for example, the process of implant placement and restoration can prove difficult, if not impossible.

The longevity of dental implants can be even more compromised in the maxilla. It has been shown that the osseointegration of implants in even a healthy and robust maxilla has lower success rates than the mandible. These success rates are even lower in the posterior maxilla compared with the anterior.[1] In patients with a severely

This article has been updated from a version previously published in *Dental Clinics of North America*, Volume 64, Issue 2, April 2020.

[a] Department of Oral and Maxillofacial Surgery, The Brooklyn Hospital Center, 121 Dekalb Avenue, Brooklyn, NY 11201, USA; [b] Department of Dentistry/Oral and Maxillofacial Surgery, The Brooklyn Hospital Center, 121 DeKalb Avenue, Brooklyn, NY 11201, USA

* Corresponding author.

E-mail address: Hdym@tbh.org

atrophic maxilla successful endosseous implant placement becomes even more challenging. Many solutions have been offered and practiced for treating such a maxilla, such as onlay bone grafting, sinus lift procedures, ridge split procedures, and even LeFort I surgical downfracture with interpositional bone grafting. In recent years, however, the advent of zygomatic implants may allow for a much simpler solution for the restoration of the dentition of a patient with an atrophic maxilla.[2]

TREATMENT OPTIONS FOR THE ATROPHIC MAXILLA

As mentioned earlier, various modalities have been used in order to aid in placement of implants into low quality and quantity of maxillary bone. The gold standard of treatment has long been bone grafting procedures, such as crestal onlay grafts, sinus lifts, and Lefort I osteotomy with interpositional bone grafting. However, bone grafting procedures are not always a viable option for many patients. Patients with cancer who have undergone head and neck radiation therapy, for example, may present with compromised vasculature, rendering bone grafting a procedure with high risk of failure. This same can be said for patients with certain metabolic disorders, congenital deformities, or those in an immunocompromised state.

Even without the aforementioned comorbidities, patients may choose not to undergo extensive bone grafting procedures due to factors such as graft donor site morbidity, increased healing time, longer surgical time, and increased chance of infection. Lower implant survival rates for grafted areas of the maxilla have also been reported, when compared with native bone.[2] Zygomatic implants offer a nongrafting option to restore the resected or atrophic maxilla.

OVERVIEW OF MAXILLARY BONE QUALITY

As previously stated, the type of bone present in the maxilla is usually of lower quality and quantity than that of the mandible. Lekholm and Zarb (1985) described 4 main bone types in the maxilla and mandible, listed as follows in descending order of density:

1. Type 1: mostly or all homogenous cortical bones
2. Type 2: bone that contains a core of densely packed cancellous bone, surrounded by at least 2 mm of cortical bone
3. Type 3: bone that contains a core of densely packed cancellous bone, surrounded by only one layer of cortical bone less than 2 mm
4. Type 4: mostly nondense cancellous bone, surrounded by only a thin layer of cortical bone

In general, the success rate of osseointegration increases in proportion to the bone density. It is thought that increased bone-implant contact and stabilization occurs in dense bone, as opposed to the loosely organized cancellous bone. A healthy maxilla will usually have type 3 bone anteriorly, changing to type 4 in the posterior. Bone density is often even further diminished in a resorbed maxilla.[3] Studies have shown that the maxilla resorbs, on average, 2 mm within the first year after tooth extraction, and then at a rate of 0.5 mm/y, compared with 0.2 mm/y in the mandible.[4]

ZYGOMATIC IMPLANTS

The Branemark System outlines a surgical technique for the intrasinus placement of zygomatic implants in 1988.[5] Zygomatic implants have been shown to be successful as support for an obturator or other larger maxillofacial prostheses for patients who had undergone maxillectomies.[6] Since then, the surgical techniques and approaches for placement of zygomatic implants have been expanded. Two main treatment designs are currently commonly used for the restoration of a patient's dentition:[7]

1. For patients with sufficient anterior maxillary bone for traditional implant placement: 1 zygomatic implant placed on each side of the posterior maxilla (2 total), and 2 or more traditional endosteal implants placed in the anterior maxilla.
2. For patients without sufficient anterior maxillary bone: 2 or more zygomatic implants on each side of the posterior maxilla.

Both designs have been shown to have high success rates when used to support a fixed dental prosthesis or overdenture. Some have documented success rates approaching 100%.[8] Although some studies have shown occasional failures, most agree that zygomatic implants have success rates of greater than 95%.[9]

ZYGOMATIC IMPLANT STABILITY

The stability and success of zygomatic implants is likely *not* due to the bone quality of the zygoma, itself. On the contrary, the zygoma is composed mainly of loose cancellous bone that, as explained earlier, is not favorable for implant osseointegration. Rather, the stability of zygomatic implants is thought to be due to the fact that the implant usually passes through 3 to 4 cortical layers of bone, compared with the single cortical layer that most traditional implants would pass through[10] (explained later in this article).

TECHNIQUE FOR PLACEMENT OF ZYGOMATIC IMPLANTS

Many techniques have been described for zygomatic implant placement. One technique, known as the intrasinus approach, is the most commonly used, which is explained later (surgical steps adapted from Dental Clinics, Clinics Review Articles, April 2020).[11] Other approaches are described as variations or modifications on the *intrasinus approach*.

- *Surgical incision and flap*: a crestal incision is made on the palatal aspect of the maxillary crest from the area of the first molar to the opposing first molar. A flap is then elevated to expose the lateral surface of the maxilla until the zygomatic process is revealed, similar to the flap used in a LeFort 1 osteotomy. The infraorbital neurovascular bundle should also be visualized. At this point, due to the placement of the incision, both the buccal and palatal aspect of the alveolar crest

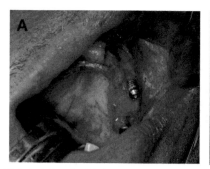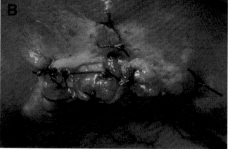

Fig. 1. (*A*) Left-sided maxillary mucoperiosteal flap raised. Implants shown were present before surgery. (*B*) Flap closure.

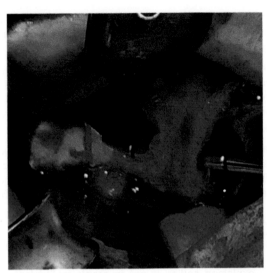

Fig. 2. Lateral sinus window osteotomy (after elevation of sinus membrane) and depth indicator to confirm appropriate implant length. (*From* Rosenstein J, Dym H. Zygomatic implants: a solution for the atrophic maxilla. Dent Clin North Am. 2020;64(2):404; with permission.)

should be fully exposed. One technique that the investigators use for this step includes an anterior midline vertical releasing incision. This allows for complete flap elevation unilaterally (**Fig. 1**A), which can be helpful for ease of flap elevation and hemostasis. Closure can be performed one side at a time or both sides simultaneously (**Fig. 1**B).

- *Lateral window*: a window should be made into the lateral aspect of the maxillary sinus, close to the inferior border of the zygomatic crest. This can be performed with a rotary handpiece and round bur, Piezo, or any such instrument that would normally be used for the osteotomy of a lateral window approach for a maxillary sinus lift. The dimensions of the window should be such that it will facilitate easy visualization of the implant drill and zygomatic implant, itself (**Fig. 2**). The suggested size is approximately 10 × 5 mm.

- *Elevation of Schneiderian membrane*: similar to the technique used for a lateral window sinus lift, the sinus membrane should be carefully elevated off of the inferior, lateral, and superior walls of the sinus (**Fig. 3**). This is to prevent perforation of the membrane by the implant drill or implant, itself. Although this is not necessary for the success of the zygomatic implant, it is ideal, as some have theorized it may decrease the chance of a persistent oroantral communication, as well as future sinus disease. Many current authors, however, are not concerned with this as a significant risk.

- *Implant osteotomy*: based on the presurgical and prosthodontic planning, often with the aid of a custom-fabricated surgical guide (**Fig. 4**), the zygomatic implant drill should be used to start the osteotomy on the alveolar crest at the point from which the head of the implant will emerge. The osteotomy should be continued in a superior-lateral-posterior direction, through the alveolar crest, into the sinus cavity, and eventually end within the superior cortical layer of the zygoma, itself. It is important to use a specialized drill guard during osteotomy formation in order to prevent contact between the shaft of the drill and surrounding soft tissue

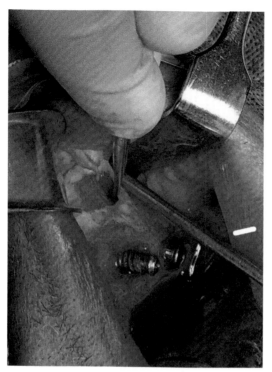

Fig. 3. Elevation of the Schneiderian membrane through lateral sinus window.

(**Fig. 5**). Just as with traditional endosteal implants, the zygomatic drill burs are used under irrigation and in ascending orders of width until the appropriate size is reached. At this point, a depth indicator is used to confirm appropriate

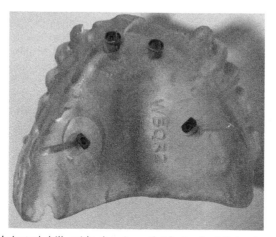

Fig. 4. Custom fabricated drill guide showing pilot holes for bilateral zygomatic implants and sleeve guides for 2 anterior maxillary implants.

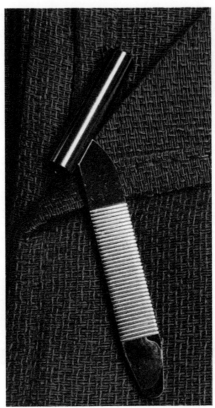

Fig. 5. Zygomatic implant drill guard. (*From* Rosenstein J, Dym H. Zygomatic implants: a solution for the atrophic maxilla. Dent Clin North Am. 2020;64(2):405; with permission.)

implant length (see **Fig. 2**). These implants are usually between 35 mm and 55 mm in length.

- *Implant placement*: once the osteotomies have been completed, and the appropriate length and angulation of the implant has been finalized, the zygomatic implant can be placed. It can be placed using the rotary handpiece at low speed or using a specialized hand driver (**Fig. 6**). The implant must be guided along the same route taken with the implant drills. It should be advanced until the apex

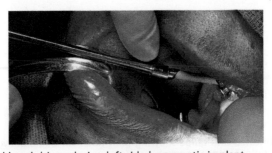

Fig. 6. Specialized hand driver placing left-sided zygomatic implant.

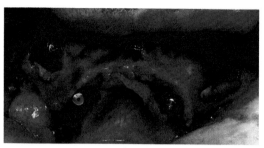

Fig. 7. Final position of bilateral zygomatic implants. (*From* Rosenstein J, Dym H. Zygomatic implants: a solution for the atrophic maxilla. Dent Clin North Am. 2020;64(2):406; with permission.)

reaches the superior cortex of the zygoma and then further rotated until the angled implant head is at the desired position at the maxillary alveolar crest (**Fig. 7**). At this point the cover screw can be placed, and the surgical flap reapproximated and closed with sutures (see **Fig. 1**B).

VARIATIONS ON THE INTRASINUS APPROACH

1. *Sinus slot procedure*: Stella and Warner have described a variation on the intrasinus procedure, known as the sinus slot procedure,[12] in which a "slot" is first drilled into the side of the malar bone. This slot should extend from 5 mm superior to the alveolar crest to the superior extent of the zygomatic buttress. The slot is then used to guide the implant drills and path of insertion of the implant, allowing the zygomatic implant to pass directly through the lateral wall of the maxillary bone on its way to the zygomatic bone. One advantage to this approach is that it obviates lateral sinus window. This decreases the chances of sinus membrane perforation and also allows for the head of the implant to emerge at the height of the alveolar crest, rather than the palatal aspect.

2. *Extrasinus approach*: in the case of a patient with a deep buccal concavity of the lateral surface of the maxilla, it may be impossible to extend the zygomatic implant through the sinus or maxillary bone into the zygoma while still having the emergence of the implant head at an appropriate location on the alveolar ridge. The extrasinus approach was developed in order to accommodate such patients. In this technique, the implant will pass from the alveolar ridge, out through the lateral surface of the maxilla, where it would otherwise have entered the sinus cavity. It will then reenter the maxilla at the zygomatic buttress and then eventually enter the zygoma itself.[13]

3. *Extramaxillary technique*: this technique was developed in order to simplify the surgical technique and to facilitate a more prosthodontically appropriate emergence of the implant head. Similar to the extrasinus approach, the extramaxillary approach does not have the path of implant insertion enter into the sinus. However, in the extramaxillary approach, the implant will *only* contact the maxilla at the height of alveolar ridge, itself, before traveling lateral-superior-posterior and then anchoring the implant apex within the zygoma. In this approach, it is said that the alveolar ridge only *accommodates* the implant, meaning that it will pass through a channel made just at the lateral surface of the alveolus, in order to allow for ideal prosthodontic placement at the height of the crest but that no actual anchorage or

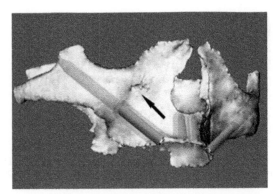

Fig. 8. Implant positions in All-on-4 hybrid situation. One standard maxillary anchored implant and one extramaxillary implant were placed bilaterally. Note extramaxillary implant placed posteriorly in inferior edge of zygoma, 3 mm from posterior vertical edge of zygomatic bone. Extramaxillary implant used exclusively zygomatic anchorage. Maxillary crest only accommodates implant, meaning that implant osseointegration only occurs in zygomatic bone. Note infraorbital foramen indicated by arrow. (*From* Maló P, Nobre M de A, Lopes I. A new approach to rehabilitate the severely atrophic maxilla using extramaxillary anchored implants in immediate function: a pilot study. J Prosthet Dent. 2008;100(5):357; with permission.)

osseointegration occurs at this location (**Fig. 8**). All of the support for the implant comes from the osseointegration occurring within the zygoma, itself.[14]

4. *Virtual surgical planning*: although not necessarily a separate technique, the advent of computer guided virtual surgical planning has provided the surgeon with novel ways to improve on the aforementioned techniques. Using a computed tomography scan of a patient's facial bones, a surgical guide (see **Fig. 4**) can be fabricated that will be able to accurately predetermine the appropriate length and width of the implant, as well as direct the implant drills and placement of the implant along a preplanned path of insertion. This can obviate the necessity for such a large lateral window in the intrasinus technique, other than for intraoperative verification of implant placement.

INDICATIONS AND CONTRAINDICATIONS

The obvious indications for zygomatic implants, as mentioned earlier, include those patients with a severely resorbed posterior maxilla who require an implant supported prosthesis. These patients may include those with systemic diseases that cause resorption of the maxilla, patients who had undergone maxillary resection or radiation therapy, immunocompromised patients, or those with congenital deformities such as severe cleft palate. More routine indications could include patients for whom bone grafting would not be desirable due to possible donor site morbidity, increased pain, longer surgical time, or even cultural/religious aversion to foreign bone material.

Contraindications and relative contraindications for zygomatic implants would be similar to those for normal dental implant placement. These include tobacco smoking addiction, past head and neck radiotherapy, and bisphosphonate therapy. Some investigators believe that zygomatic implants may increase the risk of chronic maxillary sinusitis due to the implant's passage through the maxillary sinus. For patients prone to these infections, zygomatic implants may be contraindicated.[15]

Prosthodontic concerns may also present a possible relative contraindication. Because of the necessary angulation of the zygomatic implant, the implant head will often emerge more palatally than traditional dental implants. This may make the dental prosthesis excessively bulky in this area, which can cause discomfort to selected patient. The extreme angulation of the zygomatic implant necessitates the use of angled abutments, which come in standard 25°, 35°, 45°, and 55° angulations.

COMPLICATIONS

As with any surgical procedure, there are risks and complications involved with the placement of zygomatic implants. Most of the complications associated with zygomatic implants are no different than those associated with standard dental implant placement. These can include the following:

- Bleeding
- Swelling
- Infection
- Failure of osseointegration

Other complications thought to be more strongly associated specifically with zygomatic implants include the following[2]:

- Sinusitis
- Oroantral fistula formation
- Periorbital and conjunctival hematoma or edema
- Facial pain and edema
- Epistaxis

Some of the more serious complications could even include the following:

- Paraesthesia of the infraorbital nerve (due to possible proximity of the path of zygomatic implant insertion)
- Orbital floor perforation
- Perforation into the infratemporal fossa.

In a cadaver study performed by Yuki Uchida and colleagues, in 2001, it was shown that deviation from a fairly narrow range could cause severe damage to sensitive anatomic structures. If a line were drawn from the point of ideal emergence of the zygomatic head in the alveolar bone to the point at which the temporal and frontal processes of the zygomatic bone meet (ie, jugale), it was shown that directing the implant at an angulation of 43.8° or less above this line could cause perforation of the infratemporal fossa, whereas directing the implant at an angulation of 50.6° or more above this line could cause perforation of the orbital floor.[16]

SUMMARY

Many studies have shown that zygomatic implants can be used as a successful and predictable method for supporting fixed or removable prostheses and can be used to restore the maxillary dentition in patients with a severely atrophic or resected maxilla. Zygomatic implants demonstrate high survival rates of 98.4% over the course of at least 12 years[9] and lack significant risk factors.[17] Because of the relative simplicity of zygomatic implant placement compared with the drawn out process of significant bone grafting to restore the severely atrophic or resected maxilla, zygomatic implants continue to be an ideal, stable, and viable option for many patients who would have difficulty or be unable to undergo more traumatic treatment.

CLINICS CARE POINTS

- Zygomatic implants for the first time user is best done with computer planning with a custom made surgical stent. After multiple surgical procedures, one can easily shift to placing these implants in a non-guided fashion.
- Zygomatic implants can be placed either through the maxillary sinus cavity.

DISCLOSURE

The authors have nothing to disclose.

REFERENCES

1. Meyer U, Vollmer D, Runte C, et al. Bone Loading Pattern around Implants in Average and Atrophic Edentulous Maxillae: a Finite-Element Analysis. J Craniomaxillofac Surg 2001;29:100–5.
2. Block MS, Haggerty CJ, Fisher GR. Nongrafting Implant Options for Restoration of the Edentulous Maxilla. J Oral Maxillofac Surg 2009;67:872–81.
3. Devlin H, Horner K, Ledgerton D. A Comparison of Maxillary and Mandibular Bone Mineral Densities. J Prosthet Dent 1998;79:323–7.
4. Bryant SR, Zarb GA. Outcomes of implant prosthodontic treatment in older adults. J Can Dent Assoc 2002;68:97–102.
5. Branemark PI. Surgery and fixture installation. Zygomaticus fixture clinical procedures. 1st edition. Goteborg (Sweden): Nobel Biocare AB; 1998.
6. Weischer T, Schettler D, Mohr C. Titanium implants in the zygoma as retaining elements after hemimaxillectomy. Int J Oral Maxillofac Implants 1997;12:211–4.
7. Stievenart M, Malevez C. Rehabilitation of totally atrophied by means of four zygomatic implants and fixed prosthesis: A 6-40 month follow-up. Int J Oral Maxillofac Surg 2010;39:358–63.
8. Ahlgren F, Størksen K, Tornes K. A study of 25 zygomatic dental implants with 11 to 49 months' follow-up after loading. Int J Oral Maxillofac Implants 2006;21:421–5.
9. Aparicio C, Ouazzani W, Hatano N. The use of zygomatic implants for prosthetic rehabilitation of the severely resorbed maxilla. Periodontol 2000 2008;47:162–71.
10. Nkenke E, Hahn M, Lell M, et al. Anatomic site evaluation of the zygomatic bone for dental implant placement. Clin Oral Implants Res 2003;14:72–9.
11. Rosenstein J, Dym H. Zygomatic Implants: A Solution for the Atrophic Maxilla. Surgical and Medical Management of Common Oral Problems. Dent Clin North Am 2020;64:401–11.
12. Stella J, Warner M. Sinus slot technique for simplification and improved orientation of zygomaticus dental implants: a technical note. Int J Oral Maxillofac Implants 2000;20:788–92.
13. Aparicio C, Ouazzani W, Garcia R, et al. Prospective clinical study on titanium implants in the zygomatic arch for prosthetic rehabilitation of the atrophic edentulous maxilla with a follow-up of 6 months to 5 years. Clin Implant Dent Relat Res 2006;8:114–22.
14. Maló P, Nobre Mde A, Lopes I. A new approach to rehabilitate the severely atrophic maxilla using extramaxillary anchored implants in immediate function: a pilot study. J Prosthet Dent 2008;100:354–66.
15. Ishak MI, Abdul Kadir MR. Treatment options for severely atrophic maxillae. Biomechanics in dentistry: evaluation of different surgical approaches to treat

atrophic maxilla patients. Elsevier: Journal of Oral and Maxillofacial Surgery; 2013.

16. Uchida Y, Goto M, Katsuki T, et al. Measurement of the maxilla and zygoma as an aid in installing zygomatic implants. J Oral Maxillofac Surg 2001;59:1193–8.

17. Chana H, Smith G, Bansal H, et al. A Retrospective Cohort Study of the Survival Rate of 88 Zygomatic Implants Placed Over an 18-year Period. Int J Oral Maxillofac Implants 2019;34:461–70.

Printed and bound by CPI Group (UK) Ltd, Croydon, CR0 4YY

03/10/2024

01040478-0006